A Day-by-Day Chronicle of the 2013–2016 Ebola Outbreak

Stephan Gregory Bullard

A Day-by-Day
Chronicle of the 2013–2016
Ebola Outbreak

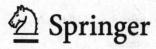 Springer

Stephan Gregory Bullard
University of Hartford
Hillyer College
West Hartford, CT, USA

ISBN 978-3-030-09523-9   ISBN 978-3-319-76565-5   (eBook)
https://doi.org/10.1007/978-3-319-76565-5

This book is dedicated to everyone directly and indirectly impacted by the 2013–2016 Ebola outbreak. It is also dedicated to my loving wife, Candace Corbeil.

Acknowledgments

This book would not have been possible without the help of numerous individuals and institutions. Research support was provided by the University of Hartford, Hillyer College, and Dean David Goldenberg. Michael Robinson and Candace Corbeil helped with editing. Copyright permission and assistance was provided by the World Health Organization, National Public Radio, Médecins Sans Frontières, National Geographic, Pardis Sabeti, Stephen Gire, and Mark McLaughlin.

Contents

Contents

About the Author

Stephan Bullard is an Associate Professor of Biology at the University of Hartford in Connecticut. He studies notable disasters. His previous books include *The Silver Bridge Disaster of 1967* and *Three Mile Island, Chernobyl and Fukushima: Curse of the Nuclear Genie*.

List of Abbreviations

BSL	Biosafety level; 4 levels are recognized, biosafety level 4 is the highest
CDC	Centers for Disease Control and Prevention
DOD	Department of Defense
ECDC	The European Center for Disease Prevention and Control
ECOWAS	Economic Community of West African States
FDA	Food and Drug Administration
HHS	Health and Human Services
MSF	Médecins Sans Frontières, known as Doctors Without Borders in English
NGO	Non-governmental organization
NHS	UK National Health Service
NIH	National Institutes of Health
PPE	Personal protective equipment
UNICEF	United Nations Children's Fund
UNMEER	United Nations Mission for Ebola Emergency Response
USAMRIID	United States Army Medical Research Institute of Infectious Diseases
WHO	World Health Organization

Chapter 1
Introduction

Abstract Ebola is one of the most frightening diseases of the modern era. The Ebola virus was discovered in 1976 when two separate species of Ebola caused outbreaks in Zaire and Sudan. Since then, several additional Ebola species have been identified. Ebola is contagious, highly fatal, and incurable. *Zaire ebolavirus* is the most dangerous species in the group. It has a fatality rate of up to 90%. The initial symptoms of Ebola are non-specific. This makes it very difficult to clinically diagnose Ebola, especially in countries with numerous endemic diseases. Laboratory tests can identify Ebola, but standard RT-PCR tests can take several days to conduct. There is no specific treatment for Ebola. Supportive care is used to assist patients. Several potential drug candidates are available, but none has been approved for general use. Many survivors experience long-term effects from the disease. Some body fluids, especially the semen, can remain Ebola RNA-positive for years after a person has recovered. This book presents a day-by-day account of the 2013–2016 *Zaire ebolavirus* outbreak. It provides a detailed case study of one of the most significant disease events of the early twenty-first century.

1.1 Introduction

Ebola was first discovered in 1976. From June to November 1976, an outbreak of an unknown pathogen took place in southern Sudan. A similar disease outbreak occurred in Yambuku, Zaire, in September and October 1976. Upon investigation, the outbreaks were found to be caused by two closely related species of virus. Both species were new to science but were similar to the previously known Marburg virus. The new viruses were eventually named *Zaire ebolavirus* and *Sudan ebolavirus*. In the media, both forms were generally referred to simply as Ebola. The disease caused by Ebola was contagious and incurable. Transmission occurred through direct contact with infected bodily fluids. The fatality rate for *Zaire ebolavirus* was close to 90%. *Sudan ebolavirus* was slightly less lethal, with a fatality rate around 50%. The new viruses caused significant concern in the medical community. Some professionals worried that Ebola could cause a major international outbreak, especially if it was spread through air travel. Few people outside the medical community were aware of the disease.

S. G. Bullard, *A Day-by-Day Chronicle of the 2013-2016 Ebola Outbreak*,
https://doi.org/10.1007/978-3-319-76565-5_1

Two events in the mid-1990s put a spotlight on Ebola and brought the disease to the public's attention. First, in 1994, Richard Preston published the highly successful book *The Hot Zone* (Preston1994). The book was written in a clear and engaging style and presented the horrors of Ebola to a general audience. Second, in 1995, a large and well-publicized Ebola outbreak took place in Kikwit, Zaire. The highly lethal and contagious nature of Ebola captured the imagination of the Western world. References to Ebola began to appear in popular TV shows like *The Simpsons* and *Gilmore Girls*. Sporadic outbreaks took place in Africa during the early 2000s. As time progressed, the medical community began to reevaluate its opinion of Ebola. As more information became available, a consensus began to form that Ebola killed too quickly to allow for widespread human-to-human transmission. It began to seem unlikely that Ebola could cause a major international outbreak. The 2013–2016 outbreak changed all that. The 2013–2016 event started as a small, "typical" Ebola outbreak. It rapidly grew, however, to encompass three West African countries. Smaller outbreaks were ignited in other parts of the world. The virus was only brought under control by the intense and concerted effort of the worldwide medical community. When the outbreak was over, Ebola had infected almost 29,000 people and had killed more than 11,000.

1.2   Ebola Virus Disease

The 2013–2016 outbreak was caused by *Zaire ebolavirus* (Baize et al. 2014). *Zaire ebolavirus* is a member of the family Filoviridae. The Filoviridae includes seven species in three genera. The species are *Marburg marburgvirus*, *Zaire ebolavirus*, *Sudan ebolavirus*, *Reston ebolavirus*, *Bundibugyo ebolavirus*, *Taï Forest ebolavirus*, and *Lloviu cuevavirus* (International Committee on Taxonomy of Viruses 2016). The Filoviridae are commonly known as thread viruses because of their elongated, hairlike shape. Many members of the group are pathogenic in humans. *Marburg marburgvirus*, *Zaire ebolavirus*, *Sudan ebolavirus*, and *Bundibugyo ebolavirus* have caused human outbreaks (Kuhn 2008; MacNeil et al. 2010). *Taï Forest ebolavirus* (formally known as *Côte d'Ivoire ebolavirus*) infected one person in 1994 and may have caused other isolated infections (Kuhn 2008). Unless otherwise stated, all references to Ebola in this book refer to *Zaire ebolavirus*.

The disease caused by the Ebola virus has been referred to as Ebola virus disease (EVD) and Ebola hemorrhagic fever (EHF). The term EVD is generally preferred because Ebola victims do not always exhibit hemorrhagic symptoms (e.g., Baize et al. 2014). EVD also allows researchers to distinguish between the virus particle itself (i.e., the Ebola virus) and the disease produced by the virus (EVD). In this book, the virus and the disease are both referred to as "Ebola." This is because Ebola is the term most familiar to the general public and the term most commonly used by news sources and government agencies.

Ebola is zoonotic. It does not normally circulate in human populations but can be passed to people from an animal reservoir. Outbreaks occur when an animal transfers the virus to a human host and human-to-human transmission begins. Fruit bats are a significant vector for Ebola but may not be the primary animal reservoir for the virus (Leroy et al. 2005, 2009; Hayman et al. 2012; Leendertz et al. 2016). The 2013–2016 outbreak is believed to have started when the human index case interacted with, or was in close proximity to, insectivorous, free-tailed bats (*Mops condylurus*) (Saéz et al. 2015).

Ebola produces extreme, debilitating illness in humans. Ebola is infectious and readily transmitted through contact with infected blood and bodily fluids. Limited airborne transmission may also occur (Osterholm et al. 2015). Fatality rates associated with *Zaire ebolavirus* can approach 90%. During the 1976 outbreak in Yambuku, Zaire, the fatality rate was 88% (International Study Team 1978). During the 1995 outbreak in Kikwit, Zaire, the fatality rate was 81% (Khan et al. 1999). Ebola victims expel large amounts of blood, diarrhea, and vomit. All of these materials are infectious, so healthcare settings and patient's homes can easily become contaminated. The incubation period for Ebola, from the time a person becomes infected until they begin to exhibit symptoms, is 2–21 days (World Health Organization 2017). Schieffelin et al. (2014) estimated that the normal incubation period in Sierra Leone was 6–12 days.

The course of an Ebola infection usually follows a typical pattern. The initial symptoms are general and non-specific (Chertow et al. 2014). These include fever, body ache, general discomfort, and fatigue. After a few days, gastrointestinal symptoms appear. Patients have nausea, vomiting, diarrhea, and abdominal pain. Around the same time, additional symptoms like conjunctivitis (reddening of the eyes), joint pain, chest pain, and hiccups may occur. By day seven patients begin to improve or continue to decline. Declining patients may fall into a coma or have reduced consciousness. Recovering patients experience decreased gastrointestinal symptoms and increased energy levels. Late stage complications, such as secondary infections may occur (Chertow et al. 2014). Numerous additional studies describe the clinical features of Ebola patients during the 2013–2016 outbreak (e.g., Bah et al. 2015; Schieffelin et al. 2014; Lado et al. 2015; Haaskjold et al. 2016).

Because the initial symptoms of Ebola are non-specific, it can be very difficult to clinically diagnose a patient in the early stages of the disease (World Health Organization 2017). This is especially true in countries with numerous endemic diseases. Laboratory tests are needed to confirm an Ebola infection. At the beginning of the 2013–2016 outbreak, a commonly used test was reverse transcriptase polymerase chain reaction (RT-PCR) (e.g., Towner et al. 2004). RT-PCR can very accurately detect the presence of virus in a patient, but it can take several days to collect and process the samples. During the 2013–2016 outbreak, speed was of the essence. Healthcare workers needed to quickly isolate Ebola patients while making sure non-Ebola patients (such as malaria patients) were not misdiagnose as having Ebola. As the outbreak progressed, rapid field tests were developed that could diagnose a patient in as little as 15 min (Boseley 2015). Though not quite as accurate as RT-PCR, the new tests allowed Ebola patients to be rapidly identified and isolated.

There is no cure for Ebola. Only supportive care is available. Most commonly, oral and intravenous hydration and nutrition are provided to Ebola patients (Kuhn

2008). Antibiotics are administered to deal with secondary infections (Kuhn 2008). Before the 2013–2016 outbreak, a variety of drug candidates were under investigation to treat Ebola. These included Avigan (Favipiravir), TKM-Ebola, and ZMapp. Transfusions with convalescent blood were also proposed as a possible Ebola treatment (Mupapa et al. 1999). The blood of Ebola survivors contains antibodies. If a survivor's blood is transfused into an infected patient, the antibodies might help the new person's immune system identify and attack the virus. During the 1995 Ebola outbreak in Kikwit, Zaire, seven of eight patients treated with convalescent blood survived (Mupapa et al. 1999). Many of these potential drugs and treatments were tried during the 2013–2016 outbreak. Results were mixed. ZMapp seemed very successful (e.g., Gupta and Dellorto 2014). Transfusions of convalescent blood plasma were ineffective (Van Griensven et al. 2016). As of 2016, no specific drug treatment had been recommended for general use.

No Ebola vaccine was available at the start of the 2013–2016 outbreak (Centers for Disease Control and Prevention 2015). Several vaccine candidates were in development, but none had completed clinical trials or been approved for general use. Vaccine trials were fast-tracked during the outbreak. Early field results were exceptionally promising (World Health Organization 2015). In late 2016 – after the outbreak had ended – the rVSV-ZEBOV was found to be 100% effective at preventing Ebola infection (Berlinger 2016; Henao-Restrepo et al. 2017).

Many Ebola survivors experience long-lasting effects from the disease. In the year following the 2013–2016 outbreak, 78% of survivors in Sierra Leone had encountered some form of disability (Jagadesh et al. 2017). The persistent, sometimes dangerous, collection of symptoms has been referred to as post-Ebola syndrome or post-Ebolavirus disease syndrome (Carod-Artal 2015; Epstein et al. 2015). Typical symptoms include joint pain, fatigue, anorexia, and vision problems. Psychiatric problems can also occur (Howlett et al. 2017). In at one case, a survivor developed Ebola-related meningitis 9 months after they had initially recovered from the disease (Jacobs et al. 2016). Work continues to determine the prevalence of post-Ebola syndrome and to find ways to treat it.

Ebola virus particles can remain in the body fluids of survivors for a long time. The semen and the aqueous humor of the eyes are particularly amenable to harboring the virus (Deen et al. 2017; Varkey et al. 2015). Early studies found that the semen of some survivors was Ebola-positive 9 months after the survivors had developed the disease (Sow et al. 2016). More recently, the semen of 11% of survivors was found to be Ebola RNA-positive 2 years after the survivors had developed the disease (Fischer et al. 2017). Ebola can almost certainly be transmitted sexually (Christie et al. 2015; Thorson et al. 2016). It is unclear, however, whether Ebola RNA-positive semen is infectious and, if so, how easily it can infect a man's sexual partners. To ensure safety, the WHO recommends that the semen of survivors be checked until it tests RT-PCR negative twice. Alternatively, survivors should abstain from sex or use condoms for at least a year after they develop Ebola symptoms (World Health Organization 2016). These recommendations were implemented as data became available and were not in place until late into the 2013–2016 outbreak.

1.3 Ebola Case Definitions

The WHO classifies Ebola cases as confirmed, probable, and suspected cases (World Health Organization 2014).

A confirmed case is a patient who has positive IgM antibody, has positive PCR, or has had virus particles isolated from their body or body fluids.

A probable case is a suspected case who has been evaluated by a clinician or a deceased suspected case with an epidemiological link to a confirmed case.

A suspected case is (1) a person who has the onset of high fever after having contact with a suspected, probable, or confirmed Ebola case; (2) a person who has the onset of high fever after having had contact with a sick or dead animal; (3) a person with high fever and at least three of the following symptoms: vomiting, diarrhea, stomach pain, difficulty swallowing, headache, loss of appetite, lethargy, aching muscles or joints, difficulty breathing, or hiccups; (4) a person with inexplicable bleeding; (5) a person who has died suddenly.

1.4 History of *Zaire ebolavirus*

The first known *Zaire ebolavirus* outbreak occurred in Zaire (now the Democratic Republic of the Congo) in 1976. Cases were centered around a Catholic Mission in the town of Yambuku. Some patients became infected when they received inoculations with reused, unsterilized syringes. A total of 318 people were infected during the outbreak, 280 of them died (International Study Team 1978). The outbreak took place during September and October, the time of the local rice harvesting season (International Study Team 1978; Kuhn 2008). At this time of year, local people do not travel very much (Kuhn 2008). Had the outbreak occurred at a different time of year, the virus might have spread more widely.

Yambuku was the first known *Zaire ebolavirus* outbreak, but Ebola may have caused earlier disease events. It has been suggested that some historical epidemics, including the Plague of Athens, may have been caused by Ebola (Scarrow 1988; Olson et al. 1996).

In 1977, one person contracted Ebola in Zaire (Kuhn 2008). No other *Zaire ebolavirus* outbreaks took place until 1994. During 1994–1997, a cluster of outbreaks occurred in Gabon (Georges et al. 1999). In all, 114 people were infected and 78 died (Kuhn 2008). When the outbreaks first started, chimpanzees and gorillas were reported to be dying in the nearby forest (Georges et al. 1999).

In 1995, there was a large Ebola outbreak in Kikwit, Zaire (Khan et al. 1999). The likely index case was a charcoal maker who died in early January 1995 (Muyembe-Tamfum et al. 1999). By mid-April, the disease had reached the local hospital, and healthcare workers began to fall sick (Muyembe-Tamfum et al. 1999). The illness was initially thought to be epidemic dysentery. Ebola was identified as the causative agent around May 9, 1995 (Khan et al. 1999). Local and international healthcare workers raced to the area to control the outbreak. The last known victim died on July 16, 1995. In all, 315 people had been infected. The fatality rate was 81% (Khan et al. 1999) (Kuhn 2008 reports 317 infections and 245 deaths).

Another cluster of Ebola outbreaks took place in Gabon and the Democratic Republic of the Congo between 2001 and 2005 (World Health Organization 2003, 2004; Kuhn 2008). The index case for the first outbreak may have been an infected hunter (Kuhn 2008). As with earlier Ebola outbreaks, large numbers of dead animals were reported in nearby forests (World Health Organization 2003; Rouquet et al. 2005). This outbreak cluster led to 324 infections and 273 deaths (Kuhn 2008).

In 2007, Ebola returned to the Democratic Republic of the Congo when the disease struck a remote part of Kasaï-Occidental province (ProMED-mail 2007; Grard et al. 2011). Due to the difficulty of obtaining samples from the region, it is unclear exactly how many people actually had Ebola. Of 264 suspected cases, there were 187 deaths (ProMED-mail 2007).

In 2008, the last *Zaire ebolavirus* outbreak to occur before the 2013–2016 event took place in the Democratic Republic of the Congo. This event occurred in the same area as the 2007 outbreak. In all, 32 people were infected and 15 died (World Health Organization 2009; Grard et al. 2011). The last victim died on January 1, 2009 (World Health Organization 2009).

Several laboratory incidents have involved Ebola. A fatal laboratory-acquired Ebola infection is reported to have occurred in Russia in 1996 (Kuhn 2008). In 2004, a female technician suffered a needlestick injury while working with infected guinea pig tissue in Koltsovo, Russia. She died 14 days after contracting Ebola. A similar incident took place at a US facility in 2004. Fortunately, the female worker in this case did not develop Ebola (Kuhn 2008).

1.5   Notes on the Text

Entries in this book are recorded in the present tense. The body of the text was written at the time of outbreak. Information was collected every day and summaries were written each evening. Data collection started on July 17, 2014. Earlier data were collected retroactively. Because the text was written while the events were taking place, the initial entries were recorded in the present tense. When the book was being prepared for publication, an effort was made to change the text into past tense. This diminished the impact of the writing and left the text feeling lifeless. As a result, present tense has been retained in the final version.

Using the present tense presents a challenge to reporting material in a strict chronological order. For example, the name of an Ebola patient was often not known when their infection was first reported. When this occurs, the patient's name is written in brackets until their identity was officially known. Strict chronological order is also a problem with epidemiologically important cases, such as the first US Ebola patient. A great deal of information about these patients often became available after their infection was first identified. In these cases, a short biography is included in the patient's first entry.

There were many false Ebola scares during the outbreak. These often occurred when travelers arrived in a western country with Ebola-like symptoms. Only a few of these cases are included in the text, mostly at the beginning of the outbreak.

Names are spelled according to the generally accepted spelling in the name's original language.

Military time is used throughout the text. 6:30 p.m. is 1830 h. Midnight is 0000 h. Unless otherwise noted, time is local time. The year is usually included with dates.

Monetary values are in US dollars. Foreign currency is converted into US dollars using the international exchange rate on the day the value was reported.

Considerable effort has been made to credit all reference sources. When all of the information in a paragraph comes from a single source, the source is credited at the end of the last sentence of the paragraph. When multiple sources are used in a single paragraph, sources are credited at the end of each sentence using the source. If a string of sentences comes from a single source, credit brackets the information; one credit is placed at the end of the first sentence that uses the source, and a second credit is placed at the end of the last sentence that uses the source.

Throughout the text, the 2013–2016 Ebola event is referred to as an "outbreak." The terms epidemic and pandemic are somewhat subjective. An epidemic is a health event that affects a large number of people in a short time (ReliefWeb 2008). A pandemic is a worldwide health event or one that affects many countries (i.e., World Health Organization 2010). The 2013–2016 Ebola event certainly affected a large number of people and affected many countries. Hence, it could be considered either an epidemic or a pandemic. Experts will likely debate the correct term for the 2013–2016 event. The nonsubjective term outbreak is used in this work.

Official WHO casualty figures are presented. The WHO started releasing tabular Ebola figures in July 2014. The agency occasionally published confusing or erroneous data. The WHO also revised its figures several times. In some cases this led to negative numbers of new cases being reported. Official WHO numbers are always reported in this book, regardless of whether they conflict with previously reported numbers.

References

Bah EI, Lamah MC, Fletcher T et al (2015) Clinical presentation of patients with Ebola virus disease in Conakry, Guinea. N Engl J Med 372:40–47

Baize S, Pannetier D, Oestereich L et al (2014) Emergence of Zaire Ebola virus disease in Guinea – preliminary report. N Engl J Med 371:1418–1425

Berlinger J (2016) Ebola vaccine gives 100% protection, study finds. CNN. http://www.cnn.com/2016/12/22/health/ebola-vaccine-study/index.html. Accessed 24 Nov 2017

Boseley S (2015) WHO approves 15-minute test for Ebola. The Guardian. http://www.theguardian.com/world/2015/feb/20/who-approves-15-minute-test-for-ebola. Accessed 20 Feb 2015

Carod-Artal FJ (2015) Post-Ebolavirus disease syndrome: what do we know? Expert Rev Anti-Infect Ther 13:1185–1187

Centers for Disease Control and Prevention (2015) Ebola (Ebola virus disease) – treatment. 22 Jul 2015

Chertow DS, Kleine C, Edwards JK et al (2014) Ebola virus disease in West Africa—clinical manifestations and management. N Engl J Med 371:2054–2057

Christie A, Davies-Wayne GJ, Cordier-Lassalle T et al (2015) Possible sexual transmission of Ebola virus-Liberia. MMWR Morb Mortal Wkly Rep 64:479–481

Deen GF, Knust B, Broutet N et al (2017) Ebola RNA persistence in semen of Ebola virus disease survivors—preliminary report. N Engl J Med 377:1428–1437

Epstein L, Wong KK, Kallen AJ et al (2015) Post-Ebola signs and symptoms in US survivors. N Engl J Med 373:2484–2486

Fischer WA, Brown J, Wohl DA et al (2017) Ebola virus ribonucleic acid detection in semen more than two years after resolution of acute Ebola virus infection. In: Open forum infectious diseases, vol 4, no 3. Oxford University Press

Georges AJ, Leroy EM, Renaut AA et al (1999) Ebola hemorrhagic fever outbreaks in Gabon, 1994–1997: epidemiologic and health control issues. J Infect Dis 179(Supplement_1):S65–S75

Grard G, Biek R, Muyembe Tamfum JJ et al (2011) Emergence of divergent Zaire ebola virus strains in Democratic Republic of the Congo in 2007 and 2008. J Infect Dis 204(Supplement_3):S776–S784

Gupta S, Dellorto D (2014) Experimental drug likely saved Ebola patients. CNN. http://www.cnn.com/2014/08/04/health/experimental-ebola-serum/. Accessed 13 Jan 2017

Haaskjold YL, Bolkan HA, Krogh KØ et al (2016) Clinical features of and risk factors for fatal Ebola virus disease, Moyamba District, Sierra Leone, December 2014–February 2015. Emerg Infect Dis 22:1537–1544

Hayman DT, Yu M, Crameri G et al (2012) Ebola virus antibodies in fruit bats, Ghana, West Africa. Emerg Infect Dis 18:1207–1209

Henao-Restrepo AM, Camacho A, Longini IM et al (2017) Efficacy and effectiveness of an rVSV-vectored vaccine in preventing Ebola virus disease: final results from the Guinea ring vaccination, open-label, cluster-randomised trial (Ebola Ça Suffit!). Lancet 389:505–518

Howlett P, Walder A, Lisk D et al (2017) Neurological and psychiatric manifestations of post Ebola syndrome in Sierra Leone. Lancet 389:S48

International Committee on Taxonomy of Viruses (2016) Family: Filoviridae. https://talk.ictvonline.org/ictv-reports/ictv_9th_report/negative-sense-rna-viruses-2011/w/negrna_viruses/197/filoviridae. Accessed 23 Oct 2017

International Study Team (1978) Ebola hemorrhagic fever in Zaire, 1976. Bull WHO 56:271–293

Jacobs M, Rodger A, Bell DJ et al (2016) Late Ebola virus relapse causing meningoencephalitis: a case report. Lancet 388:498–503

Jagadesh S, Sevalie S, Fatoma R et al (2017) Disability among Ebola survivors and their close contacts in Sierra Leone: a retrospective case-controlled cohort study. Clin Infect Dis 66:131–133

Khan AS, Tshioko FK, Heymann DL et al (1999) The reemergence of Ebola hemorrhagic fever, Democratic Republic of the Congo, 1995. J Infect Dis 179(Supplement_1):S76–S86

Kuhn JH (2008) Filoviruses; a compendium of 40 years of epidemiological, clinical, and laboratory studies. Springer-Verlag/Wien, New York

Lado M, Walker NF, Baker P et al (2015) Clinical features of patients isolated for suspected Ebola virus disease at Connaught Hospital, Freetown, Sierra Leone: a retrospective cohort study. Lancet Infect Dis 15:1024–1033

Leendertz SA, Gogarten JF, Düx A et al (2016) Assessing the evidence supporting fruit bats as the primary reservoirs for Ebola viruses. EcoHealth 13:18–25

Leroy EM, Kumulungui B, Pourrut X et al (2005) Fruit bats as reservoirs of Ebola virus. Nature 438:575–576

Leroy EM, Epelboin A, Mondonge V et al (2009) Human Ebola outbreak resulting from direct exposure to fruit bats in Luebo, Democratic Republic of Congo, 2007. Vector Borne Zoonotic Dis 9:723–728

MacNeil A, Farnon EC, Wamala J et al (2010) Proportion of deaths and clinical features in *Bundibugyo Ebola virus* infection, Uganda. Emerg Infect Dis 16:1969–1972

Mupapa K, Massamba M, Kibadi K et al (1999) Treatment of Ebola hemorrhagic fever with blood transfusions from convalescent patients. J Infect Dis 179(Suppl 1):S18–S23

Muyembe-Tamfum JJ, Kipasa M, Kiyungu C et al (1999) Ebola outbreak in Kikwit, Democratic Republic of the Congo: discovery and control measures. J Infect Dis 179(Supplement_1):S259–S262

Olson PE, Hames CS, Benenson AS et al (1996) The Thucydides syndrome: Ebola deja vu? (or Ebola reemergent?). Emerg Infect Dis 2:155–156

Osterholm MT, Moore KA, Kelley NS et al (2015) Transmission of Ebola viruses: what we know and what we do not know. MBio 6:e00137–e00115

Preston R (1994) The hot zone. Random House, New York

ProMED-mail (2007) Ebola hemorrhagic fever – Congo DR, 21 Nov 2007. http://www.promed-mail.org/pls/apex/f?p52400:1000. Accessed 24 Oct 2017

ReliefWeb (2008) Glossary of humanitarian terms. http://www.who.int/hac/about/reliefweb-aug2008.pdf?ua=1. Accessed 27 Oct 2017

Rouquet P, Froment JM, Bermejo M et al (2005) Wild animal mortality monitoring and human Ebola outbreaks, Gabon and Republic of Congo, 2001–2003. Emerg Infect Dis 11:283–290

Saéz AM, Weiss S, Nowak K et al (2015) Investigating the zoonotic origin of the West African Ebola epidemic. EMBO Mol Med 7:17–23

Scarrow GD (1988) The Athenian plague: a possible diagnosis. Anc Hist Bull 2:4–8

Schieffelin JS, Shaffer JG, Goba A et al (2014) Clinical illness and outcomes in patients with Ebola in Sierra Leone. N Engl J Med 371:2092–2100

Sow MS, Etard JF, Baize S et al (2016) New evidence of long-lasting persistence of Ebola virus genetic material in semen of survivors. J Infect Dis 214:1475–1476

Thorson A, Formenty P, Lofthouse C et al (2016) Systematic review of the literature on viral persistence and sexual transmission from recovered Ebola survivors: evidence and recommendations. BMJ Open 6:e008859

Towner JS, Rollin PE, Bausch DG et al (2004) Rapid diagnosis of Ebola hemorrhagic fever by reverse transcription-PCR in an outbreak setting and assessment of patient viral load as a predictor of outcome. J Virol 78:4330–4341

Van Griensven J, Edwards T, De Lamballerie X et al (2016) Evaluation of convalescent plasma for Ebola virus disease in Guinea. N Engl J Med 374:33–42

Varkey JB, Shantha JG, Crozier I et al (2015) Persistence of Ebola virus in ocular fluid during convalescence. N Engl J Med 372:2423–2427

World Health Organization (2003) Outbreak(s) of Ebola haemorrhagic fever, Congo and Gabon, October 2001–July 2002. Wkly Epidemiol Rec 78:223–228

World Health Organization (2004) Ebola haemorrhagic fever in the Republic of the Congo – update 6. 6 Jan 2004

World Health Organization (2009) End of Ebola outbreak in the Democratic Republic of the Congo. 17 Feb 2009

World Health Organization (2010) What is a pandemic? 24 Feb 2010

World Health Organization (2014) Case definition recommendations for Ebola or Marburg Virus Diseases. 9 Aug 2014

World Health Organization (2015). World on the verge of an effective Ebola vaccine. 31 Jul 2015

World Health Organization (2016) Interim advice on the sexual transmission of the Ebola virus disease. 21 Jan 2016

World Health Organization (2017) Ebola virus disease. June 2017

Chapter 2
Initial Outbreak Period (December 2013– May 22, 2014)

Abstract The 2013–2016 Ebola outbreak began in a small Guinean village. A 2-year-old boy contacted Ebola, most likely after coming into contact with free-tailed bats, possibly by playing with them. The epidemiology of the outbreak initially followed the course of previous Ebola outbreaks. A small number of people were infected and local officials and international aid agencies worked to identify and isolate patients. Significant concern was raised when Ebola cases began to appear in Guinea's capital, Conakry, and in the neighboring country of Liberia. The disease was also thought to have spread to Sierra Leone, although no positive samples were collected from that country. By the middle of May 2014, it appeared that the outbreak had run its course. No new cases had been seen for some time, and all known patients had either recovered or died. What was not known was that undetected transmission chains remained. Ebola continued to spread, helped by local customs such as traditional burial practices where the body of the deceased is washed and touched. The stage was set for the rapid expansion of Ebola that would occur in the late spring and early summer of 2014.

2.1 Day-by-Day Outbreak Entries (December 2013–May 22, 2014)

December 2, 2013 (Monday)
Emile Ouamouno, the first known victim of the 2013–2016 Ebola outbreak, becomes ill (Baize et al. 2014; Yan and Kinkade 2014). His symptoms include fever, black stools, and vomiting (Baize et al. 2014; Yan and Kinkade 2014). Retroactive epidemiological analysis suggests that this child is the index case for the subsequent Ebola outbreak (Baize et al. 2014). Ouamouno was a 2-year-old boy who lived in the village of Meliandou, Guinea. The village is located about 6 miles northeast of the town of Guéckédou. Ouamouno probably became infected while playing near a hollow tree that housed a colony of insectivorous, free-tailed bats (species *Mops condylurus*) (Saéz et al. 2015). The tree stood about 50 m from his house. Children from the community frequently played near the tree and often captured and played with bats (Saéz et al. 2015).

December 6, 2013 (Friday)
Emile Ouamouno dies (Baize et al. 2014).

March 10, 2014 (Monday)
The Guinean Ministry of Health is notified about the outbreak of an unidentified, highly fatal disease in the south-central part of the country (Baize et al. 2014).

March 12, 2014 (Wednesday)
MSF is notified about the unidentified, deadly disease in Guinea (Baize et al. 2014).

March 14, 2014
The Guinean government dispatches a team to Guéckédou to investigate the recent disease outbreak (Baize et al. 2014).

March 22, 2014 (Saturday)
Ebola is officially identified as the disease causing the outbreak in Guinea (Médecins Sans Frontières 2014a). This is the first time Ebola has occurred in West Africa. To date, six Ebola cases have been confirmed and 49 suspected cases have been identified. At least 29 people have died (Médecins Sans Frontières 2014a). Disturbingly, the disease does not seem to be confined to a single area. Three of the suspected cases have occurred in Conakry, Guinea's capital city, about 250 miles from Guéckédou (Lazuta 2014a). The disease might also be in neighboring Sierra Leone. Medical personnel in Sierra Leone are working to determine if a 14-year-old boy has died from Ebola in the town of Buedu in the eastern Kailahun District (Samb 2014).

   MSF has set up an isolation hospital in Guéckédou, Guinea and is in the process of setting up a second clinic in Macenta, Guinea. Guéckédou, a city of ~220,000, appears to be the epicenter of the outbreak. MSF plans to airlift additional medical personnel and 33 tons of supplies to the area to compliment the 24 MSF medical staff already in Guinea (Médecins Sans Frontières 2014a).

March 23, 2014 (Sunday)
UNICEF confirms that Ebola has spread to Guinea's capital, Conakry (Bah 2014). This is a serious turn of events and raises concerns that the outbreak could quickly become considerably worse. Conakry has a population of about two million, and sanitation in the city is generally poor (UNICEF n.d.; Lazuta 2014b). These factors could allow the disease to spread rapidly among the urban population.

   As of March 22, 2014, there have been 49 Ebola cases and 29 deaths in Guinea (Disease Outbreak News 2014a).

March 25, 2014 (Tuesday)
Guinea has banned the sale and consumption of bats to try to curb the spread of Ebola (BBC 2014a). Bats, especially fruit bats, are thought to be a reservoir for the Ebola virus. Local residents enjoy eating bats, which they often prepare in a spicy pepper soup (BBC 2014a).

March 26, 2014 (Wednesday)
Ebola is believed to have reached Liberia. Eight suspect cases, including five deaths, have been recorded by Liberian health officials. Most of the cases have been in people who are thought to have come to Liberia from Guinea (Reuters 2014a).

The WHO reports a total of 86 suspected Ebola cases, including 59 deaths in southeast Guinea (Reuters 2014a).

March 27, 2014 (Thursday)
There are now 103 suspected Ebola cases in Guinea (Lupkin 2014). Red Cross volunteers are disinfecting the homes and bodies of Guinean Ebola victims, while medical teams track down contacts of known Ebola cases (Reuters 2014e).

Two Ebola deaths are believed to have occurred in Sierra Leone (Reuters 2014b).

March 29, 2014 (Saturday)
The Ebola strain circulating in West Africa appears to be *Zaire ebolavirus*. This is an exceptionally dangerous species of Ebola. In past outbreaks, *Zaire ebolavirus* has had a fatality rate of up to 90% (Camara and Marone 2014).

Guinea's Ministry of Health says that eight people have tested positive for Ebola in Conakry and one person has died. The Ministry asks that citizens report any suspected Ebola cases and requests that people avoid touching anyone who might have the disease. Due to the public health risk posed by the virus, Ebola patients in Conakry are being treated free of charge (Lazuta 2014b).

There are six suspected Ebola cases in Sierra Leone, including five deaths (Lazuta 2014b).

Senegal has closed its border with Guinea to try to keep Ebola from entering (Camara and Marone 2014).

March 30, 2014 (Sunday)
The WHO confirms that two blood samples from Liberia have tested positive for Ebola (Auerbach 2014). One of the Liberian victims was a 35-year-old woman who died on March 21, 2014. She was the wife of a Guinean man who had recently returned to Liberia after becoming sick while visiting Guinea. The second victim is the woman's sister (Auerbach 2014). Since at least March 26, 2014, officials have suspected that Ebola has been in Liberia, but these are the first confirmed cases in the country.

Youssou Ndour, a Senegalese music performer, has canceled a weekend concert in Conakry, Guinea because of the Ebola outbreak. He is worried that bringing a large number of people together could help spread the disease (Auerbach 2014).

April 1, 2014 (Tuesday)
In the past 3 days, 19 new suspected Ebola cases have been identified in Guinea. This brings the total number of suspected cases in the country to 122 (UN News Service 2014). Even so, the WHO stresses that the current West African Ebola event should be considered an outbreak, not an epidemic (Schlein 2014). WHO spokesmen Gregory Härtl says that it is vital to break the chains of transmission and to conduct thorough contact tracing of all suspected cases. He also says that while the spread of Ebola to Conakry, Guinea is a serious development, it is not necessarily

unusual for Ebola to affect major cities. For example, cases occurred in Libreville, Gabon in the late 1990s (Schlein 2014).

The Ebola outbreak has started to affect social customs in Guinea. People no longer shake hands, and relatively few people attend funerals (BBC 2014b).

People in Liberia did not initially believe that Ebola posed a real danger. Many thought that local officials were using the threat of the disease to obtain funds. As more information has become available, however, this belief is starting to change. At one point, Liberian schools were closed, but they have now reopened (BBC 2014b).

The government of Sierra Leone has banned people from bringing corpses from Guinea into Sierra Leone for burial. It is hoped that this will reduce the risk of importing Ebola into Sierra Leone (BBC 2014b).

April 2, 2014 (Wednesday)
A single Ebola victim seems to have initiated the outbreak in Conakry, Guinea. A sick man came to Conakry from Dabola, Guinea, for treatment. All subsequent cases in Conakry are linked to this initial victim. To date, there have been 12 suspected Ebola cases in Conakry and 4 deaths. One of the deaths was the initial victim (Samb and Nebehay 2014).

Due to the outbreak, some mining companies in Guinea have locked down operations and withdrawn international staff (Samb and Nebehay 2014).

Suspected Ebola cases have been reported in The Gambia. These reports have been refuted by the country's director of Health Promotion and Education. He says that an elderly man was tested for the disease but tested negative (Samb and Nebehay 2014).

April 3, 2014 (Thursday)
Firmin Bogon of Guéckédou, Guinea recently lost ten relatives to Ebola. His sister returned ill from Sierra Leone on February 27, 2014. She was taken to the hospital where she was diagnosed with typhoid fever. She actually had Ebola. Not realizing she was highly contagious, her family took care of her at home. She died around March 3, 2014 and was given a traditional burial. A few days later, the people who had treated her began to fall ill. Since Bogon's sister death, nine other people have died, including Bogon's wife (BBC 2014c).

Medical experts are trying to reassure the public about Ebola. They point out that compared with other diseases, like influenza, Ebola is relatively easy to contain. Ebola is not airborne, and transmission requires direct contact with bodily fluids. They also say that even though cases have been found in several countries, most of the victims have come from a very small geographic area. Hence, the outbreak is not as widely distributed as it might seem (Sheets 2014).

Foreign traffic to Ebola-affected areas is slowing. A Brussels Airlines flight traveling between Brussels, Belgium and Conakry, Guinea arrived in Guinea today with 55 passengers. It left with 200 (Reuters 2014c).

April 5, 2014 (Saturday)
A mob attacked an Ebola clinic in Macenta, Guinea today (Associated Press 2014a; Reuters 2014c). They accused the MSF staff of bringing Ebola into the country. Rocks were thrown at staff members, but no one was hurt. In response, MSF has evacuated all of their personnel and closed the clinic (Reuters 2014c). At least 14 people have died from Ebola in Macenta since the outbreak began.

Dr. Michel Van Herp of MSF says the current Ebola outbreak is of an unprecedented scale. Other outbreaks have been relatively localized, but this one is spread among a variety of communities in three separate countries (Cobiella 2014).

Ebola may have reached Mali. Three suspected cases have been isolated in the country and are undergoing tests (Reuters 2014c).

April 7, 2014 (Monday)
Airport checkpoints have been set up in Guinea to screen passengers for Ebola before they leave the country (Vibes 2014). Travelers are observed for signs of illness, and their temperatures are taken before they are allowed to board outgoing planes (Quist-Arcton 2014a). Two recent cases have occurred where passengers have left Guinea with Ebola-like symptoms. In late March, a Canadian man was isolated in Saskatoon with an Ebola-like illness. Officials have not said what illness the patient actually had, but he did not have Ebola (Associated Press 2014b). On March 31, 2014, a man became sick in Minnesota after returning from West Africa. He tested positive for Lassa fever (Minnesota Department of Health 2014). Although neither of these patients had Ebola, the events demonstrate that air travel could help spread the disease.

April 9, 2014 (Wednesday)
To date, 158 Ebola cases have been reported, including 101 deaths (Sonricker Hansen 2014).

Despite Ebola's high fatality rate, some people survive the disease. At least seven people in Guinea have recovered and been released from isolation centers. Dr. Marie-Claire Lamah, an MSF doctor in Conakry, Guinea, says that their whole team was cheering when the first patients were released. The very first survivor was an 18-year-old woman named Rose Komano. She was released from a medical ward in Guéckédou (Mazumdar 2014).

April 10, 2014 (Thursday)
Aid groups are working to increase Ebola awareness across Africa. Agencies such as UNICEF, the Red Cross, and the WHO are using text messaging, robocalls, radio shows, TV programs, and door-to-door contacts to distribute information about Ebola. UNICEF is also providing soap, chlorine, and gloves to people affected by the outbreak (UNICEF 2014).

April 11, 2014 (Friday)
Challenges are being faced by Ebola survivors when they attempt to integrate back into their communities. When a survivor returns home, they are often shunned by neighbors who are afraid the survivor is still contagious. Henry Gray, the MSF

coordinator in Guinea, stresses that survivors pose no risk. However, it is hard to get community members to accept this (Quist-Arcton 2014b).

April 14, 2014 (Monday)
The US Department of Defense has opened a laboratory in Monrovia, Liberia, to test Liberian samples for Ebola. Previously, Liberian samples were sent to Guinea for testing (Reuters 2014d).

Institutions across the world are working to develop Ebola treatments. Currently, only supportive treatments such as hydration and fluid replacement are available for Ebola patients. San Diego-based Mapp Biopharmaceutical has developed a cocktail of monoclonal antibodies that help a patient's body identify and attack the virus (Thompson 2014).

April 15, 2015 (Tuesday)
Officials in Guinea believe that the Guinean Ebola outbreak is almost under control. A government spokesmen says that the number of new cases has fallen rapidly. Once no new cases emerge, the official says the outbreak can be considered controlled (Reuters 2014d).

The Gambia has banned flights from Guinea, Sierra Leone, and Liberia from landing in its territory. The ban is in place as of today, but The Gambia apparently began preparing the ban earlier. A letter about the ban was issued to airlines on April 10, 2014 (AFP 2014a).

April 16, 2014 (Wednesday)
The Ebola virus circulating in West Africa is 97% similar to the *Zaire ebolavirus* strain that caused the recent outbreaks in the Democratic Republic of the Congo and Gabon (Baize et al. 2014). The strain is genetically different enough to suggest that it has evolved separately from other Ebola strains. The case fatality rate in the current outbreak is 86% among confirmed cases (Baize et al. 2014). Baize et al. (2014) also appear to have identified Emile Ouamouno as the first known case. Their first case, identified as patient S1, was a 2-year-old boy who became ill on December 2, 2013, and died on December 6, 2013. Emile Ouamouno had not yet been identified by the media as the likely index case.

Nigeria is concerned that Ebola may reach the country. It has begun a public education campaign to help inform citizens about the virus (Christian Today 2014).

April 17, 2014 (Thursday)
A senior Guinean health official says the government will no longer release Ebola death toll numbers because they might frighten the country's citizens. The Guinean government has previously said that 106 people have died from Ebola in Guinea (Al Jazeera 2014).

April 18, 2014 (Friday)
Sixteen patients are being treated for Ebola at Donka Hospital in Conakry, Guinea. Eleven are being treated in Guéckédou, Guinea. Overall, Donka Hospital has 40 beds available for Ebola patients. Guéckédou has 20 beds (Médecins Sans Frontières 2014b).

April 22, 2014 (Tuesday)
There have been 208 clinical cases of Ebola, including 139 deaths, in Guinea through April 20, 2014. In Liberia, 34 clinical cases have occurred through April 21, 2014. The last confirmed Liberian case appeared on April 10. In Sierra Leone, there have been 19 clinical cases. However, as of yet, no Sierra Leone samples have tested positive for Ebola (Disease Outbreak News 2014b).

Fear of Ebola is mounting in Conakry, Guinea. Passengers recently abandoned a bus in the city when a pregnant woman vomited (Diallo 2014).

April 23, 2014 (Wednesday)
One anonymous Guinean Ebola survivor has seen nine family members contract Ebola. Only three have survived, including the informant. The survivor says his first symptoms were headache, backache, diarrhea, and vomiting. He was initially diagnosed with malaria but was later determined to have Ebola. MSF doctors at a clinic comforted him and provided him with moral support. Unfortunately, when people in the clinic died, the doctors had to collect the bodies and sterilize the area, while other patients watched. As the informant started to get better, he began to tolerate food and water again. Soon his diarrhea stopped. He felt exhilarated when he officially recovered from Ebola and was released from the hospital (BBC 2014d).

April 28, 2014 (Monday)
Faith healer Finda Nyuma, locally known as Mendinor, becomes ill (AFP 2015). Nyuma was a significant Ebola vector. Numerous woman who attended her funeral became sick and spread the disease (AFP 2015; Gire et al. 2014; Menezes 2014). Nyuma was a well-known and respected healer who lived near the border of Guinea and Sierra Leone. She claimed that she could heal Ebola and was visited by patients seeking a cure (AFP 2015). There is some confusion about the timing of Nyuma's illness and debate about the role she played in spreading the disease. The most commonly accepted account – that Nyuma became ill at the end of April 2014 and her funeral led to additional Ebola infections – is presented here. Sack et al. (2014) say that Nyuma became ill at the end of March 2014 and died around April 8, 2014. Others (e.g., Blayden 2015) strongly deny that Nyuma helped ignite the subsequent outbreak.

Ebola survivors continue to be stigmatized when they return to their communities. Because of this, the Guinean Ministry of Health is no longer naming the neighborhoods with suspected Ebola cases (Lazuta 2014c).

April 30, 2014 (Wednesday)
Guinea believes its Ebola outbreak is under control. Guinean President Alpha Condé expressed confidence that disease was being contained and said there have been no new cases in recent days (AFP 2014b).

Finda Nyuma dies of Ebola (AFP 2015).

May 1, 2014 (Thursday)
There is currently one Ebola patient in Conakry, Guinea, three in Guéckédou, and none in Macenta (Médecins Sans Frontières 2014c).

May 2, 2014 (Friday)
The West African Ebola outbreak may be winding down. Only a few confirmed cases remain in Guinea, and no new cases have been reported from Liberia in over 3 weeks. With the decline in cases, a MSF Ebola clinic in Macenta, Guinea, has been placed on standby (Médecins Sans Frontières 2014c). The incubation period for Ebola is 21 days (World Health Organization 2015). The outbreak will be considered officially over once two incubation periods (42 days) have passed without a new case appearing (World Health Organization 2015).

May 6, 2014 (Tuesday)
Senegal reopened its border with Guinea at 0800 h this morning (Reuters 2014e).

May 7, 2014 (Wednesday)
Guinea has reported a total of 231 Ebola cases and 155 deaths. Liberia has reported 13 cases (Smith 2014).

May 14, 2014 (Wednesday)
There have been no new Ebola cases in Conakry, Guinea, since April 26, 2014 (AFP 2014c).

The Gambia has lifted its flight bans for Sierra Leone and Liberia. The ban on flights from Guinea presumably remains in effect. The Gambia says that it will reevaluate its bans as the situation warrants (AFP 2014c).

May 15, 2014 (Thursday)
Guinea reports two new Ebola deaths. This brings the total number of fatalities in the country to 157 (Watts 2014).

References

AFP (2014a) Gambia bans flights from Ebola-hit nations. AFP, Sydney Morning Herald. http://www.smh.com.au/world/gambia-bans-flights-from-ebolahit-nations-20140415-zqv75.html. Accessed 20 Aug 2014

AFP (2014b) Ebola outbreak under control, says Guinea president. AFP, Borneo Post. http://www.theborneopost.com/2014/05/01/ebola-outbreak-under-control-says-guinea-president/. Accessed 19 Dec 2016

AFP (2014c) Gambia lifts flight bans as Guinea says Ebola spread slowed. AFP, NDTV. http://www.ndtv.com/article/world/gambia-lifts-flight-bans-as-guinea-says-ebola-spread-slowed-523828. Accessed 20 Aug 2014

AFP (2015) Sierra Leone marks grim Ebola anniversary. AFP, Times Live. http://www.timeslive.co.za/africa/2015/05/25/Sierra-Leone-marks-grim-Ebola-anniversary. Accessed 25 May 2015

Al Jazeera (2014) Ebola continues to spread through West Africa, stoking fears of epidemic. Al Jazeera. http://america.aljazeera.com/articles/2014/4/17/ebola-west-africa.html. Accessed 20 Aug 2014

Associated Press (2014a) Ebola clinic in Guinea evacuated after attack. CBC. http://www.cbc.ca/news/world/ebola-clinic-in-guinea-evacuated-after-attack-1.2599555. Accessed 19 Aug 2014

Associated Press (2014b) Man in Canadian hospital with Ebola-like symptoms after travel to Africa. Fox News. http://www.foxnews.com/health/2014/03/25/man-in-canadian-hospital-with-ebola-like-symptoms-after-travel-to-africa/. Accessed 19 Aug 2014

Auerbach T (2014) Outbreak of deadly flesh-eating Ebola virus has now spread to three countries and already killed 78. Daily Mail. http://www.dailymail.co.uk/news/article-2593035/2-cases-deadly-Ebola-virus-confirmed-Liberia.html. Accessed 19 Aug 2014

Bah M (2014) Ebola epidemic spreads to Guinea's capital: UNICEF. http://reliefweb.int/report/guinea/ebola-epidemic-spreads-guineas-capital-unicef. Accessed 19 Aug 2014

Baize S, Pannetier D, Oestereich L et al (2014) Emergence of Zaire Ebola virus disease in Guinea – preliminary report. N Engl J Med 371:1418–1425

BBC (2014a) Guinea Ebola outbreak: bat-eating banned to curb virus. BBC. http://www.bbc.com/news/world-africa-26735118. Accessed 19 Aug 2014

BBC (2014b) Eyewitness: Ebola outbreak fears. BBC. http://www.bbc.com/news/world-africa-26844105. Accessed 20 Aug 2014

BBC (2014c) I lost 10 relatives to Ebola. BBC. http://www.bbc.com/news/world-africa-26868674. Accessed 19 Aug 2014

BBC (2014d) I caught Ebola in Guinea and survived. BBC. http://www.bbc.com/news/world-africa-27112397. Accessed 19 Aug 2014

Blayden SO (2015) Facebook. https://www.facebook.com/soblyden/posts/1051156204914188. Accessed 28 Aug 2017

Camara O, Marone S (2014) Ebola death toll in Guinea rises to 70 as Senegal closes border. Bloomberg. http://www.bloomberg.com/news/2014-03-29/ebola-virus-death-toll-in-guinea-outbreak-rises-to-70-people.html. Accessed 18 Aug 2014

Christian Today (2014) Ebola virus outbreak in Nigeria? Nation is on high alert as nearby countries struggle with virus. Christian Today. http://www.christiantoday.com/article/ebola.outbreak.nigeria.the.nation.high.alert.nearby.countries.struggle.virus/36821.htm. Accessed 20 Aug 2014

Cobiella K (2014) Ebola breaks out on a scale never seen before. CBS News. http://www.cbsnews.com/news/ebola-breaks-out-on-a-scale-never-seen-before/. Accessed 20 Aug 2014

Diallo M (2014) Ebola: facing down fear to save lives in Guinea. IFRC. https://www.ifrc.org/en/news-and-media/news-stories/africa/guinea/ebola-facing-down-fear-to-save-lives-in-guinea-65710/. Accessed 20 Aug 2014

Disease Outbreak News (2014a) Ebola virus disease in Guinea. World Health Organization. 23 March 2014

Disease Outbreak News (2014b) Ebola virus disease, West Africa – update. World Health Organization. 22 April 2014

Gire SK, Goba A, Andersen KG et al (2014) Genomic surveillance elucidates Ebola virus origin and transmission during the 2014 outbreak. Science 345(6202):1369–1372

Lazuta J (2014a) Emergency Ebola intervention launched in Guinea. VOA News. http://www.voanews.com/content/deadly-ebola-virus-confirmed-in-guinea/1877059.html. Accessed 19 Aug 2014

Lazuta J (2014b) Guinea Ebola outbreak spreads to Conakry, poses new challenges. VOA News. http://www.voanews.com/a/ebola-outbreak-spreads-to-conakry-poses-new-challenges/1882132.html. Accessed 19 Aug 2014

Lazuta J (2014c) Ebola victims face stigma in West Africa. VOA News. http://www.voanews.com/content/ebola-victims-face-stigma-in-west-africa/1902587.html. Accessed 20 Aug 2014

Lupkin S (2014) 4 Health care workers among 66 dead in Ebola outbreak. ABCNews. http://abcnews.go.com/blogs/health/2014/03/27/4-health-care-workers-among-66-dead-in-ebola-outbreak/. Accessed 19 Aug 2014

Mazumdar T (2014) Guinea Ebola outbreak: 'Some patients recovering.' BBC. http://www.bbc.com/news/health-26963083. Accessed 20 Aug 2014

Médecins Sans Frontières (2014a) Guinea: Ebola epidemic declared, MSF launches emergency response. MSF. http://www.msf.org/article/guinea-ebola-epidemic-declared-msf-launches-emergency-response. Accessed 19 Aug 2014

Médecins Sans Frontières (2014b) MSF continues Ebola response in Guinea and Liberia. MSF. http://www.doctorswithoutborders.org/news-stories/field-news/msf-continues-ebola-response-guinea-and-liberia. Accessed 19 Aug 2014

Médecins Sans Frontières (2014c) Guinea MSF remains vigilant in Ebola outbreaks in Guinea and Liberia. MSF. http://www.msf.org/article/guinea-msf-remains-vigilant-ebola-outbreaks-guinea-and-liberia. Accessed 19 Aug 2014

Menezes A (2014) Faith healer helped spread Ebola in Sierra Leone: report. International Business Times. http://www.ibtimes.com/faith-healer-helped-spread-ebola-sierra-leone-report-1663694. Accessed 20 Aug 2014

Minnesota Department of Health (2014) Lassa fever confirmed in traveler returning to Minnesota from West Africa. http://content.govdelivery.com/accounts/MNMDH/bulletins/af26a6. Accessed 14 Dec 2016

Quist-Arcton O (2014a) The Ebola outbreak 3 weeks in: dire but not hopeless. NPR. http://www.npr.org/blogs/health/2014/04/08/300509073/the-ebola-outbreak-three-weeks-in-dire-but-not-hopeless. Accessed 20 Aug 2014

Quist-Arcton O (2014b) The Ebola survivors: reborn but not always embraced. NPR. http://www.npr.org/blogs/health/2014/04/11/301439165/the-ebola-survivors-reborn-but-not-always-embraced. Accessed 21 Aug 2014

Reuters (2014a) W Africa scrambles to prevent Ebola spread. Reuters, Aljazeera. http://www.aljazeera.com/news/africa/2014/03/w-africa-scrambles-prevent-ebola-spread-201432622029370444.html. Accessed 19 Aug 2014

Reuters (2014e) Guinea says Ebola outbreak contained death toll rises. Reuters, Fox News. http://www.foxnews.com/health/2014/03/27/guinea-says-ebola-outbreak-contained-death-toll-rises/. Accessed 19 Aug 2104

Reuters (2014b) UPDATE 2-Mob attacks Ebola treatment in Guinea, suspected cases reach Mali. Reuters. http://in.reuters.com/article/2014/04/04/guinea-ebola-mali-idINL-5N0MW2AG20140404. Accessed 19 Aug 2014

Reuters (2014c) Guinea says Ebola outbreak nearly under control. Reuters, Fox News. http://www.foxnews.com/health/2014/04/15/guinea-says-ebola-outbreak-nearly-under-control/. Accessed 19 Aug 2014

Reuters (2014d) Senegal reopens border with Guinea as Ebola threat eases. Reuters. http://www.reuters.com/article/2014/05/06/us-ebola-senegal-guinea-idUSKBN0DM0SE20140506. Accessed 20 Aug 2014

Sack K, Fink S, Belluck P, Nossiter A (2014). How Ebola roared back. New York Times. https://www.nytimes.com/2014/12/30/health/how-ebola-roared-back.html?mcubz=0. Accessed 28 Aug 2017

Saéz AM, Weiss S, Nowak K et al (2015) Investigating the zoonotic origin of the West African Ebola epidemic. EMBO Mol Med 7:17–23

Samb S (2014) Ebola kills dozens in Guinea may have spread To Sierra Leone. The Huffington Post. http://www.huffingtonpost.com/2014/03/22/ebola-guinea_n_5014500.html. Accessed 19 Aug 2014

Samb S, Nebehay S (2014) Miners in lock-down as Ebola death toll hits 83 in Guinea. Reuters. http://www.reuters.com/article/2014/04/02/guinea-ebola-idUSL5N0MU2ZT20140402. Accessed 20 Aug 2014

Schlein L (2014) WHO: Ebola in Guinea an outbreak, not an epidemic. VOA News. http://www.voanews.com/content/who-ebola-in-guinea-an-outbreak-not-an-epidemic/1883860.html. Accessed 20 Aug 2014

Sheets CA (2014) Fears of Ebola outbreak spreading from Guinea unfounded, Health Officials Say. International Business Times. http://www.ibtimes.com/fears-ebola-outbreak-spreading-guinea-unfounded-health-officials-say-1566750. Accessed 20 Aug 2014

Sierra Leone marks grim Ebola anniversary. AFP, Times Live. http://www.timeslive.co.za/africa/2015/05/25/Sierra-Leone-marks-grim-Ebola-anniversary. Accessed 25 May 2015

Smith M (2014) Ebola outbreak slowing down in West Africa. Med Page Today. http://www.medpagetoday.com/InfectiousDisease/GeneralInfectiousDisease/45652. Accessed 19 Aug 2014

Sonricker Hansen AL (2014) Ebola updates and an interview. http://healthmap.org/site/disease-daily/article/ebola-updates-and-interview-41114. Accessed 21 Aug 2014

Thompson D (2014) As African Ebola outbreak spreads hopes for vaccine remain years away. HealthDay. http://consumer.healthday.com/infectious-disease-information-21/misc-infections-news-411/as-african-ebola-outbreak-spreads-hopes-for-vaccine-remain-years-away-686731.html. Accessed 19 Aug 2014

UN News Service (2014) Guinea: UN Health Agency working to contain Ebola outbreak in Guinea. UN News Service, All Africa. http://allafrica.com/stories/201404020989.html. Accessed 19 Aug 2014

UNICEF (2014) Life-saving information helps reduce spread of Ebola across West Africa. UNICEF. http://www.unicef.org/media/media_73037.html. Accessed 21 Aug 2014

UNICEF (n.d.) Fact sheet wash. https://www.unicef.org/wcaro/wcaro_GUI_factsheet_wash_09.pdf. Accessed 12 Dec 2016

Vibes J (2014) Ebola cases suspected in US and Canada, airports in Guinea begin health checkpoints. The Daily Sheeple. http://www.thedailysheeple.com/ebola-cases-suspected-in-us-and-canada-airports-in-guinea-begin-health-checkpoints_042014. Accessed 21 Aug 2014

Watts AG (2014) Two more Ebola deaths reported in Guinea despite waning outbreak. https://followtheoutbreak.wordpress.com/2014/05/15/two-more-ebola-deaths-reported-in-guinea-despite-waning-outbreak/comment-page-1/. Accessed 19 Dec 2016

World Health Organization (2015) Criteria for declaring the end of the Ebola outbreak in Guinea, Liberia or Sierra Leone. 7 May 2015

Yan H, Kinkade L (2014) Ebola: who is patient zero? Disease traced back to 2 year old in Guinea. CNN. http://www.cnn.com/2014/10/28/health/ebola-patient-zero/. Accessed 28 Oct 2014

Chapter 3
Escalation (May 23, 2014–August 31, 2014)

Abstract By the middle of May 2014, the West African Ebola outbreak appeared to be under control. Then suddenly and unexpectedly, new cases began to emerge. First as a trickle, and then as a flood, the number of confirmed and suspected cases increased rapidly. West African medical facilities did their best to cope with the outbreak. Initially they were able to handle the onrush of cases, but soon resources were stretched thin. Then doctors began to die from the disease. In some cities, corpses of Ebola victims lay in the streets. Rural areas were also hard-hit. Reporters described finding whole communities decimated by the virus. In a desperate bid to contain the outbreak, countries closed their borders and issued travel bans. Despite these efforts, Ebola continued to spread. By the end of August 2014, there were active Ebola cases in Guinea, Liberia, Sierra Leone, Nigeria, and Senegal. In addition, a small number of Western healthcare workers had become infected and been transported to the United States, Spain, and the United Kingdom for treatment. Overall, more than 3000 people had contracted Ebola. More alarmingly, the number of new cases continued to grow exponentially.

3.1 Day-by-Day Outbreak Entries (May 23, 2014–August 31, 2014)

May 23, 2014 (Friday)
Guinea has confirmed two new Ebola cases. The discovery of these new patients is disturbing. They not only represent a reemergence of Ebola, but they also come from the town Telimele in a part of the country that has not yet been affected by the outbreak. The victims both attended a woman's funeral (possibly Finda Nyuma's). However, the deceased woman's body has not been tested, so it is unclear if she died from Ebola. Both patients have been isolated, and the government is monitoring 41 people who had contact with the new victims (Hussain and Samb 2014).

May 24, 2014 (Saturday)
In Sierra Leone, a pregnant woman who attended Finda Nyuma's funeral arrives at Kenema Hospital (Gire et al. 2014; Hammer 2015; Vogel 2014). She has symptoms of hemorrhagic fever but tests negative for Lassa (Hammer 2015). She is the hospital's first Ebola patient (Hammer 2015 states the woman arrived on May 23, 2014).

May 25, 2014 (Sunday)
Scientists have confirmed the first two cases of Ebola in Sierra Leone (Gire et al. 2014). Both patients arrived at the same treatment facility in Kenema yesterday. They were confirmed as having Ebola today. One of the patients is a pregnant woman; the other is an older housewife (AFP 2015; Gire et al. 2014; Vogel 2014). There were suspected cases of Ebola in Sierra Leone before, but these are the first confirmed cases.

May 26, 2014 (Monday)
Sierra Leone's health ministry confirms that Ebola is present in the country (Al Jazeera 2014a). One recent death has been confirmed as being caused by Ebola. Three other deaths are under investigation. Eleven people have been admitted to Koindu community health center with Ebola-like symptoms (Al Jazeera 2014a). The WHO is sending six experts to the region (Reuters 2014a).

Guinea says a person has died from Ebola in the town of Telimele (Diallo and Roy-MacCaulay 2014).

May 27, 2014 (Tuesday)
A family has removed a female Ebola patient from a healthcare center in Koindu, Sierra Leone (Reuters 2014b; Gbandia 2014a). Medical workers strongly protested the patient's removal, but the family did not trust the medical officials. Healthcare workers had planned to transfer the patient to the hospital in Kenema, but her family thought she would die if she was moved. Officials are concerned the sick woman will infect others in the community (Reuters 2014b).

In a separate incident, villagers in eastern Sierra Leone threw stones at medical workers who were trying to inspect the bodies of two suspected Ebola victims. The attack might have occurred because the medical staff did not properly introduce themselves to the villagers or explain what they were doing before they started their work (Gbandia 2014a).

Two Liberians have composed a song entitled "Ebola in Town" (Mark 2014a; Poole 2014). It has a catchy beat and is becoming popular in West Africa. The lyrics are intended to increase Ebola awareness. The song describes ways to avoid catching the disease, such as not eating bushmeat and not shaking hands (Poole 2014).

May 28, 2014 (Wednesday)
Two new Ebola cases have been identified in Conakry, Guinea. They are the first cases in the city in over a month. Government official Aboubacar Sidiki Diakité says that the flare-up might have occurred because families are hiding patients so they can treat them with traditional methods (Nebehay and Samb 2014).

Families have aggressively removed a total of six Ebola patients from treatment facilities in Koindu, Sierra Leone (Guardian 2014a).

May 29, 2014 (Thursday)
One of the patients who was removed from the healthcare center in Koindu, Sierra Leone, has died. Many people in rural Sierra Leone think cholera is affecting the

region, not Ebola. As a result, they are not concerned about interacting with infected patients (Cooper 2014).

May 30, 2014 (Friday)
Ten new Ebola cases and seven new deaths have occurred in Guinea since May 28, 2014. A total of 50 clinical cases have been reported from Sierra Leone. Liberia has reported one suspected case which is still under investigation. The Liberian case involves a person who died in the Foya District of Liberia and had their body transported to Sierra Leone for burial (Disease Outbreak News 2014a).

May 31, 2014 (Saturday)
Computational biologist Pardis Sabeti has been working in a medical laboratory in Kenema, Sierra Leone. She has been running PCR tests to determine if patients are infected with Ebola (Sabeti 2014). She describes the working conditions of the laboratory staff and the challenges of using full-body PPE in a tropical environment:

> Entering the lab requires a ten-minute ritual of donning a full-body protective suit, complete with built in booties and head cap. I put on two sets of gloves, making sure to tuck them into the sleeves of my suit so that no skin was showing. I bring up the hood cap and tuck my hair underneath, wiping the sweat that has already formed on my forehead. It's at least 85 °F where we dress to enter the lab. I will be in this suit for the next four hours as I process suspected Ebola cases with fellow lab members...
>
> As the day moves on, the heat finally takes its toll. I feel exhausted and my concentration wanes. I push the feeling aside, but I quickly start losing basic reasoning skills. I stare at my lab notebook, but I can't make sense of what's on the page. I have to get out: I am of no use to anyone in this condition. It's ironic, almost; our protective equipment is supposed to keep us safe, but now it's putting me at risk. I quickly decon out of the lab and remove my gear.
> (Sabeti 2014)

June 3, 2014 (Tuesday)
MSF is setting up an Ebola treatment center in Koindu, Sierra Leone (Médecins Sans Frontières 2014a).

The British firm, London Mining, has evacuated some nonessential staff from Sierra Leone. However, the company says that production at its iron ore mine in Marampa, Sierra Leone is unaffected (BBC 2014a).

June 4, 2014 (Wednesday)
There were 37 new Ebola cases and 21 deaths in Guinea between May 29, 2014 and June 1, 2014. During the same period, there were 13 new cases, but no deaths in Sierra Leone. Overall, a total of 214 deaths have been attributed to the outbreak, 208 in Guinea and 6 in Sierra Leone (Disease Outbreak News 2014b).

MSF reports receiving 20 new Ebola cases at its Guinean treatment centers during the past week. Bart Janssens, the director of MSF operations, says the large number of new cases clearly shows the outbreak is not under control (Look 2014).

To help educated people about Ebola and explain why some unfamiliar protective protocols are necessary, Sierra Leone's Health Ministry posted a series of FAQs about Ebola on its website. Several of the questions include (transcribed verbatim):

Question: How should I greet people, if the hand shake is not recommended?

Answer: Hand shaking should be avoided as it is a risk during the outbreak or before a potential outbreak. You can greet people by waving to them or acknowledge by shaking your head. Washing your hands with soap and clean water regularly is also recommended.

Question: Why am I told not to eat bush meats?

Answer: People are advised not to eat bush meats during an Ebola outbreak as current evidence suggests that those animals may be the sources of the virus. Monkeys, chimpanzees, bats or dead animals found in the bush MUST be avoided during and before the outbreak. People can resume eating the meat once the government declares the outbreak to be over.

Question: In rainy season, bats feed on mangoes. Do I stop eating mangoes?

Answer: No, you can continue eating mangos but they properly need to be washed before eating. However, you should avoid the mangoes which bat has bitten (bat mot).

Question: Can I call a hotline to report suspicious cases?

Answer: Yes, call toll free 117 to report any suspicious case and to get more information on Ebola Virus Disease. You should also report any suspicious cases to the nearest health facility as soon as possible. (Sierra Leone Ministry of Health and Sanitation 2014)

June 5, 2014 (Thursday)

Sierra Leone has reinstated its ban on citizens traveling to Guinea to attend funerals (Al Jazeera 2014a).

June 7, 2014 (Saturday)

The Lancet published a short note describing the current Ebola outbreak and explaining why it has been so hard to contain. Some of the key issues identified by the report are (1) the poor healthcare infrastructure of the affected countries, (2) the lack of experience local healthcare workers have with the virus (this is the first time Ebola has occurred in West Africa), (3) the widespread geographical nature of the outbreak, (4) the lack of trust local communities have for healthcare workers, and (5) the high mobility of people in the infected communities. In regard to this last point, Michel Van Herp of MSF says that even the dead in the region move. This refers to the common West African practice of transporting bodies for burial (Lancet 2014).

June 8, 2014 (Sunday)

Ebola has reached the town of Mambolo in Northern Sierra Leone. Mambolo is about 20 miles northwest of Port Loko. The Disease Surveillance Officer for the Kambia District says the disease arrived when an infected driver returned to Mambolo from Koindu. The driver began exhibiting symptoms after he returned and subsequently infected his wife. Both the driver and his wife have tested positive for Ebola. The infected driver traveled widely, and it is feared he might have spread the disease to other parts of the country (Awareness Times 2014).

June 9, 2014 (Monday)

Sierra Leone reports 42 confirmed Ebola cases and 12 deaths (Fofana 2014a). One of the victims was a nurse named Messie Konneh (Awareness Times 2014). Konneh became ill in Koindu, but Ebola was not suspected. As she became sicker, her husband took her to the town of Bombohun for treatment. Eventually he started to move her toward Kenema, but nurse Konneh died on the way. Her body was washed and prepared according to traditional customs. Since her death, her mother and sisters who helped prepared her body have all died. Some of the healthcare workers who assisted her in Bombohun have also died (Awareness Times 2014). Messie Konneh's husband, Sheku Konneh, was also thought to have died from Ebola. However, on June 11, 2014, he suddenly reappeared and said that he had gone into hiding once he realized his wife had died from Ebola (Samba 2014).

The ECDC released a rapid risk assessment of the Ebola outbreak today. It confirms the outbreak now involves Guinea, Liberia, and Sierra Leone. It also says that there is cause for concern because of the recent surge in cases and because the geographic area affected by the disease is expanding (ECDC 2014).

June 10, 2014 (Tuesday)
Two healthcare workers in Kailahun District, Sierra Leone, have died from Ebola (Butty 2014a).

June 11, 2014 (Wednesday)
Sierra Leone has closed its borders with Guinea and Liberia. It has also ordered the closure of schools, movie theaters, nightclubs, and trade fairs in Kailahun District. Checkpoints will be installed around the district, and any travelers passing through will be screened. The schools were ordered closed when a 9-year-old tested positive for Ebola after both of their parents had died from the disease. The government is requesting that residents notify them of all deaths. Health officials will attend the funerals of anyone thought to have died from Ebola (Reuters 2014c).

Rumors accuse medical personnel of spreading Ebola in West Africa (Diallo 2014). The rumors say the disinfectant being sprayed by workers is actually a poison that helps spread Ebola (Diallo 2014). This type of mistrust is a major problem and is making controlling the outbreak very difficult.

June 14, 2014 (Saturday)
Ebola has reached Liberia's capital, Monrovia. There have been seven suspected cases in New Kru Town, a suburb west of the city. Six victims have died and four of their bodies have tested positive for Ebola. The first case was a woman who had left Kailahun District, Sierra Leone and moved in with relatives in New Kru Town (APA 2014).

Sierra Leone has released its first Ebola survivor (AFP 2014a). Victoria Yillah, about 30 years old and pregnant, was discharged from the hospital in Kenema. She is the first person in Sierra Leone to recover from Ebola (AFP 2014a). Yillah's exact release date is unclear. She may have been discharged on June 8, 2014 (Johnson 2014). It is also unclear what effect, if any, Ebola has had on Yillah's unborn infant.

June 18, 2014 (Wednesday)
Since the beginning of the outbreak, there have been 398 Ebola cases in Guinea, 97 in Sierra Leone, and 33 in Liberia. Of these 528 cases, 337 (63.8%) have been fatal (Disease Outbreak News 2014c).

Liberia has reactivated its national task force for Ebola and has reopened its Ebola isolation unit (Lazuta 2014a).

Virologist Robert Garry of Tulane University has just returned from West Africa. He says that many villages in Sierra Leone have been heavily hit by Ebola. His group found 25 corpses in one village, including one house that contained seven bodies (Doucleff 2014).

June 19, 2014 (Thursday)
Many people in West Africa have more faith in traditional healers than Western medicine. Residents often think that diseases are caused by curses, so they do not believe Western medicine will help (Economist 2014). This is a problem because patients often avoid medical personnel or refuse to help them.

June 20, 2014 (Friday)
Bart Janssens, director of operations for MSF, says the agency is stretched to the limit with its Ebola relief efforts. He also says the epidemic is experiencing a second wave and appears to be out of control (DiLorenzo 2014).

Rumors continue to persist that healthcare workers are harming patients, not fighting Ebola. Some people in Guinea think Ebola is not real. Instead, they believe healthcare workers are harvesting the organs from the supposed Ebola victims (Ruble 2014).

June 21, 2014 (Saturday)
Pierre Formenty of the WHO was asked about the resurgence of Ebola and how the disease is currently spreading. He said that by the end of April 2014, there was a decrease in cases. This may have led to reduced vigilance in teams on the ground. Because people in West Africa travel a great deal, the disease spreads easily from place to place. It appears that transmission often occurs when people go to Conakry, Guinea, or Monrovia, Liberia, for healthcare (AFP 2014b).

June 23, 2014 (Monday)
Ebola has now been identified in 60 separate locations in Guinea, Sierra Leone, and Liberia (Jones 2014).

Phebe Hospital in Bong County, Liberia, has received its first Ebola patient. The patient, a middle-aged woman, arrived this evening. She has a high fever and is vomiting, but because Ebola has not yet been seen at the hospital, Ebola is not suspected. It is only later learned that she has the disease. Seven of the nurses who helped her contracted Ebola, six of them died (Levine 2014).

June 24, 2014 (Tuesday)
There are a total of 618 confirmed and suspected Ebola cases in West Africa (World Health Organization 2014a). This number includes 273 fatal cases in Guinea, 47 in Sierra Leone, and 37 in Liberia (World Health Organization 2014a). The WHO is organizing a meeting about the outbreak with regional Health Ministers, technical experts, and stakeholders. The meeting will be held July 2–3, 2014, in Accra, Ghana (Disease Outbreak News 2014d).

Many people in Sierra Leone still deny the existence of Ebola. In Kenema, where mortality among Ebola patients has been very high, some believe that medical staff in the Ebola wards are killing patients with lethal injections (Estrada 2014).

June 27, 2014 (Friday)
The WHO does not believe the Ebola outbreak is out of control (United Nations News Center 2014). The agency says it is working with the governments of the three affected countries to contain the disease (United Nations News Center 2014). The WHO does, however, caution that travelers could spread the virus throughout the region (Reuters 2014d; Voice of America News 2014a). It also warns that sickened people in rural areas might spread the disease when they travel to cities for treatment (Reuters 2014d).

A Guinean man on a flight from Morocco to Spain started exhibiting Ebola-like symptoms. He has been isolated in Valencia, Spain, and is being tested for Ebola (Live Press 2014).

June 28, 2014 (Saturday)
President of Liberia Ellen Johnson Sirleaf addressed the Liberian nation about the Ebola outbreak (Sirleaf 2014). She declared the outbreak a national public health emergency. She stressed that Ebola is very real and described the ways the disease can spread. She also promised to prosecute people who hid Ebola victims. She said:

> Major issues confronting the response teams include but not limited to keeping sick people in healing centers, prayer homes and other non medical centers. These practices create public health hazards to families, neighbourhoods and other innocent people. It is illegal under our public health law to expose the people to health hazard such as Ebola. Let this warning go out, anyone found or reported to be holding suspected Ebola cases in homes or prayer house will be prosecuted under the laws of Liberia. (Sirleaf 2014)

WHO spokesperson, Daniel Epstein, says that some Ebola workers in West Africa have been chased out of villages, had stones thrown at them, or been threatened with machetes (Lazuta 2014b).

Dr. Hilde De Clerck of MSF says the normal social customs of West Africa can help spread Ebola. For example, people in the region often have very large social networks and travel extensively. Because of the long incubation time of Ebola, infected people can unknowingly spread the disease as they travel (Lazuta 2014b).

June 30, 2014 (Monday)
Patients have been fleeing from Ebola isolation wards in Sierra Leone. The reasons patients leave vary, but they are generally related to being suspicious of the medical staff or being scared of the disease. At least 57 Ebola patients are currently missing from Sierra Leone clinics. In one case, a patient left a Kenema isolation ward. Messages about him were broadcast on the radio, and he was eventually located in Freetown. People he had contact with while he was out of the ward, including a nurse who thought he had typhoid and was treating him, are now being monitored. His mother is still missing (Fofana 2014b).

July 1, 2014 (Tuesday)

Total cases: 759   Total fatalities: 467 (Disease Outbreak News 2014e)

The WHO has begun providing tabular data about Ebola cases and deaths. The data are being published in *Disease Outbreak News* and represent the most recent figures available at the time of publication. By necessity, this means the data are at least 1 day old. For example, today's Disease Outbreak News (2014e) tallies data through June 30, 2014. The total reported cases include all confirmed, probable, and suspected cases. The 759 total cases reported today include 544 confirmed, 140 probable, and 75 suspected cases (Disease Outbreak News 2014e).

Dr. Samuel Muhumuza Mutoro has died from Ebola at John F. Kennedy Medical Centre in Monrovia, Liberia. Dr. Mutoro was a Ugandan doctor working at Redemption Hospital near Monrovia. He is believed to have become infected after he volunteered to treat a sick colleague (Muhindo and Bwambale 2014).

July 2, 2014 (Wednesday)
The West African countries affected by Ebola are urgently requesting funds to help fight the disease. Underscoring the need, the President, Vice President, and all cabinet ministers of Sierra Leone have promised to donate half of their salaries to Ebola-fighting efforts (Kpodo 2014).

Denial and fear are causing some locals to act aggressively toward medical workers in West Africa. In one case, Red Cross workers were threatened by knife-wielding residents in Guéckédou, Guinea. In response, the Red Cross has removed some international workers from the area (Hussain 2014a).

Health officials from 11 African countries began meeting in Accra, Ghana, today for a 2-day conference about the Ebola outbreak (Thompson 2014). Separately, Dr. Peter Piot, co-discoverer of the Ebola virus, called the current outbreak unprecedented (Krever 2014). He believes that more rigorous control measures, including intense military and community involvement, are needed to stop the disease (Krever 2014).

July 3, 2014 (Wednesday)

Total cases: 779 (20 new)   Fatalities: 481 (14 new)
                             (Disease Outbreak News 2014f) (new cases are
                             the cases added since the last officially reported
                             numbers; in this case, new cases represent the cases
                             added since July 1, 2014)

MSF says that at least 1500 people known to have had contact with Ebola victims still need to be traced (Pflanz 2014). In addition, there are 20 Guinean communities where MSF no longer operates because of hostility from the local residents (Dixon 2014).

Given that there are no current treatments or vaccines for Ebola, Jeremy Farrar, of the humanitarian group Wellcome Trust, has suggested that patients be offered experimental drugs. In response, Bart Janssens of MSF said that this was an interesting idea, especially because of Ebola's high fatality rate. However, he cautioned that there could be some significant challenges to actually providing experimental drugs to Ebola patients (Dixon 2014).

West African cultural practices may play a major role in the transmission of Ebola. For example, when a member of the Kissi ethnic group dies, the body is kept at home for several days (Mark 2014b). During this time mourners touch the corpse, especially around the head (Mark 2014b). Because secretions from deceased victims are infectious, these practices are very dangerous.

Some Liberians think Ebola is not actually in the country. Rather, they think the government is using the fear of Ebola to distract people from recent political scandals. To help counteract these ideas, newspapers have been publishing graphic photographs of dead Ebola victims. At the other end of the spectrum, the fear of Ebola has caused some survivors to be stigmatized. Aissata Bangoura's husband died of Ebola in March 2014. She has been declared virus-free but is generally avoided by community members. During her husband's wake, she was left by herself because people were afraid to get close to her (Mark 2014b).

July 4, 2014 (Thursday)

Kenema, Sierra Leone, has been hard-hit by Ebola. One anonymous man says that one of his female relatives became sick and was taken to the hospital. Doctors misdiagnosed her as having typhoid, and her family visited her. By the time it was clear she had Ebola, seven other family members were infected. Four of them have died (Trenchard 2014).

Medical experts think it is unlikely that Ebola will cause a large outbreak in North America. If the virus does reach the United States or Canada, perhaps in the form of an infected traveler, it is thought that the patient and their contacts will be quickly isolated and the disease rapidly contained (Schwartz 2014).

July 7, 2014 (Monday)

MSF is operating out of three medical facilities in Guinea. They have treated 59 patients in Conakry, of whom 33 have recovered. In Guéckédou, they have treated 130 patients, with 31 recovering. In Telimele, they have treated 21 patients, with 16 recovering. Operations in Telimele are being closed because there have been no new cases at the site in 21 days. In Sierra Leone, MSF is working in Kailahun, Kenema, Koindu, and Daru and has a treatment center in Kailahun. In Liberia, MSF has people working in Monrovia and Foya (Médecins Sans Frontières 2014b).

July 8, 2014 (Tuesday)

Total cases: 844 (65 new)   Fatalities: 518 (37 new)
                      (Disease Outbreak News 2014g)

In response to a question about the resurgence of Ebola after it was apparently contained in mid-May, Dr. Hilde de Clerck of MSF commented:

> Just a few weeks ago, there were only two villages left in Guinea that MSF still had to monitor for 'contact' people—anyone who had been in contact with confirmed or suspected cases of Ebola. As a result, we were quite hopeful that we were witnessing the end of the epidemic.
>
> But then, all at once, we received calls from three different sites in Guinea. Within five minutes, everything changed. It emerged that several cases had also appeared in villages in

neighboring Sierra Leone that are very close to the Guinean border. (Médecins Sans Frontières 2014c)

She continued by describing the difficulty of building trust with local residents:

In Macenta, Guinea, one family lost 15 people to the Ebola virus. MSF was able to treat the head of the family and his wife, who both survived. As a result, we were confident that those two successfully treated parents would then have a lot of influence on the rest of the family about the critical need to seek treatment immediately if anyone experienced Ebola-like symptoms. Yet, a few days later, a small boy from this same family fell ill. His aunt fled with him to another village and the child died a few days later.

Often, convincing one member of the family is simply not enough. To control the chain of disease transmission it seems we have to earn the trust of nearly every individual in an affected family. This is a mammoth task, which is why greater involvement from the religious and political authorities in raising awareness about the disease is crucial. (Médecins Sans Frontières 2014c)

West African beliefs can make it difficult for Western healthcare workers to control the virus. MSF is working with anthropologists to foster better communication between medical workers and local communities (Médecins Sans Frontières 2014c).

July 10, 2014 (Thursday)

Total cases: 888 (44 new)   Fatalities: 539 (21 new)
                             (Disease Outbreak News 2014h)

Samaritan's Purse, a Christian relief agency, has taken over responsibility for the Ebola center in Foya, Liberia, from MSF (Zaimov 2014). The Liberian government is encouraging citizens to take sick people to treatment centers instead of caring for them at home or taking them to prayer groups or witch doctors (Quist-Arcton 2014a).

Nigeria will contribute $3.5 M to help fight Ebola (BBC 2014b).

July 11, 2014 (Friday)

MSF emergency coordinator Anja Wolz is worried that many Ebola victims in Sierra Leone are going undetected. If so, officials may only be seeing the tip of the iceberg in terms of case numbers (BBC 2014b). Regional UNICEF director Manuel Fontaine echoed these concerns and appealed for more aid to fight the disease (UNICEF 2014). He said that in addition to providing basic medical care, healthcare workers also urgently need to earn the trust of the population (UNICEF 2014).

July 12, 2014 (Saturday)

Ebola has reached Sierra Leone's capital, Freetown (Gbandia 2014b). An infected Egyptian national came to Freetown from Kenema, Sierra Leone, and checked into a clinic (Gbandia 2014b). When it was determined he had Ebola, he was returned to the Ebola center in Kenema (Besser 2014).

July 13, 2014 (Sunday)

Many West African residents mistrust healthcare workers. Throughout the region, patients avoid treatment centers because they believe going to the hospital is a death sentence. Some families hide victims. Other patients hide in the forest until medical personnel leave their community. Marc Poncin of MSF says that villages in Guinea are sealing themselves off. In one case, villagers dismantled a bridge so healthcare workers could not reach their community. Local responses are sometimes violent. An armed mob recently chased healthcare workers away from a village in Lofa County, Liberia (Samb and Bailes 2014).

July 14, 2014 (Monday)
Dr. Bernice Dahn, Deputy Minister for Health Services, in Monrovia, Liberia, says there are many challenges to dealing with Ebola victims. The first problem is denial. Once a patient has been identified, major logistical issues then have to be overcome to deal with the situation. The patient has to be taken to an isolation ward. Then, all of the victim's contacts need to be identified and traced. Finally, if a patient dies, special burial teams have to handle their body (Filou 2014).

July 15, 2014 (Tuesday)
The Ivory Coast has prevented 400 Ivory Coast refugees from returning home. The people had crossed into Liberia to avoid political unrest in the Ivory Coast. The Ivory Coast is now worried that if the refugees return, they could bring Ebola with them (Gladstone 2014).

July 16, 2014 (Wednesday)
A 70-year-old woman died from Ebola on July 14, 2014 near Kailahun, Sierra Leone (Silver 2014a). Her family wanted to bury her behind their house, but the local chief stopped them and had them bury her in the adjacent jungle instead (Beaubien 2014a) (it is unclear if this happened today or during one of the last 2 days). When interviewed, some of the local residents were found to have misconceptions about the foreign medical staff who helped with the burial (Silver 2014a). One said that when they first arrived, he thought the healthcare workers were cannibals who had come to steal body parts. On a more positive note, it seems that the residents are following the no-touching recommendations made by NGOs working in the area (Silver 2014a).

July 17, 2014 (Thursday)

Total cases: 982 (94 new)   Fatalities: 613 (74 new)
                            (Disease Outbreak News 2014i)

Some confusion exists over patient admission protocols in Monrovia, Liberia. One man says that he recently took his sick brother to JFK Medical Center. The two tried to enter the main gate but were redirected to a separate cholera unit. When they got there, the man's brother, who was profusely vomiting blood, was not immediately admitted. It is thought that the delay occurred because the brothers did not call the established Ebola hotline to report the case (AllAfrica 2014a).

The Minister of Tourism and Cultural Affairs in Sierra Leone is worried that news about the Ebola outbreak is scaring away tourists. He says that between January and June 2014, there were 21% fewer tourists in Sierra Leone than during the same period in 2013. He asks that journalists report about the outbreak in a responsible and objective manner (Tommy 2014).

Store and restaurant owners in Ebola-affected areas face slumping business and economic hardship. One Sierra Leone restaurant owner is unable to sell bushmeat and is having trouble getting supplies of regular food. Drivers of motorcycle taxis are also being hard-hit. Few passengers want to ride on motorcycles because they have to ride pressed against the driver; they worry that the driver may have been exposed to Ebola (Beaubien 2014b).

Ebola survivors continue to face challenges when they return home. Some survivors have lost jobs because their employers are afraid that they are contagious (Bax 2014).

July 18, 2014 (Friday)
A major challenge facing medical workers in Ebola-affected areas is convincing locals the disease is real. Many people do not think Ebola exists. Others think it can be treated with local remedies. For example, some people believe eating two large onions can cure Ebola (Hogan 2014a).

July 19, 2014 (Saturday)

Total cases: 1048 (66 new)   Fatalities: 632 (19 new)
                              (Disease Outbreak News 2014j)

In Liberia, a student group calling itself the "Concern [sic] Students of the United Methodist University against the Spread of Ebola in Liberia" has organized (AllAfrica 2014b).

July 20, 2014 (Sunday)
Ebola has been introduced to Nigeria, though at present no one knows it. Patrick Sawyer, a 40-year-old Liberian and a consultant for the Liberian Finance Ministry, collapsed after arriving at the airport in Lagos, Nigeria, today (Onuah and Miles 2014). He was very ill and taken to the First Consultant Hospital (AFP 2014c; Onuah and Miles 2014). Sawyer was conscious when he arrived at the hospital and denied having contact with Ebola patients (Odunsi 2014). The staff began treating him for malaria (Odunsi 2014). No one knew that Sawyer was infected with Ebola. Patrick Sawyer was a naturalized US citizen (Wilson 2014a). His wife and three daughters live in Coon Rapids, Minnesota (Wilson 2014a). Sawyer's sister had died from Ebola on July 8, 2014, and he likely caught the disease from her (Satellite 2014a; Onuah and Miles 2014). Sawyer may have suspected that he had Ebola. He had previously told his employer that he had been exposed to virus (Ibekwe 2014a; Satellite 2014b). On the flight from Liberia, he was acting strange, looked sad, and was trying to avoid bodily contact with people (Ibekwe 2014b). As the hospital staff treated him, they became increasingly concerned when Sawyer began to develop symptoms of hemorrhagic illness (Odunsi 2014). It will be several days before Sawyer is diagnosed with Ebola.

Researchers at USAMRIID think Ebola might have been present in West Africa at low levels for years (Fox 2014a). The researchers tested archived blood samples from the region. The blood had been collected from patients who were thought to have Lassa fever but who tested negative for Lassa fever. They found that 19 of 220 specimens (8.6%) tested positive for Ebola antibodies (Schoepp et al. 2014). This suggests that some of these earlier patients had undiagnosed Ebola infections.

July 21, 2014 (Monday)

Nurse Mbalu Fonnie, head of the Lassa fever unit and Ebola management center at Kenema Hospital in Sierra Leone, died today. Several other nurses from the facility (possibly as many as four) also died today (Moriba 2014).

Four nurses working at Phebe Hospital in Suakoko, Liberia, have contracted Ebola. They have been transferred to Monrovia for treatment (New Vision 2014).

To help reduce the marketing of bogus Ebola cures, the Liberian Assistant Health Minister for Preventive Services requests that people report to the police anyone who is providing or selling medicines claimed to prevent Ebola. In particular, he stresses that *Garcinia kola*, also known as bitter kola, does not cure Ebola. This product has been recently touted as a possible cure for Ebola (AllAfrica 2014c).

The UN warns that wild animals harvested for the bushmeat trade could be infected with Ebola and could pass the disease on to hunters or consumers. The collection of fruit bats and primates is of particular concern because these animals are believed to be natural reservoirs for the Ebola virus. The sale of bushmeat is part of the West African underground economy. It is generally carried out by individuals, so it is difficult to determine the overall scale of the business. However, bushmeat is very widely sold and is thought to generate millions of dollars in revenue each year (Caulderwood 2014).

Possible Ebola cases have been reported from the Aru region of the Democratic Republic of the Congo. Samples from the area are being tested to see if the victims are suffering from Ebola (Baguma 2014).

July 22, 2014 (Tuesday)

Sierra Leone's head Ebola doctor, a 39-year-old virologist Dr. Sheik Umar Khan, has contracted Ebola (Reuters 2014e) (his name is sometimes reported as Dr. Sheik Humarr Khan e.g., Wilson 2014b). Sierra Leone's Health Minister called Dr. Khan a national hero and vowed to do everything possible to make sure he recovers (Reuters 2014e). Dr. Khan may have become infected when he conducted a quick physical exam on a nurse without using proper PPE (Hammer 2015). He and the nurse, Alex Moigboi, had just finished a shift in the Ebola ward and had removed their PPE when Moigboi said he was not feeling well. Dr. Khan quickly assessed Moigboi, which included touching Moigboi around the eyes. Moigboi tested positive for Ebola the next day and died several days later (Hammer 2015).

Nancy Writebol, a 59-year-old missionary working with Samaritan's Purse at an Ebola care unit in Mornovia, Liberia, begins feeling ill (CBS News 2014a). She has a fever, fatigue, and malaise (Lyon et al. 2014). She hopes it is malaria, but she has been helping staff working with Ebola patients don and doff their PPE. She has also been helping decontaminate staff when they finish their shifts (Lyon et al. 2014).

Though she does not know it yet, Writebol has Ebola. Writebol is the first natural-born American citizen to contract Ebola during the 2013–2016 outbreak.

Healthcare workers in Kenema, Sierra Leone, are demanding that the Ebola unit be moved out of the local hospital and that MSF to take over operation of the Ebola facility. The medical personnel do not think the clinic is being managed properly. They have several other concerns, including the fact that they lack adequate PPE (Moriba 2014).

July 23, 2014 (Wednesday)

Dr. Kent Brantly, a 33-year-old American, begins feeling ill in Monrovia, Liberia. He wakes up this morning with fever and fatigue (Lyon et al. 2014). Dr. Brantly is the medical director for Samaritan's Purse Ebola Consolidated Case Management Center in Monrovia (Sutton and Yan 2014). This is the same facility where Nancy Writebol has been working. Dr. Brantly has been treating Ebola patients since June 11, 2014 (Lyon et al. 2014). Though he has not yet been diagnosed, Dr. Brantly has Ebola. He is the second American to contract the disease.

The United Methodist Hospital in Ganta, Liberia, has recorded its first Ebola death. The victim was a 36-year-old man from Monrovia (Doloquee 2014).

July 24, 2014 (Thursday)

Total cases: 1093 (45 new)   Fatalities: 660 (28 new)
                              (Disease Outbreak News 2014k)

A Liberian man in his 40s [Patrick Sawyer] is being tested for Ebola in Lagos, Nigeria (Onuah and Miles 2014; Reuters 2014f).

July 25, 2014 (Friday)

Ebola has officially reached Nigeria. Patrick Sawyer died in Lagos, Nigeria, at 0650 h this morning (Channels Television 2014). Tests conducted after his death confirm that he had Ebola (Onuah and Miles 2014). His body was cremated (Odunsi 2014). Officials are now trying to trace his contacts (Awoniyi 2014).

A female Ebola patient has been forcibly removed from an isolation ward in King Harman hospital in Freetown, Sierra Leone, by her family (Fofana 2014c, d). Saudatu Koroma, 32 years old, tested positive for Ebola yesterday. Her family then stormed the hospital and removed her. Radio stations have been announcing her flight and are asking for help in locating her (Fofana 2014c).

Thousands of people marched against the main hospital in Kenema, Sierra Leone, after a former nurse said cannibalism was occurring in the Ebola ward. Police dispersed the crowd with tear gas (Reuters 2014g).

July 26, 2014 (Saturday)

Two Americans, Dr. Kent Brantly and Nancy Writebol, have tested positive for Ebola in Liberia (Lyon et al. 2014; Williams 2014). They are the first Americans to contract the virus during the outbreak. It is unclear exactly when Writebol tested positive. Lyon et al. (2014) say a sample obtained on the fifth day of her illness (i.e., July 26, 2014) was positive, but they do not specifically say what day the sample was tested.

Dr. Samuel Brisbane died from Ebola today (AllAfrica 2014d). Dr. Brisbane was a Liberian doctor and the Chief Medical Doctor at JFK Medical Center in Monrovia, Liberia. During an emergency situation in June 2014, he helped move the hospital's first Ebola patient. Dr. Brisbane was only wearing a pair of gloves at the time (Davis 2014). He became sick a little over a week later (Davis 2014). His body will be buried in a mass grave with other Ebola victims (McCray 2014).

Missing Ebola patient Saudatu Koroma has been found (Reuters 2014g). She was hiding in the home of a traditional healer in Freetown, Sierra Leone (Reuters 2014g). Her family did not want officials to take her and a struggle developed, but she was removed. She died in the ambulance on the way to the hospital (Fofana 2014d).

Two types of Ebola victims are handled by the Red Cross Society's Dead Body Management Team in Kailahun, Sierra Leone: those who die in treatment centers and those who die in the community. Bodies in treatment centers are disinfected before the team recovers them. The team asks family members if they would like the body returned, or if they would prefer the victim be buried in a special Ebola cemetery. Most choose the cemetery. Ebola victims who die outside of treatment centers are more challenging to recover. The team must decontaminate the bodies before they move them. This requires a great deal of care and forces team members to wear considerable PPE. Any items associated with a body, such as soiled bedding or clothing, are collected and buried with the victim (Mueller 2014).

Nigeria has started screening arriving airline passengers for Ebola. Airports in Nigeria are also preparing holding rooms to isolate Ebola patients (Associated Press 2014a).

July 27, 2014 (Sunday)

Total cases: 1201 (108 new)   Fatalities: 672 (12 new)
(Disease Outbreak News 2014l)

Liberia has closed most of it borders to prevent travelers from importing or exporting Ebola (Reuters 2014h). A special statement released by Liberian President Sirleaf says in part:

> All borders of Liberia will be closed with the exception of major entry points including the Roberts International Airport, James Spriggs Payne Airport, Foya Crossing, Bo Waterside Crossing, Ganta Crossing. At these entry points, preventive and testing centers will be established, and stringent preventive measures to be announced will be scrupulously adhered to. (Republic of Liberia n.d.)

A group of armed youths stood guard outside the village of Kolo Bengou in Guinea to prevent MSF workers from entering. The youths think MSF personnel will bring Ebola into the village (Nossiter 2014a).

Nigeria's Arik Air has suspended flights to Liberia and Sierra Leone (Godwin 2014).

July 28, 2014 (Monday)
Nigeria has closed and quarantined First Consultant Hospital in Lagos, the hospital that treated Patrick Sawyer. Decontamination efforts are underway, and some of the healthcare workers who assisted Sawyer have been isolated. Officials are also trying to locate all of the passengers who were on Sawyer's flight from Liberia (Cocks 2014).

Dr. Daniel Bausch, associate professor at the Tulane School of Public Health and Tropical Medicine and the head of the Virology and Emerging Infections Department at the United States Naval Medical Research Unit No. 6 in Lima, Peru, has been assisting with the Ebola outbreak in Guinea and Sierra Leone. At one point, he and one other physician were the only healthcare workers available to assist 55 Ebola patients in Kenema, Sierra Leone. He says the two focused their efforts on the most important tasks and helped those who had a chance of survival. He also says it was common to find patients who had fallen out of bed and were soiled with vomit, blood, and stool (Grady 2014a).

July 29, 2014 (Tuesday)
Dr. Sheik Umar Khan died from Ebola in Sierra Leone today (Wilson 2014b). He was buried behind Kenema Government Hospital (Hammer 2015). During his illness, there had been considerable debate about how to treat Dr. Khan. One idea was to give him the experimental Ebola drug ZMapp. Three vials of the drug were available in Kailahun, Sierra Leone, where Dr. Khan was being treated, but the drug had never been tested on humans. On July 25, 2014, health officials decided not to use ZMapp (Hammer 2015). Officials also considered flying Dr. Khan to a health facility in a more developed country, such as Germany, for treatment (Huggler 2014). This was ruled out because of Dr. Khan's precarious health (Hammer 2015). These decisions were very difficult to make and were made in good faith (Pollack 2014). Later in the outbreak, however, the decisions not to use ZMapp or to air evacuate Dr. Khan were heavily criticized when these techniques were used to successfully treat other Ebola patients.

Dr. Kent Brantly has been given a unit of whole blood from a 14-year-old male Ebola survivor (Lupkin 2014a; Lyon et al. 2014). It is hoped that antibodies in the survivor's blood will help Dr. Brantly fight the disease.

Two North Carolina Christian aid groups, Samaritan's Purse and Serving in Mission, are removing about 60 nonessential personnel from West Africa due to the Ebola outbreak (Spain 2014).

The emergency department at the Carolinas Medical Center in Charlotte, North Carolina, briefly closed this evening because of an Ebola scare. The staff became concerned when an ill patient arrived at the ED after having been in an Ebola-affected country. It was soon clear that the patient's symptoms and history were not consistent with Ebola (Fox and Edwards 2014).

July 30, 2014 (Wednesday)
Sierra Leone has declared a state of emergency due to the Ebola outbreak (Fofana 2014e; Government of Sierra Leone 2014). In announcing the action, President Ernest Bai said that the scale of the outbreak is too large for any one country to deal

with. He listed some of the specific control measures that will be implemented in Sierra Leone:

> All epicenters of the disease will be quarantined;
> The police and the military will give support to health officers and NGOs to do their work unhindered and restrict movements to and from epicenters;
> Localities and homes where the disease is identified will be quarantined until cleared by medical teams;
> Public meetings and gatherings will be restricted with the exception of essential meetings related to Ebola sensitization and education;
> Active surveillance and house-to-house searches shall be conducted to trace and quarantine Ebola victims and suspects;
> Parliament is recalled to promote MPs leadership at constituency levels;
> Paramount chiefs are required to establish bye-laws that would complement other efforts to deal with the Ebola outbreak;
> Mayors, chairmen of councils and councilors are hereby required to support Ebola control measures in their local government areas;
> All deaths must be reported authorities before burial;
> New protocols for arriving and departing passengers have been instituted at the Lungi International Airport;
> Cancellation of all foreign trips by ministers and other government officials except absolutely essential engagements. (Government of Sierra Leone 2014)

July 31, 2014 (Thursday)

Total cases: 1323 (122 new)   Fatalities: 729 (57 new)
(Disease Outbreak News 2014m)

The experimental drug ZMapp arrived in Liberia this morning for use on American Ebola patients Dr. Kent Brantly and Nancy Writebol (Gupta and Dellorto 2014). Several frozen vials of the drug arrived, but they needed to thaw before they could be used. Initially, Dr. Brantly asked that the first available vial be given to Writebol (Lupkin 2014a). However, Dr. Brantly suddenly became gravely ill and was having difficulty breathing. He then requested to use the first vial himself (Gupta and Dellorto 2014). Within an hour of having ZMapp administered, Dr. Brantly's condition remarkably improved and his breathing difficulties disappeared (Gupta and Dellorto 2014). Writebol also received a dose of ZMapp, but she did not experience as dramatic an improvement in her condition as Brantly (Lyon et al. 2014).

Airports in Ghana have started checking the temperatures of travelers arriving from West Africa. Ghana is also monitoring 11 passengers who flew with Patrick Sawyer (Fofana 2014e).

The CDC has issued a Level 3 travel warning for Guinea, Liberia, and Sierra Leone (Centers for Disease Control and Prevention 2014a). A Level 3 warning is the highest warning issued by the agency. It means that travelers are at high risk of infection and that all unnecessary travel to the affected region should be avoided (Centers for Disease Control and Prevention n.d. a).

August 1, 2014 (Friday)

West African officials have announced that an Ebola isolation zone will be imposed at the junction of Guinea, Liberia, and Sierra Leone. The plan is to cordon off and quarantine the Mano River Union region where about 70% of Ebola cases have occurred. The military and police will enforce the quarantine and supplies will be delivered to the people in the zone (AFP 2014d).

Dr. Kent Brantly and Nancy Writebol will be evacuated from Liberia and returned to the United States for treatment (Hasting and Hutchison 2014). They will be flown to the United States in a private jet equipped with a quarantine pod. Emory University Hospital in Atlanta, Georgia, says they expect to receive one patient within the next several days (CBS News 2014b; Hasting and Hutchison 2014). It is unclear if the second patient will also go to Emory. Some people think bringing Ebola-infected people to the United States is a bad idea. They worry that it could cause an Ebola outbreak in America (Edwards 2014).

Various US entry points, including Newark Liberty Airport in New Jersey and John F. Kennedy Airport in New York, have trained health officials on site to identify and isolate travelers with Ebola-like symptoms (CBS New York 2014).

August 2, 2014 (Saturday)

Dr. Kent Brantly has returned to the United States (Fieldstadt et al. 2014). The plane carrying him landed at Dobbins Air Reserve Base at 1120 h today. From the airport, Dr. Brantly was taken to Emory University Hospital. He arrived at Emory around 1250 h and walked into the hospital under his own power. Dr. Brantly was wearing a hooded biocontainment suit and was assisted by a PPE-covered worker (Fieldstadt et al. 2014; Snyder S 2014). Security at the hospital was tight during his arrival (Blinder and Grady 2014).

Six missionaries, including Father Miguel Pajares, a 75-year-old Roman Catholic priest from Spain, have been quarantined at Saint Joseph Hospital in Monrovia, Liberia (AFP 2014e). The hospital director died today from Ebola. The missionaries have been quarantined because they had contact with the director (AFP 2014e).

Dubai-based Emirates airline has suspended flights to Guinea (AFP 2014f). The airline does not operate in Sierra Leone or Liberia.

August 3, 2014 (Sunday)

The bodies of two Ebola victims were found lying in the streets of Clara Town, Liberia today. Clara Town is a slum in Monrovia. Both men had been bleeding and vomiting before they collapsed and died. It is unclear how long the bodies were in the streets before officials learned of them. Some residents say they had been there for several days. Others say they were there for a few hours. Both bodies have now been removed (Reuters 2014i).

The bodies of 37 Ebola victims have been abandoned in a cemetery in Kparpeh's Town, Liberia. The Ministry of Health and Social Welfare had purchased land to bury the bodies. When the burials began, however, it was quickly discovered that the area was too marshy to dig in, and the burial team's backhoe became stuck. Some of the bodies were buried, but others were simply left on the ground in body bags. A few bodies were found floating in uncovered, water-filled graves. Residents of the community are outraged and have barricaded the road leading to the cemetery (Kollie 2014).

Nancy Writebol has been given a second dose of ZMapp (Gupta and Dellorto 2014; Lyon et al. 2014).

August 4, 2014 (Monday)

Total cases: 1603 (280 new)   Fatalities: 887 (158 new)
(Disease Outbreak News 2014n)

Nigeria has confirmed a second Ebola case. The doctor who treated Patrick Sawyer has contracted the virus. Three other people who helped Sawyer have also developed Ebola-like symptoms. They are being tested. Currently about 70 people are under surveillance in Nigeria (Adigun 2014a).

Sierra Leone is deploying troops to help contain the Ebola outbreak. About 750 Sierra Leone troops are being transported to affected parts of the country as part of Operation *Octopus*. The troops will stage out of the town of Bo and move to isolated villages to set up quarantines (Fofana and MacDougall 2014a).

Liberia has ordered that the bodies of all Ebola victims be cremated (BBC 2014c). Twelve bodies were cremated in the country today (MacDougall and Flynn 2014). Liberia is also deploying troops throughout the country to help deal with the crisis (Fofana and MacDougall 2014a).

Saudi Arabia will not allow Haj pilgrims from Liberia, Sierra Leone, or Guinea to enter Saudi Arabian territory (Sophia 2014).

A 72-year-old woman collapsed and died at Gatwick Airport in the United Kingdom after arriving from Sierra Leone. Her sudden death sparked considerable fear at the airport. Officials closed the jet bridge she used and quarantined the aircraft. However, it does not appear that the woman had Ebola (Doherty 2014).

A man who recently returned from West Africa is being tested for Ebola at Mount Sinai Hospital in New York City. Officials do not think he has Ebola, but the fact that he is being tested has nearby residents on edge (Schram 2014).

August 5, 2014 (Tuesday)

The bodies of some Ebola victims are being dumped in the streets of Monrovia, Liberia. People are worried that they will be quarantined if the government knows one family member has died from Ebola. So, instead of notifying officials about a death, some families are leaving the bodies of the dead in the streets (MacDougall and Flynn 2014). It is unclear if the two bodies reported on August 3, 2014 had been abandoned in this manner.

One of the Nigerian nurses who helped treat Patrick Sawyer has died from Ebola (Mark 2014c). Six other Nigerians who had contact with Sawyer now have Ebola-like symptoms (Mazen 2014).

Nancy Writebol has arrived in the United States (McClam 2014). Like Dr. Kent Brantly before her, she arrived at Dobbins Air Reserve Base and was transported to Emory University Hospital (Copeland and Stanglin 2014). Unlike Brantly, she was much weaker and could not walk into the hospital on her own. Instead, she was wheeled in on a gurney (Copeland and Stanglin 2014).

Spanish priest, Father Miguel Pajares, has tested positive for Ebola in Liberia (AFP 2014e). Two of the African missionaries quarantined with him have also tested positive (Govan 2014). The Spanish government plans to transport Father Pajares to Spain for treatment (AFP 2014e). Father Pajares is the first European to contract Ebola during the outbreak.

British Airways will suspend all flights to Sierra Leone and Liberia starting August 6, 2014. The ban will last until at least August 31, 2014 (Freeman and Akkoc 2014).

August 6, 2014 (Wednesday)

Total cases: 1711 (108 new)   Fatalities: 932 (45 new)
                                (Disease Outbreak News 2014o)

Liberia has declared a 90-day state of emergency due to the Ebola outbreak (BBC 2014d; NBC News 2014a). The country has also shut down Saint Joseph Catholic Hospital in Monrovia where Spanish priest, Father Miguel Pajares, was infected (Snyder D 2014).

Radios and loudspeakers in Freetown, Sierra Leone, are broadcasting Ebola awareness announcements. It is hoped this will help convince skeptics that Ebola is real and is a major health emergency (Quist-Arcton 2014b).

A 2-day UN emergency meeting on the Ebola outbreak has started in Geneva, Switzerland (Shinkman 2014).

The United States has granted permission for an experimental Ebola test to be used. The test, called DoD EZ1 Real-time RT-PCR Assay, has not yet been approved by the Food and Drug Administration. The emergency authorization will let the test be used during the current crisis (Chiacu 2014). It is unclear how widely available the test will be, but it could help quickly identify Ebola patients.

August 7, 2014 (Thursday)

Infected Spanish priest, Father Miguel Pajares, has arrived in Spain. He was flown to the country on a specially equipped Airbus A310. Father Pajares flew into Torrejón Air Base and was taken to Carlos III Hospital in Madrid (Kassam 2014; NBC News 2014b). The entire sixth floor of the hospital was cleared for him (Fofana and MacDougall 2014b). All of the other patients were released or transferred to other facilities before his arrival. Father Pajares is currently in stable condition (Kassam 2014). Father Pajares is the first Ebola patient to arrive on European soil during the outbreak.

Operation *White Shield* is the name for the Liberian military response to Ebola. It should be fully in place by August 8, 2014. As part of the operation, checkpoints are being set up outside of Monrovia (Fofana and MacDougall 2014b).

Many Ebola victims in Kenema, Sierra Leone, are avoiding the hospital and dying at home (Nossiter 2014b). A member of the hospital's burying team says about four people are dying at the hospital each day, while five or six people die in the community (Nossiter 2014b). People are generally avoiding medical facilities throughout the country. Many tropical diseases have symptoms similar to Ebola. People with other diseases, such as malaria, are afraid if they go to the hospital, they will be misidentified as having Ebola and placed in an Ebola ward (Kitamura and Gbandia 2014). Separately, Kenema, Sierra Leone, has instigated a 1900 h curfew (Nossiter 2014b).

The CDC has issued a Level 1 response for the Ebola outbreak (Stanglin 2014). A Level 1 response means that the agency will assign the largest possible staff to work on the crisis (Centers for Disease Control and Prevention n.d. b). CDC Director Dr. Thomas Frieden says the CDC has more than 200 people working on the outbreak in Atlanta. Additionally, more than 50 experts will be deployed to West Africa (Reuters 2014j).

The US Department of State has ordered the families of US embassy personnel to leave the Liberia because of the outbreak (US Department of State 2014a).

August 8, 2014 (Friday)

Total cases: 1779 (68 new)   Fatalities: 961 (29 new)
(Disease Outbreak News 2014p)

The WHO has declared the Ebola outbreak a public health emergency of international concern (World Health Organization 2014b).

Ebola is significantly affecting the social fabric of West Africa. In Monrovia, Liberia, people are lining up at banks and hoarding food. In Sierra Leone, the cost of basic goods is rising. The price of rice is up to 30% since the beginning of the outbreak. The price of salt doubled over one 24 h period (Sullivan and Moyer 2014).

Nigerian President Goodluck Jonathan has requested that citizens avoid public gatherings and refrain from moving the corpses of Ebola victims. He has also approved $11.7 M to fight Ebola in Nigeria (Reuters 2014k).

August 9, 2014 (Saturday)
Guinea has closed its borders with Sierra Leone and Liberia. This is expected to slow some cross-border traffic, but it will be very difficult to prevent people from crossing the borders in remote rural areas (Guardian 2014b).

Zambia will deny entry to travelers from Ebola-affected countries and will prevent its citizens from traveling to countries with Ebola outbreaks (Bariyo 2014).

Disease experts believe they have identified patient zero for the outbreak. The victim was a 2-year-old boy [Emile Ouamouno] who died on December 6, 2013, in Guéckédou, Guinea. One week after the boy's death, his mother, grandmother, and 3-year-old sister all became ill. Mourners at the grandmother's funeral and healthcare workers were then infected (Grady and Fink 2014).

Riot police have broken up a demonstration in Monrovia, Liberia. People were protesting the slow pace of body collection. In the town of Weala, Liberia, several bodies have been lying in the streets for 2 days (Weise 2014).

The economic toll of the outbreak continues to rise. The World Bank has lowered its estimate for Guinea's 2014 economic growth from 4.5% to 3.5%. Several corporations, including Caterpillar Inc., have started to remove workers from Ebola-affected areas (Wiseman 2014).

A traveler has been isolated in Brampton Civic Hospital in Ontario, Canada. The person had recently been in Africa and has Ebola-like symptoms (NBC News 2014c).

August 10, 2014 (Sunday)

Spain has authorized the use of the experimental drug ZMapp on infected priest Father Miguel Pajares (Lewis 2014).

A suspected Ebola case has appeared in Hong Kong. A 31-year-old Nigeria man complained of feeling ill and having diarrhea. After going to Queen Elizabeth Hospital, he was transferred to the Infectious Disease Centre at Princess Margaret Hospital (South China Morning Post 2014).

August 11, 2014 (Monday)

Total cases: 1848 (69 new)   Fatalities: 1013 (52 new)
                              (Disease Outbreak News 2014q)

The United States has agreed to send ZMapp to Liberia to treat Liberian doctors. Mapp Biopharmaceutical Inc., the maker of ZMapp, says its supply of the drug is now exhausted and that it has provided ZMapp free of charge to those who have needed it (Loftus 2014).

The village of Njala Ngiema in Sierra Leone has been hard-hit by the outbreak. To date, 61 people have died in the community out of a population of about 500. In one house 16 people have died. In another five have died. In many cases, the clothing and household items used by the dead victims remain where they left them. People are afraid to touch or remove the items (Nossiter 2014c).

Survivors are released from the Ebola treatment center in Kenema, Sierra Leone, around 1500 h each day. As they leave, survivors are given transportation money, a clean set of clothes, and a certificate saying they no longer have Ebola (Sahara Reporters 2014a).

A Roman Catholic Church in Freetown, Sierra Leone, ends each Mass with an Ebola prayer:

> *Hear our humble cry and save our country from the Ebola disaster. By the power of your divine touch, heal all those who have been affected by the Ebola virus and totally free them from the clutches of the evil one.* (Silver 2014b)

American universities are trying to determine how to respond to the West African Ebola outbreak. Most schools are playing it safe. They are suspending study abroad and cultural exchange programs to West Africa. For example, New York University has decided not to send students to Ghana in the fall (Weintraub 2014).

August 12, 2014 (Tuesday)

Spanish priest, Father Miguel Pajares, died in Madrid's Carlos III Hospital today. It is unclear whether he had been given ZMapp before his death. His body will be cremated (Cheng and Giles 2014).

Guinea-Bissau has closed its southern and eastern borders with Guinea. The borders will remain closed until further notice (Voice of America News 2014b).

Due to Ebola's high mortality and lack of effective treatments, the WHO has given its support to treating Ebola patients with experimental drugs. Separately, the Assistant Director-General of the WHO, Marie-Paule Kieny, leveled criticism at pharmaceutical companies for not developing Ebola treatments before the crisis. It is thought that drug makers did fully research treatments for the disease because the countries normally affected by Ebola are poor. Since people in these countries would have little money to spend on treatments, there was little economic incentive for companies to develop Ebola medications (Bacon and Weintraub 2014).

August 13, 2014 (Wednesday)

Total cases: 1975 (127 new)   Fatalities: 1069 (56 new)
                              (Disease Outbreak News 2014r)

Guinea has declared the Ebola outbreak a public health emergency (Shankar 2014). Guinean President Alpha Condé says large amounts of medical supplies and personnel are headed to Guinea's borders with Liberia and Sierra Leone (Voice of America News 2014c).

Officials are worried that an infected nurse may have spread Ebola to the eastern part of Nigeria. The nurse contracted Ebola while treating Patrick Sawyer. She then traveled to Enugu (about 120 miles northeast of Port Harcourt) with her husband, became sick, and checked into a hospital. The nurse has since been transported back to Lagos and been isolated (AFP 2014g).

In a surprising move, Nigeria has suspended all of its resident doctors. Resident doctors have been on strike since July 1, 2014 over training and funding issues. They make up ~90% of the doctors in Nigerian teaching hospitals (Ibeh 2014). This suspension could significantly affect the country's Ebola-fighting efforts.

Sierra Leone has lost another high-level doctor to Ebola (Roy-Macaulay and Cheng 2014). Dr. Modupeh Cole died today in Kailahun. The 56-year-old Dr. Cole is believed to have become infected at Connaught Hospital in Freetown while treating a patient (Nossiter 2014d). After being diagnosed with Ebola, he was transferred to Kailahun for treatment (Roy-Macaulay and Cheng 2014).

Ebola burials are conducted in Kailahun, Sierra Leone, by workers of the Red Cross Dead Body Management Team between 2000 and 0000 h each day. Bodies are enclosed in two body bags, buried 6 feet deep, and sprayed with large amounts of bleach (Haglage 2014).

Several doses of ZMapp have arrived in Liberia (MacDougall 2014a). Health officials plan to treat Liberian doctors at the JFK Medical Center with the drug (AllAfrica 2014e).

In the village of Ballajah, Liberia, 51-year-old Abdulah Sherrif, his 43-year-old wife Seidia Passawee, and their 12-year-old daughter Fatu have all died from Ebola. Abdulah became sick on July 20, 2014. By the time he died, his wife and child were infected. None of the people in the village were willing to help the family, and their house was shuttered; it is unclear if the house was sealed by the village or the family. The mother died on August 10, and the little girl remained inside with the body. Her cries for help were ignored. She died during the night of August 11–12, 2014. Only the family's 15-year-old son Barnie remains alive. He is currently living alone in an abandoned house (Dossa 2014).

The WHO reports that between 94% and 98% of Ebola contacts have been traced in Guinea, Nigeria, and Sierra Leone. Thus, most of the people who had contact with Ebola victims have been identified and tracked in these countries. Efforts in Liberia are not yet as well coordinated (Disease Outbreak News 2014r).

Germany is urging all of its nationals, except medical workers and diplomatic staff, to leave Guinea, Sierra Leone, and Liberia (Voice of America News 2014b).

Throughout West Africa, there are many rumors about potential Ebola preventatives and cures. One rumor says that drinking or bathing in salt water can fight the disease. Unfortunately, using these unfounded remedies can have severe consequences. Two people died in Nigeria recently after drinking large quantities of salt water (Aliyu and Nanlong 2014).

August 14, 2014 (Thursday)

The WHO says their Ebola casualties estimates may vastly underestimate the true scale of the outbreak (World Health Organization 2014c). This is likely true given that little information is available from isolated parts of West Africa.

The US Department of State has ordered the families of US embassy personnel to leave Sierra Leone (US Department of State 2014b).

MSF is building a major 120-bed Ebola isolation ward in Monrovia, Liberia. Currently two isolation centers are operating in the country. MSF coordinator Lindis Hurum says the outbreak is escalating rapidly and more personnel are needed to help with the situation (NPR 2014a).

The Ebola outbreak is having a disproportionate impact on women. Overall, 55–60% of Ebola victims are women. In Liberia, women make up 75% of infected cases. Women are usually the family caregivers in West Africa, and traditional healers are often women. Thus, women may be more exposed to the virus than men (Hogan 2014b).

There is great concern that quarantined areas may be suffering from food shortages. Local farmers have died and truckers are reluctant to take food into the isolated zones. International groups are thinking about sending emergency air drops of food to the quarantined regions (Dawson 2014).

Some unscrupulous people have found ways to take advantage of the Ebola outbreak. In Liberia, one man crushed tomatoes and placed the juice in his ears and nose. He then approached a store clerk and yelled "I'm bleeding!" When the clerk ran away, the man stole all the money from the cash register (Beaubien 2014c).

Kenya is a major African transportation hub and could serve as a vector for Ebola cases. Because of this, Korean Air Lines will suspend services to Nairobi, Kenya, starting August 20, 2014 (Al Jazeera 2014b).

Science writer Laurie Garrett is concerned about the Ebola outbreak. She worries that Westerners have become accustomed to the idea that the "the government" is capable of handling any disease threat. Through movies, books, and popular media, people have come to believe that "the government" has access to vast high-tech resources that can be used to quickly halt an outbreak. She notes that this is not the case. Instead, she says that considerable on-the-ground support is needed in West Africa and is needed quickly (Garrett 2014).

August 15, 2014 (Friday)

Total cases: 2127 (152 new)   Fatalities: 1145 (76 new)
                               (Disease Outbreak News 2014s)

Three infected African healthcare workers have started treatment with ZMapp (MacDougall 2014b). Two Liberian doctors, Dr. Zukunis Ireland and Dr. Abraham Borbor, and Nigerian doctor, Dr. Aroh Cosmos, have received the drug (MacDougall 2014b). Before the medication was administered, each recipient signed consent forms stating that they understood the risks involved and released all parties from liability (Fink 2014a). The President of Liberia, Ellen Johnson Sirleaf, expressed gratitude for the drug. She said that even though only a few doses were available, the fact that they were being used to treat Africans was inspiring (Fink 2014a).

Liberian Ebola centers are filling extremely rapidly. One 80-bed facility filled as soon as it opened (Adigun 2014b).

An 80-bed hospital in Kailahun, Sierra Leone, has so far admitted 204 confirmed Ebola cases. Of these, 53 (25.9%) have survived. Kailahun remains under a military quarantine (NPR 2014b).

Dr. Oliver Johnson of King's Health Partners describes what it is like when a new Ebola patient arrives at Connaught Hospital in Sierra Leone. Patients are screened by a nurse and moved into an isolation unit. When they enter the ward, the patients are often disoriented and scared, partly because the healthcare workers are in full PPE. To comfort them, staff sit and talk with them (Early 2014).

To date, four people have died from Ebola in Nigeria. These are Patrick Sawyer, two nurses who cared for him, and a Nigerian ECOWAS protocol officer whose job was to welcome ECOWAS ambassadors. There are currently six confirmed Ebola patients in the country and 169 people under surveillance (AllAfrica 2014f).

The Nigerian government is seeking medical staff willing to fight Ebola. They are offering $185 a day to doctors who work with infected patients. So far, relatively few have accepted. Many are afraid they will be stigmatized if people know they are working with Ebola victims (Grady 2014b).

Cameroon has suspended all flights to Sierra Leone, Liberia, Guinea, and Nigeria (Al Jazeera 2014c).

At the Youth Olympic Games in Nanjing, China, the International Olympic Committee has announced that athletes from Ebola-affected countries will not be allowed to compete in contact sports or swim in the swimming pool. These moves will affect three athletes. In addition, all team members from Ebola-affected countries will be subject to temperature checks and physical assessments throughout the games (Keith 2014).

Online marketers are selling a variety of false Ebola cures and preventatives. One such product is Garcinia Cambogia [sic] powder. In addition to fighting Ebola, this miracle item also apparently helps with weight loss, cholesterol, colds, flu, etc. (Duhaime-Ross 2014).

August 16, 2014 (Saturday)
An armed mob broke into an Ebola clinic in the West Point slum of Monrovia, Liberia, today and liberated some patients (AFP 2014h; Associated Press 2014b). Several hundred local residents chanting "No Ebola in West Point" chased away an Ebola burial team who had come to collect some bodies (AFP 2014h). The crowd then forced open an Ebola isolation ward and allowed some patients to leave. Between 20 and 29 patients are believed to have left the facility (AFP 2014h; BBC 2014e). The attackers then looted the clinic. A police official said that many people were seen running off with items taken from sick Ebola patients, including blood-stained sheets and mattresses (Associated Press 2014b). There is major concern that this will cause an explosive Ebola outbreak in West Point.

Nigeria is training 800 volunteers to assist Ebola patients and conduct contact tracing. The country will also pull its athletes from the Youth Olympics in China due to the restrictions imposed by event organizers (Al Jazeera 2014d).

Some West Africans still think aid workers are cannibalizing Ebola victims or stealing their organs. Healthcare workers are working hard to build trust and dispel these rumors. In Guinea, the families of some Ebola victims are allowed to watch the burials at a distance. In other cases, family members are given PPE and taken to see the body of their relative. In these ways, the families can see that the bodies are intact and have not been desecrated (Fink 2014b).

Kenya will close its borders to travelers from Liberia, Guinea, and Sierra Leone starting on August 19, 2014 (AFP 2014i). Kenya Airways will suspend flights to Liberia and Sierra Leone (Reuters 2014l). Gambia Bird Airlines will stop flights to Liberia, Sierra Leone, and Nigeria (Paye-Layleh and Larson 2014).

Dr. Kent Brantly and Nancy Writebol continue to recover from Ebola. They are both improving (McKay 2014).

August 17, 2014 (Sunday)
Operation *White Shield* continues in Liberia. It is unclear what conditions are like in the quarantined areas, but there are concerns that not enough supplies are reaching the isolated communities. Indeed, inhabitants seem to have been left to fend for themselves. Aid workers are worried that residents will try to flee if they do not get enough supplies. If they do flee, this could further spread the disease (Farge 2014a).

A second Ebola treatment center named ELWA-3 has opened in Monrovia, Liberia (Dossa 2015; Sifferlin 2014). The new center has 120 beds and compliments an existing 80-patient facility in Monrovia (Paye-Layleh and Larson 2014).

A Nigerian woman traveling to the United Arab Emirates became ill on her flight and died in Abu Dhabi. Medics found signs of possible Ebola. However, the woman was on her way for cancer treatment, and she likely died from issues related to her cancer. In a separate incident, a 48-year-old British woman collapsed and died in

Austria after traveling from Nigeria. Her body is being tested for Ebola (Blake and Hall 2014).

August 18, 2014 (Monday)

The WHO does not support trade or travel bans against any of the Ebola-affected countries. Instead, the agency thinks screening airline passengers is an effective way to prevent the spread of Ebola (Jansen 2014).

The West Point slum in Liberia could be an ideal site for Ebola magnification. West Point is located on a sandy peninsula about 800 m long by 550 m wide (Silver 2014c). There are two paved roads in the community. Houses are typically one-story, made of plywood or cement, and have corrugated metal roofs (Silver 2014c). The slum is very crowded. Often seven or more people live in a single small dwelling (McCoy 2014a). Sanitation is poor. In 2009, only four public toilets were available for 70,000 residents. It costs three cents a visit to use the toilets. Many residents use the nearby beach for toilet purposes instead of paying the fee (McCoy 2014a).

Medical workers assisting Ebola patients in West Africa often work 14 h shifts, 7 days a week. Despite these efforts, a large proportion of their patients die. One morning, Cokie Van der Velde, a sanitation specialist with MSF, discovered the bodies of four victims who had died during the night. One man had crawled to the door of the ward, the others appeared to have fallen out of their beds. Blood and feces were scattered around the room (Cheng 2014).

A 30-year-old New Mexico woman is being tested for Ebola after visiting Sierra Leone. She is currently in the University of New Mexico Hospital in stable condition (Cruz 2014).

August 19, 2014 (Tuesday)

Total cases: 2240 (113 new)   Fatalities: 1229 (84 new)
                              (Disease Outbreak News 2014t)

Liberia has ordered the West Point slum quarantined (Paye-Layleh 2014a; Associated Press 2014c). Security forces will prevent anyone from entering or leaving the community. A nighttime curfew from 2100 to 0600 h will be enforced (Paye-Layleh 2014a). The coast guard will patrol the waters around the community to prevent residents from leaving the area in canoes (Associated Press 2014c). To help increase Ebola awareness in West Point, the government will send representatives door-to-door to describe the symptoms of Ebola and explain why patients need to be isolated (MacDougall and Nebehay 2014). All of the Ebola patients that were liberated from the West Point Clinic on Saturday, August 16, 2014, have been located and are now back in treatment at the JFK medical facility (MacDougall and Nebehay 2014).

John Moore, a photographer for Getty Images, says there still isn't a sense of panic in Monrovia, Liberia. Many people continue to believe that Ebola is a hoax or a conspiracy cooked up by the government (Katz 2014).

One 30-year-old woman in Liberia is now the only adult caregiver for six small children, not all her own. The woman's mother died on Monday, August 11, 2014.

On Tuesday the parents of one of the children died. On Wednesday the woman's husband died (MacDougall 2014c).

The three West African doctors treated with ZMapp are showing considerable signs of improvement (MacDougall and Nebehay 2014).

Nigeria is optimistic that it has contained the Ebola outbreak started with Patrick Sawyer. Five people who developed Ebola have recovered and been released from the hospital (NPR 2014c). One hundred eighty-nine people are under surveillance in Lagos; six are under surveillance in Enugu (Chiejina 2014). Contact tracing of people who interacted with infected individuals is reported to be 94–98%. A man, who visited an airport on Monday, August 18, 2014, says he saw officials taking passenger's temperatures, asking how they felt, and finding out where they had been (Chiejina 2014).

American missionary Nancy Writebol has recovered from Ebola and been released from Emory University Hospital. She quietly left the hospital today without fanfare. Her departure was not publically reported until Thursday, August 21, 2014 (Garloch and Funk 2014).

August 20, 2014 (Wednesday)

Total cases: 2473 (233 new)   Fatalities: 1350 (121 new)
                               (Disease Outbreak News 2014u)

Residents of the West Point slum in Liberia have responded violently to the quarantine of their community. Inhabitants attempted to storm the government barriers but were repulsed by soldiers firing live ammunition (MacDougall and Giahyue 2014; Onishi 2014a). The shots were reportedly fired into the air, but at least one person, a 15-year-old boy named Shakie Kamara, was wounded – he was shot in the legs (Onishi 2014a). The head of national police operations, Lieutenant Colonel Abraham Kromah, arrived at the scene soon after the shooting. He was dismayed that Kamara had been shot and said that at least one of his officers had been wounded by the crowd (Onishi 2014a). Around the time the violence was occurring, the District Commissioner of West Point, Miata Flowers, and her family were evacuated from the community (McCoy 2014b; Sim 2014). Conditions in the center of West Point are unclear. It is reported that the price of goods has doubled (Paye-Layleh and Williams 2014). To help alleviate the situation, authorities have started delivering rice and cooking oil to the residents (MacDougall and Giahyue 2014).

Five new suspected Ebola cases have been isolated in Lagos, Nigeria (Kay and Ibukun 2014).

Air France crews are requesting that flights to Conakry, Guinea, and Freetown, Sierra Leone, be stopped immediately. Crews can refuse to work on the flights, but the union would like the airlines to stop flying the routes altogether. At present, Air France flies to these cities four times per week. There are protocols in place to deal with an in-flight Ebola emergency. These include isolating a suspected case in the airplane's restroom (RT 2014).

About ten people, including four healthcare workers, have died with Ebola-like symptoms in the town of Boende in the Democratic Republic of the Congo. A team of government experts is on its way to investigate and see if the disease event is related to the current West African Ebola outbreak (Reuters 2014m). Boende is rather far from West Africa. It is located about 2200 miles southeast of Monrovia, Liberia.

Vietnam and Myanmar have isolated three travelers from Africa with Ebola-like symptoms (AFP 2014j).

August 21, 2014 (Thursday)

West Point, Liberia was calm today (Paye-Layleh 2014b). However, residents are very concerned about the availability of food, and prices of commodities continue to climb. Rice normally costs about $0.30 a cup in West Point. It now costs $0.90 (McCoy 2014b). Hundreds of residents lined up at the government's food distribution point to receive rations (Associated Press 2014d). Shakie Kamara, the 15-year-old boy who was shot during the violence yesterday, died from hypovolemic shock at Redemption Hospital (Onishi 2014b); it is unclear whether he died yesterday or today.

Senegal has closed its border with Guinea. It will also no longer allow aircraft or ships from Ebola-affected countries to land in its territory (Wilson 2014c; Farge 2014b). Because of this closure, a UN flight carrying aid workers was not allowed to land in Dakar today (Farge 2014b). The plane was flying from Liberia but had made stops in the capitals of all of the affected countries (Farge 2014b). The closure of Senegal's borders is potentially very significant. Dakar is a regional transit hub, and most of the aid coming into the Ebola zone has passed through it (BBC 2014f).

Dr. Kent Brantly has recovered from Ebola and been released from Emory University Hospital (Brumfield and Wilson 2014). Officials say that Dr. Brantly and Nancy Writebol (who was released on August 19, 2014) do not pose a risk to the community (Fox 2014b). During a press conference held today to cover his release, Dr. Brantly received numerous hugs from the medical workers who treated him. The hugs were not only an emotional response from the participants, but they also helped demonstrate to the public that the Ebola survivors are not contagious (Lupkin 2014b).

Doctors in West Africa think the official WHO Ebola figures are lower than the actual number of cases. One doctor estimated that the official numbers may be off by about 20%. Barbara Knust, an epidemiologist with the CDC, says that one of the main reasons the numbers could be off is because it takes some time for case information to be entered into the official database (Greenfieldboyce 2014).

Business leaders worry about the effect Ebola is having on West African economies. Small businesses have been feeling the economic pinch for some time. Prices continue to rise and goods keep getting harder to find. Large businesses are also affected. In Sierra Leone, rice, cocoa, and banana crops are not being harvested because many of the farmers have died. Some companies are paying workers to stay home. The goal is to try to keep their workers from getting Ebola, so they will be available to work after the outbreak is over (Bax et al. 2014).

The South African Cabinet has issued an entry ban for residents of Ebola-affected countries. The Cabinet also requests that South African citizens avoid nonessential travel to Ebola-affected countries (Times Live 2014).

A survey conducted between August 13 and 17, 2014, finds that 39% of Americans are worried that a large Ebola outbreak will occur in the United States. Twenty six percent are concerned that they or someone in their family will contract Ebola during the next year (Harvard T.H. Chan School of Public Health 2014).

August 22, 2014 (Friday)

Total cases: 2615 (142 new)   Fatalities: 1427 (77 new)
                          (Disease Outbreak News 2014v)

The WHO is developing a comprehensive Ebola-fighting strategy. The plan is being called "the roadmap." The roadmap will outline the steps needed to fight Ebola over the next 6–9 months. It should be released early next week (Nebehay and MacDougall 2014).

The WHO says there are "shadow zones" in Ebola-affected regions (World Health Organization 2014d). These are areas that are thought to have the disease, but which cannot be reached, or which will not allow medical personnel to enter. The agency also says there are many hidden Ebola victims, even in developed areas:

In parts of Liberia, a phenomenon is occurring that has never before been seen in an Ebola outbreak. As soon as a new treatment facility is opened, it is immediately filled with patients, many of whom were not previously identified. This phenomenon strongly suggests the existence of an invisible caseload of patients who are not being detected by the surveillance system. (World Health Organization 2014d)

Jatu Harris, a resident of West Point, Liberia, says the government distributed 300 bags of rice today. This is helpful, but it is not nearly enough for all of the people in West Point's six zones. She also says the rice that was provided was rotten (Butty 2014b).

In the community of Mount Barclay, outside of Monrovia, Liberia, dogs have been seen pulling Ebola victims from shallow graves and feeding from the bodies (Daygbor 2014).

Two new Ebola cases have been detected in Nigeria. The new victims, a man and a woman, did not have direct contact with Patrick Sawyer. They are the spouses of healthcare workers who assisted Sawyer. Both healthcare workers died from Ebola (Associated Press 2014e).

Ivory Coast has closed its land borders with Liberia and Guinea (BBC 2014g).

If Ebola maintains its current rate of infection, by September 1, 2014, the death toll from the current Ebola outbreak will surpass the total number of deaths caused by the disease in all previous outbreaks combined (Lynch 2014). Before this outbreak, 1548 people had died from Ebola (Lynch 2014). To date, 1427 people have died during this outbreak (Disease Outbreak News 2014v).

August 23, 2014 (Saturday)
Sierra Leone's government has passed legislation making it illegal to hide Ebola patients. Violators will face up to 2 years in prison. The measure is not yet law, but the President is expected to quickly sign the bill (Roy-Macaulay 2014a).

At the government hospital in Kenema, Sierra Leone, only three nurses remain from the original staff present before the outbreak. At least 15 nurses have died from Ebola. Senior nurse Josephine Finda Sellu says the losses were incredibly rapid. Three nurses died one day, four the next, etc.(Nossiter 2014e).

People in Sierra Leone are often afraid of the healthcare workers assisting Ebola victims. Some nurses have been abandoned by their husbands; one returned home to find all of her belongings on the sidewalk. Kandeh Kamara is one of the "burial boys" in Kailahun. His job is to find and bury Ebola victims. He says that he only does the job because he does not think anyone else will do it(Nossiter 2014e).

A British volunteer nurse [William Pooley] has contracted Ebola in Kenema, Sierra Leone (BBC 2014h; Best and Endley 2014). He will be air evacuated back to Britain on August 24, 2014 (Walters and Adams 2014). Professor Sir Bruce Keogh, medical director for the NHS, says the nurse will not pose a risk to the general public (Walters and Adams 2014). The 29-year-old Pooley is from Eyke, Suffolk. He had specifically asked to work with Ebola patients while in Sierra Leone (Gardner 2014; Siddique 2014). He is the first British citizen to contract Ebola during the outbreak (Siddique 2014).

The Philippines is withdrawing 115 peacekeepers from Liberia because of the outbreak (Fonbuena 2014).

The Democratic Republic of the Congo reports that Ebola is present in its Equateur Province (Reuters 2014n). Two patients have tested positive for the disease. One tested positive for *Sudan ebolavirus*, the other for a mixture of *Sudan ebolavirus* and *Zaire ebolavirus* (Reuters 2014n). This suggests that this is a new outbreak not related to the current West African epidemic. The virus causing in the West African outbreak is *Zaire ebolavirus* (Baize et al. 2014).

August 24, 2014 (Sunday)
A Senegalese epidemiologist working for the WHO has contracted Ebola in Kailahun, Sierra Leone (Fofana and Coulibaly 2014; Joseph et al. 2014). This is the first time someone directly associated with the WHO has become infected.

The infected British nurse [William Pooley] has been airlifted from Sierra Leone to Britain (BBC 2014h). The RAF flew him to Northolt airport in the western part of London. He arrived in a C-17 equipped with an isolation tent. He was driven to the Royal Free Hospital in Hampstead in a specially adapted ambulance (BBC 2014h; Collins 2014).

Nigerian doctors have suspended their strike so they can fight the Ebola outbreak (Roy-Macaulay 2014b). Separately, First Consultant Hospital and the families of some Nigerian Ebola victims may sue Liberia for allowing Patrick Sawyer to leave Liberia (Okolie 2014).

The Philippines plans to conduct the mandatory repatriation (i.e., forced withdraw) of 3500 workers currently in Guinea, Sierra Leone, and Liberia (ABS-CBN 2014).

August 25, 2014 (Monday)
Infected Liberian doctor, Dr. Abraham Borbor, has died at ELWA Hospital in Monrovia (AllAfrica 2014g; BBC 2014i). He was one of the three African doctors treated with ZMapp. Dr. Borbor had been showing signs of improvement but began to deteriorate yesterday (BBC 2014i). The current Ebola outbreak has been particularly hard on healthcare workers. To date, 240 health workers have contracted Ebola; 120 of them have died (World Health Organization 2014e).

William Pooley has been identified as the infected British nurse. He has started treatment with ZMapp (Rayner 2014).

Due to border closing and travel bans, people in Sierra Leone worry about being trapped in the Ebola zone. The few remaining flights out of Freetown are booked solid (Frankel 2014a).

The economic impact of Ebola continues to increase. Before the outbreak, one fair-trade clothing manufacturer in Liberia had been working to expand its business. The company signed contacts with American buyers and opened a new factory near West Point, Monrovia. The firm hired 303 people, obtained new equipment, and had large orders waiting to be filled. Ebola has thrown these plans into flux. Three weeks ago the company staged a 2-week shutdown to give the Ebola situation time to stabilize. On August 19, 2014, West Point was quarantined. Now, most of the workforce is trapped in the slum (Foote 2014).

Fujifilm Corporation has offered to provide the experimental drug Avigan (also known as Favipiravir) to treat Ebola patients. The drug was designed to treat influenza but may also work against Ebola. Fujifilm Corporation currently has ~20,000 doses on hand and can make more. It is waiting for the WHO to approve the drug for general use, but a company spokesman says that Fujifilm is already willing to respond to urgent individual requests for the drug (Ryall 2014).

The CDC released a document entitled "Guidance for safe handling of human remains of Ebola patients in U.S. hospitals and mortuaries" (Centers for Disease Control and Prevention 2014b). It recommends that Ebola victims should not be autopsied or embalmed. Instead:

> At the site of death, the body should be wrapped in a plastic shroud. Wrapping of the body should be done in a way that prevents contamination of the outside of the shroud. Change your gown or gloves if they become heavily contaminated with blood or body fluids. Leave any intravenous lines or endotracheal tubes that may be present in place. Avoid washing or cleaning the body. After wrapping, the body should be immediately placed in a leak-proof plastic bag not less than 150 μm thick and zippered closed. The bagged body should then be placed in another leak-proof plastic bag not less than 150 μm thick and zippered closed before being transported to the morgue. (Centers for Disease Control and Prevention 2014b)

August 26, 2014 (Tuesday)

CDC Director Thomas Frieden is in Liberia evaluating the outbreak. His assessment is dire. He says that the outbreak is an absolute emergency. No one has ever seen anything of this magnitude before with Ebola. He says a massive global emergency response is needed to control the outbreak (Atlanta Journal-Constitution 2014).

As part of Liberia's state of emergency, the Liberian President had ordered all top government officials to return to the country. Several cabinet ministers and other high-level officials were fired today because they refused to return to the country during the outbreak (Paye-Layleh 2014c).

The WHO will close its testing laboratory in Kailahun, Sierra Leone (Fofana and Coulibaly 2014). This is the site where the Senegalese epidemiologist was infected (Fofana and Coulibaly 2014). Separately, Canada is withdrawing a three-person health team from Sierra Leone because three people at the hotel where they are staying have been diagnosed with Ebola (CBC News 2014).

A 65-year-old woman has died with Ebola-like symptoms in the city of Mbandaka in the Democratic Republic of the Congo (Fofana and Coulibaly 2014). MSF is sending personnel to help with the Ebola outbreak in the Democratic Republic of the Congo (Médecins Sans Frontières 2014d). Given its full commitment to West Africa, however, the agency can offer only limited assistance (Médecins Sans Frontières 2014d).

August 27, 2014 (Wednesday)

A third top Sierra Leone doctor, Dr. Sahr Rogers, has died from Ebola. He became infected while working in Kenema (Roy-Macaulay 2014c).

The infected Senegalese doctor working for the WHO has been evacuated from Sierra Leone to Germany (Hille 2014). He flew to Hamburg on a private plane and will be treated at the University Hospital Hamburg-Eppendorf (Hille 2014). Separately, the CDC has evacuated a staff member from Sierra Leone who had a low-risk exposure to the virus (Associated Press 2014f). The person had worked about 3 ft away from an international worker who developed Ebola (presumably the Senegalese WHO worker). The CDC staffer arrived in Atlanta today. They will remain at home and will be monitored for symptoms for 21 days (Associated Press 2014f).

Nigerian schools will remain closed until October 13, 2014. Schools were supposed to open September 1, 2014, but the opening will be delayed due to the Ebola outbreak. On a more positive note, the Nigerian government says that only one confirmed Ebola case remains in the country (BBC 2014j).

Ebola is affecting West African economies at many scales. Donald Kaberuka, chief of the African Development Bank, estimates that Sierra Leone's GDP will decline by 4% because of the outbreak (Olu-Mammah and Fofana 2014). At a smaller scale, many farmers are unable to hire field hands because the workers do not want to touch their employer's money (Mark 2014d). In Freetown, Sierra Leone, one hotel has only 8 of 34 rooms filled (Mark 2014d).

France is requesting that all of its citizens leave the Ebola zone. It has also asked Air France to stop flying to Freetown, Sierra Leone (Associated Press 2014g).

British Airways has suspended flights to Sierra Leone and Liberia until December 31, 2014 (Kitching 2014). In contrast, Brussels Airlines is resuming flights to Guinea, Liberia, and Sierra Leone (Olu-Mammah and Fofana 2014). Brussels Airlines made this decision because many people would like to leave the Ebola-affected countries and because there are 50 tons of medical supplies in Brussels waiting to be delivered to the countries (Olu-Mammah and Fofana 2014).

August 28, 2014 (Thursday)

Total cases: 3069 (454 new)   Fatalities: 1552 (125 new)
(Disease Outbreak News 2014w)

The WHO has released its Ebola response roadmap. The goal of the plan is to stop Ebola transmission in the currently affected countries in 6–9 months and prevent the international spread of the disease. The plan assumes that the current casualty figures are too low and that there are actually two to four times more Ebola cases than presently reported. It also assumes that there may be 20,000 cases over the next 9 months. The plan has three primary objectives. The first is to achieve full geographic coverage of Ebola response activities in countries with active Ebola outbreaks. The second is to immediately implement control actions as soon as Ebola appears in a new country. The third is to increase Ebola preparedness in all countries, especially those that border Ebola-affected countries and those that serve as major transportation hubs. It is estimated that $490 M will be needed to implement the plan over the next 6 months (World Health Organization 2014f).

Significant flaws are present in the West Point, Liberia, quarantine. Residents can move into and out of the restricted area with relative ease. Some people sneak away; others bribe their way out. One escaping couple says they paid $10.25 to leave – $6.00 for the man and $4.25 for the woman. Conditions inside West Point continue to deteriorate. Long lines form for rice and water. Running water is generally not available in the slum, and few residents have the money to pay for a hot bath (Onishi 2014c).

Body collection units recover the corpses of Ebola victims in and around Monrovia, Liberia. Members are paid $1000 per month. One three-man unit includes a 21-year-old artist, a 23-year-old university student, and a (presumably older) government worker. On a recent run, the team recovered the body of Rachel Wleh. Wleh's husband, a doctor, had also recently died of Ebola. When the squad recovered Wleh's body, she was in bed with blood draining out of her mouth. On the day they recovered Wleh, the team collected and transferred a total of seven bodies to the crematorium (Aizenman 2014).

Nigeria confirms that a doctor died from Ebola in Port Harcourt on August 22, 2014 (Cocks and Payne 2014; Premium Times 2014). This is the first known death from the virus outside of Lagos. The doctor did not treat Patrick Sawyer but treated a patient who had contact with Sawyer. Seventy people who had contact with the doctor are now under surveillance. Good Heart Hospital, where the doctor worked, has been closed (Cocks and Payne 2014; Premium Times 2014).

Gire et al. (2014) describe the origin of the Ebola outbreak and the mechanisms of transmission. Genome sequencing suggests that the outbreak started when a single human being [Emile Ouamouno] was infected from a natural reservoir (i.e., an animal, such as a bat). All subsequent transmission has been human to human. Two different strains of the virus entered Sierra Leone from Guinea at essentially the same time. The two strains appear to have infected people who attended a single funeral in Guinea (likely Finda Nyuma's). The outbreak is currently expanding exponentially with a doubling time of 34.8 days (Gire et al. 2014). Remarkably, five of the paper's 58 authors have died from Ebola.

The United Kingdom says all nonessential travel to Sierra Leone, Guinea, and Liberia should be avoided. It also warns British nationals already in the affected countries that if they wait too long, they may have a hard time getting out because of the increasing number of travel bans (Mundasad 2014).

The UN World Food Program is increasing its efforts in Ebola-affected countries. There is great concern that a food crisis could occur as crops are abandoned and travel in the region becomes more difficult. The cost of goods continues to rise. In Freetown, Sierra Leone, the cost of a 110 pound bag has increased from $37.50 to 45.40 since the start of the outbreak (Szabo 2014).

An experimental Ebola vaccine developed by GlaxoSmithKline is ready for fast-tracked human trials. The vaccine is made from one of the seven proteins that make up the Ebola virus. It is hoped that the vaccine will activate the recipient's immune system and prevent infection. Initial tests of the vaccine's safety should be completed by the end of 2014 (Kollewe 2014).

August 29, 2014 (Friday)
Ebola has reached Senegal (Dione 2014). The country confirms that a 21-year-old male university student from Guinea [Mamadou Alimuo Diallo] is infected with the virus (Camara 2014; Monnier 2014). Diallo was reluctant to tell officials about his exposure to Ebola or the route he took to reach Dakar, Senegal (Farge and Oberstadt 2014). It was well into September 2014 before the details of his case were known. Diallo arrived in Dakar sometime after August 15, 2014 (Farge and Oberstadt 2014). He had come to see his uncle and find out about attending school in Senegal (Camara 2014). His brother had died from Ebola, and his mother and sister were sick (Farge and Oberstadt 2014). Two days after he reached Dakar, Diallo himself began to feel ill (Camara 2014; Farge and Oberstadt 2014). His condition worsened over several days, and he eventually went to the hospital (Camara 2014). When he said that he had contact with Ebola victims, he was isolated and confirmed with having Ebola (Camara 2014; Dione 2014). Guinea appears to have been aware of Diallo and had been trying to track his movements. On Wednesday, August 27, 2014, Guinean officials warned Senegal that a person infected with Ebola (Diallo) had reportedly traveled to Senegal (Dione 2014).

Liberia says it will lift the quarantine of the West Point slum. The cordon will be removed at 0600 h August 30, 2014. Residents of the community celebrated the news. Unfortunately, some of the citizens seem to have drawn the wrong conclusion about why the quarantine is being lifted. One resident says he thinks the quarantine is being lifted because the government has not found anyone with Ebola in West Point (Onishi 2014d).

Liberia's Ebola hotline number is 4455. Ninety operators answer the phones. They receive about 3000 calls per day. Dispatchers summon an ambulance for the sick or a coroner's truck for the dead. Unfortunately there are only six ambulances and six coroner's trucks in Monrovia. As a result, calls often go unanswered, or the response time is exceptionally long. Sick people are commonly seen on the streets. Not all of the visibly sick people have Ebola. It's the rainy season and malaria is common (Hinshaw and McKay 2014).

Residents in Guinea's second largest city, Nzérékoré, rioted because disinfectant was being sprayed to control Ebola. Locals were apparently afraid that the spray was being used to spread Ebola, not control it. In a blend of mixed messages, individuals in the crowd also shouted that Ebola was not real. The crowd was dispersed with tear gas (BBC 2014k).

Qiu et al. (2014) find that ZMapp reverses the effects of Ebola and eliminates the disease in rhesus macaques. One hundred percent of macaques survived ($n = 18$) if they were given ZMapp up to 5 days after they were infected with Ebola (Qiu et al. 2014). The strain of Ebola used in the study was not the same as the one circulating in West Africa, but the antibodies in ZMapp appear to recognize the strain causing the outbreak (Geisbert 2014).

Ignorance about African geography has made many Westerners afraid to travel to any part of the continent out of fear of Ebola. Many Westerners do not realize how large Africa is. Consequently, they are simply avoiding the entire continent rather than just staying away from areas near the Ebola-affected countries (McGregor and Mokhema 2014).

Some US universities plan to monitor newly arriving West African students for signs of Ebola. Students will be assessed for fevers and have their temperatures taken for 21 days after they arrive at school (Associated Press 2014h).

August 30, 2014 (Saturday)
The quarantine of West Point, Liberia, has been lifted. Residents danced in the streets and chanted "we are free" (Giahyue and Samb 2014). Separately, the two surviving Liberian doctors who were treated with ZMapp have recovered and been released from isolation (Elbagir and Berlinger 2014).

Five additional 100-bed Ebola treatment centers are being built in Liberia (Hussain 2014b).

Crew members will not be allowed to disembark from ships arriving at any of Liberia's four ports (Yahoo News 2014).

Medical workers at Kemena Hospital, Sierra Leone, have gone on strike. The government has not paid their salaries and supplies are low (Fofana and Giahyue 2014).

In Freetown, Sierra Leone, surgical gloves are now selling for $1 each. The Lighthouse Hotel, which caters to the wealthy, is running at 15% occupancy (Frankel 2014b).

Senegal is responding to the risk posed by the infected Guinean student. Workers have disinfected the student's home and a grocery store near his house (Giahyue and Samb 2014).

The WHO thinks six countries are at high risk of having Ebola cases. These are Benin, Burkina Faso, Côte d'Ivoire, Guinea-Bissau, Mali, and Senegal. All of the countries share a border with an affected country or are a major transportation hub (Newsroom America 2014).

The government of Sudan has banned local media from reporting on Ebola (Amin 2014). Presumably this has been done to reduce the fear of the virus.

August 31, 2014 (Sunday)
The WHO says it considers the arrival of Ebola in Senegal a top priority emergency (Associated Press 2014i). The student who brought the disease to the country [Mamadou Alimuo Diallo] appears to be improving and is expected to recover. Twenty people who had contact with him are under surveillance, and officials are working hard to identify other contacts he may have had (Monnier 2014). In Dakar, due to heavy demand, pharmacies are only allowing customers to buy one bottle of hand sanitizer at a time (Associated Press 2014i).

Healthcare workers in Guinea are having a hard time obtaining medical supplies. At Donka Hospital, staff members are given only one pack of gloves per week. As a result, many workers are buying their own PPE. Some of the items they buy may have stolen from aid shipments (Bah 2014).

Nigerian diplomat Olubukun Koye may face manslaughter charges for bringing Ebola to Port Harcourt, Nigeria (Nigerian Bulletin 2014). Koye had tested positive for Ebola and had been told not to travel. However, he left quarantine in Lagos and traveled to Port Harcourt. The doctor who treated him in Port Harcourt, Dr. Iyke Enemuo, has since died. The deceased doctor's wife has also tested positive for Ebola and has been moved to Lagos for treatment (Vanguard 2014). Officials are now conducting contract tracing to identify other people who may have had contact with the infected victims. Over 200 people are under surveillance, including the morticians who embalmed Dr. Enemuo's body (Sahara Reporters 2014b). The WHO has compiled a detailed analysis of Dr. Enemuo's illness and actions; the agency is very concerned that additional cases could develop in Port Harcourt:

> *After onset of symptoms, on 11 August, and until 13 August, the physician continued to treat patients at his private clinic, and operated on at least two. On 13 August, his symptoms worsened; he stayed at home and was hospitalized on 16 August.*
>
> *Prior to hospitalization, the physician had numerous contacts with the community, as relatives and friends visited his home to celebrate the birth of a baby.*
>
> *Once hospitalized, he again had numerous contacts with the community, as members of his church visited to perform a healing ritual said to involve the laying on of hands. During his 6 day period of hospitalization, he was attended by the majority of the hospital's health care staff.*

On 21 August, he was taken to an ultrasound clinic, where 2 physicians performed an abdominal scan. He died the next day.

The additional 2 confirmed cases are his wife, also a doctor, and a patient at the same hospital where he was treated. Additional staff at the hospital are undergoing tests.

Given these multiple high-risk exposure opportunities, the outbreak of Ebola virus disease in Port Harcourt has the potential to grow larger and spread faster than the one in Lagos. (World Health Organization 2014g)

Karolinska University Hospital in Stockholm, Sweden, has isolated a suspected Ebola case. The patient is a feverish man who recently traveled to a "risk area" (Reuters 2014o).

References

ABS-CBN (2014) Mandatory repatriation eyed for Pinoys in Ebola hit nations. ABS-CBN News. http://www.abs-cbnnews.com/nation/08/24/14/mandatory-repatriation-eyed-pinoys-ebola-hit-nations. Accessed 24 Aug 2014

Adigun B (2014a) Nigeria confirms doctor as 2nd Ebola case. ABC News. http://abcnews.go.com/Health/wireStory/liberia-orders-cremation-ebola-victims-24830289. Accessed 4 Aug 2014

Adigun B (2014b) Ebola centers fill faster than they can be opened. ABC News. http://abcnews.go.com/International/wireStory/nigeria-confirms-ebola-case-24975247. Accessed 15 Aug 2014

AFP (2014a) Pregnant woman Victoria Yillah first to survive Ebola in Sierra Leone. AFP, News Corps Australia. http://www.news.com.au/lifestyle/health/pregnant-woman-victoria-yillah-first-to-survive-ebola-in-sierra-leone/story-fneuz9ev-1226954032393. Accessed 22 Aug 2014

AFP (2014b) Ebola spread due to 'relaxation' of efforts. AFP, New Vision. http://www.newvision.co.ug/news/656806-ebola-spread-due-to-relaxation-of-efforts.html. Accessed 22 Aug 2014

AFP (2014c) Nigeria fears Ebola spread to east by infected nurse. AFP, Yahoo News. https://www.yahoo.com/news/nigeria-fears-ebola-spread-east-infected-nurse-232441108.html?ref=gs. Accessed 9 Jan 2017

AFP (2014d) Ebola-hit African states seal off outbreak epicenter. AFP, Yahoo News. http://news.yahoo.com/african-states-launch-100mn-ebola-response-plan-170858040.html. Accessed 1 Aug 2014

AFP (2014e) Spain evacuating missionary sick with Ebola. AFP, Yahoo News. https://www.yahoo.com/news/spanish-missionary-liberia-tests-positive-ebola-182039710.html?ref=gs. Accessed 15 Jan 2017

AFP (2014f) Emirates suspends Guinea flights over Ebola. AFP, Aljazeera. http://www.aljazeera.com/news/africa/2014/08/emirates-suspends-guinea-flights-over-ebola-20148342526985793.html. Accessed 3 Aug 2014

AFP (2014g) Nigeria fears Ebola spread to east by infected nurse. AFP, Yahoo News. https://www.yahoo.com/news/nigeria-fears-ebola-spread-east-infected-nurse-232441108.html?ref=gs. Accessed 9 Jan 2017

AFP (2014h) Report: armed men attack Liberia Ebola clinic, freeing patients. CBS News. http://www.cbsnews.com/news/report-armed-men-attack-liberia-ebola-clinic-freeing-patients/. Accessed 17 Aug 2014

AFP (2014i) Ebola: Kenya bars travellers from worst-hit countries. AFP, Channel News Asia. http://www.channelnewsasia.com/news/health/ebola-kenya-bars/1316588.html. Accessed 16 Aug 2014

AFP (2014j) Vietnam, Myanmar test three patients for Ebola. Yahoo News. https://news.yahoo.com/vietnam-myanmar-test-patients-ebola-065852689.html. Accessed 20 Aug 2014

AFP (2015) Sierra Leone marks grim Ebola anniversary. Times Live. http://www.timeslive.co.za/africa/2015/05/25/Sierra-Leone-marks-grim-Ebola-anniversary. Accessed 25 May 2015

Aizenman N (2014) They are the body collectors: a perilous job in the time of Ebola. NPR. http://www.npr.org/sections/goatsandsoda/2014/08/28/343479917/they-are-the-body-collectors-a-perilous-job-in-the-time-of-ebola. Accessed 29 Jan 2017

Al Jazeera (2014a) Ebola kills more than 200 in Guinea. Aljazeera. http://www.aljazeera.com/news/africa/2014/06/ebola-guinea-world-health-organisation-200-dead-20146593739135838.html. Accessed 20 Aug 2014

Al Jazeera (2014b) Korean Air suspends Kenya flights over Ebola. Aljazeera. http://www.aljazeera.com/news/africa/2014/08/korean-air-suspends-kenya-flights-over-ebola-20148141050240159.html. Accessed 14 Aug 2014

Al Jazeera (2014c) Ebola virus threatens Liberian slum after residents raid quarantine center. Aljazeera. http://america.aljazeera.com/articles/2014/8/17/liberia-quarantinebreak.html. Accessed 17 Jan 2017

Al Jazeera (2014d) Nigeria trains 800 volunteers to fight Ebola. Aljazeera. http://www.aljazeera.com/news/africa/2014/08/nigeria-trains-800-volunteers-fight-ebola-2014816164320740296.html. Accessed 16 Aug 2014

Aliyu A, Nanlong M-T (2014) Ebola: two dead, 20 others hospitalised over excessive salt consumption. Vanguard. http://www.vanguardngr.com/2014/08/ebola-two-die-drinking-salt-water-jos/. Accessed 16 Jan 2017

AllAfrica (2014a) Liberia: running from Ebola – in Liberia, medics reject suspected cases. AllAfrica, Front Page Africa. http://allafrica.com/stories/201407170961.html?viewall=1. Accessed 17 Jul 2014

AllAfrica (2014b) Liberia: taking lead – students, youths enter Ebola fight. AllAfrica, Front Page Africa. http://allafrica.com/stories/201407200025.html. Accessed 24 Aug 2014

AllAfrica (2014c) Liberia: 'bitter kola' does not cure Ebola. AllAfrica, The Inquirer. http://allafrica.com/stories/201407212656.html. Accessed 22 Jul 2014

AllAfrica (2014d) Ebola claims life of JFK Chief Medical Doctor, Samuel Brisbane. AllAfrica. http://www.frontpageafricaonline.com/index.php/health-sci/2461-ebola-claims-life-of-jfk-chief-medical-doctor-samuel-brisbane. Accessed 26 March 2016

AllAfrica (2014e) Liberia: Zmapp arrives – Liberia gets test drug for two doctors. AllAfrica, Front Page Africa. http://allafrica.com/stories/201408140758.html. Accessed 16 Jan 2017

AllAfrica (2014f) 21 days after Sawyer's death, his sojourn claims another life. AllAfrica, This Day. http://allafrica.com/stories/201408150851.html. Accessed 17 Jan 2017

AllAfrica (2014g) Liberia quick burial for Borbor – JFK buries Deputy Chief Medical Doctor. AllAfrica, Front Page Africa. http://allafrica.com/stories/201408261007.html?aa_source=sptlgt-grid. Accessed 26 Aug 2014

Amin M (2014) Sudan prohibits media coverage about Ebola transmission to the country. Daily Nation. http://www.nation.co.ke/news/1056-2435794-mdosg5z/index.html. Accessed 2 Feb 2017

APA (2014) Liberia: fresh Ebola outbreak in Monrovia. Star Africa. http://en.starafrica.com/news/liberia-fresh-ebola-outbreak-in-monrovia.html. Accessed 22 Aug 2014

Associated Press (2014a) Nigeria begins screening airline travelers for Ebola after visitor dies of the disease. Penn Live. http://www.pennlive.com/midstate/index.ssf/2014/07/nigeria_begins_screening_airli.html. Accessed 26 Jul 2014

Associated Press (2014b) Ebola spread fears rise as clinic looted, Liberian officials say. Fox News. http://www.foxnews.com/health/2014/08/17/liberia-expands-ebola-treatment-centers-as-more-airlines-halt-flights-to.html. Accessed 18 Jan 2014

Associated Press (2014c) Liberia security forces quarantine Monrovia slum in effort to stop Ebola. Fox News. http://www.foxnews.com/health/2014/08/20/liberia-security-forces-quarantine-monrovia-slum-in-effort-to-stop-ebola/. Accessed 20 Aug 2014

Associated Press (2014d) Liberia gives food in slum sealed to stop Ebola. Yahoo News. http://news.yahoo.com/officials-visit-liberian-ebola-clinics-102715410.html. Accessed 22 Aug 2014

Associated Press (2014e) Ebola makes worrying advance in Nigeria. CBS News. http://www.cbsnews.com/news/ebola-spreads-in-nigeria-2-new-cases-unconnected-to-patrick-sawyer/ Accessed 22 Aug 2014

Associated Press (2014f) CDC staffer who worked with Ebola victim monitored for symptoms. The Guardian. http://www.theguardian.com/society/2014/aug/28/cdc-staffer-ebola-victim-monitored. Accessed 28 Aug 2014

Associated Press (2014g) Amid Ebola fears French government asks Air France to stop Freetown flights. U.S. News and World Report. http://www.usnews.com/news/business/articles/2014/08/27/amid-ebola-fears-air-france-urged-to-stop-flights. Accessed 27 Aug 2014

Associated Press (2014h) US colleges screen some students for Ebola. Fox News. http://www.foxnews.com/health/2014/08/29/us-colleges-screen-some-students-for-ebola/. Accessed 29 Aug 2014

Associated Press (2014i) WHO says Senegal Ebola case a 'top priority emergency'. Fox News. http://www.foxnews.com/health/2014/09/01/who-says-senegal-ebola-case-top-priority-emergency.html. Accessed 3 Feb 2017

Atlanta Journal-Constitution (2014) Ebola outbreak 'worse than we'd feared,' CDC chief says on visit to West Africa. Atlanta Journal-Constitution. http://www.ajc.com/news/ebola-outbreak-worse-than-feared-cdc-chief-says-visit-west-africa/l8wLCAELQrrafLO3dofQYL/. Accessed 27 Jan 2017

Awareness Times (2014) Sierra Leone News Ebola hits Mambolo, Kambia as Kailahun weeps from its effects. Awareness Times. http://news.sl/drwebsite/publish/article_200525533.shtml. Accessed 22 Aug 2014

Awoniyi O (2014) Liberian with Ebola-like symptoms dies in Nigeria. Yahoo News. http://news.yahoo.com/liberian-ebola-symptoms-dies-nigeria-official-132822550.html. Accessed 25 Jul 2014

Bacon J, Weintraub K (2014) UN endorses use of untested Ebola medicines. USA Today. http://www.usatoday.com/story/news/world/2014/08/12/priest-ebola-dies/13939545/. Accessed 16 Aug 2014

Baguma R (2014) Uganda alert after Ebola reports in DRC. New vision. http://www.newvision.co.ug/news/657793-uganda-alert-after-ebola-reports-in-drc.html. Accessed 21 Jul 2014

Bah M (2014) Ebola epidemic decimating health workers in Guinea. Yahoo News. https://uk.news.yahoo.com/ebola-epidemic-decimating-health-workers-guinea-145519233.html#bdyFw0f. Accessed 31 Aug 2014

Baize S, Pannetier D, Oestereich L et al (2014) Emergence of Zaire Ebola virus disease in Guinea – preliminary report. N Engl J Med 371:1418–1425

Bariyo N (2014) Zambia blocks travelers from Ebola-hit nations. The Wall Street Journal. http://online.wsj.com/articles/zambia-blocks-travelers-from-ebola-hit-nations-1407571648. Accessed 9 Aug 2014

Bax P (2014) Ebola survivor shunned as a zombie joins fight against virus. Bloomberg. http://www.bloomberg.com/news/2014-07-17/ebola-survivor-shunned-as-a-zombie-joins-fight-against-disease.html. Accessed 17 Jul 2014

Bax P, Gbandia S, Zoker E (2014) Ebola threatens to hobble three countries $13 billion in GDP. Business Week. http://www.businessweek.com/articles/2014-08-21/ebola-outbreak-west-african-economies-face-devastation. Accessed 21 Aug 2014

BBC (2014a) UK employees leave Sierra Leone over Ebola threat. BBC. http://www.bbc.com/news/uk-27675747. Accessed 20 Aug 2014

BBC (2014b) Ebola deaths mount in Sierra Leone and Liberia. BBC. http://www.bbc.com/news/world-africa-28268430. Accessed 24 Aug 2014

BBC (2014c) Liberia orders Ebola victims' bodies to be cremated. BBC. http://www.bbc.com/news/world-africa-28640745. Accessed 15 Jan 2017

BBC (2014d) Liberia declares state of emergency over Ebola virus. BBC. http://www.bbc.com/news/world-28684561. Accessed 15 Jan 2017

BBC (2014e) Ebola crisis: confusion as patients vanish in Liberia. BBC. http://www.bbc.com/news/world-africa-28827091. Accessed 17 Aug 2014

BBC (2014f) Ebola crisis: Senegal defends Guinea border closure. BBC. http://www.bbc.com/news/world-africa-28893835. Accessed 22 Aug 2014

BBC (2014g) Ebola crisis: Ivory Coast closes land borders. http://www.bbc.com/news/world-africa-28913253. Accessed 21 Jan 2017

BBC (2014h) British Ebola patient flying to UK for hospital treatment. BBC. http://www.bbc.com/news/uk-28919831. Accessed 24 Aug 2014

BBC (2014i) Ebola kills Liberia doctor despite ZMapp treatment. BBC. http://www.bbc.com/news/world-africa-28925491. Accessed 25 Aug 2014

BBC (2014j) Ebola outbreak: Nigeria closes all schools until October. BBC. http://www.bbc.com/news/world-africa-28950347. Accessed 27 Aug 2014

BBC (2014k) Ebola: Guineans riot in Nzerekore over disinfectant. BCC. http://www.bbc.com/news/world-africa-28984259. Accessed 29 Aug 2014

Beaubien J (2014a) West African villagers fear Ebola will escape from the grave. NPR. http://www.npr.org/2014/07/16/331899920/west-african-villagers-fear-ebola-will-escape-from-the-grave. Accessed 17 Jul 2014

Beaubien J (2014b) Ebola wreaks economic woe in West Africa. NPR. http://www.npr.org/2014/07/17/332351578/ebola-wreaks-economic-woe-in-west-africa. Accessed 18 Jul 2014

Beaubien J (2014c) A fiasco at the burial ground, a prank at the shop: covering Ebola. NPR. http://www.npr.org/sections/goatsandsoda/2014/08/14/340153946/a-fiasco-at-the-burial-ground-a-prank-at-the-shop-covering-ebola. Accessed 15 Dec 2014

Besser Y (2014) Ebola epidemic spreads to Freetown. Guardian Liberty Voice. http://guardianlv.com/2014/07/ebola-epidemic-spreads-to-freetown/. Accessed 19 Aug 2014

Best J, Endley K (2014) First Brit to contract Ebola is 'medic working on the front line against deadly virus'. The Mirror. http://www.mirror.co.uk/news/uk-news/first-brit-contract-ebola-medic-4096038. Accessed 22 Jan 2017

Blake M, Hall A (2014) British woman tested for Ebola 'as a precaution' after collapsing and dying following journey from Nigeria to Austria. The Daily Mail. http://www.dailymail.co.uk/news/article-2727826/British-woman-tested-Ebola-precaution-collapsing-dying-following-journey-Nigeria-Austria.html. Accessed 18 Aug 2014

Blinder A, Grady D (2014) American doctor with Ebola arrives in U.S. for treatment. New York Times. http://www.nytimes.com/2014/08/03/us/kent-brantley-nancy-writebol-ebola-treatment-atlanta.html?_r=0. Accessed 3 Aug 2014

Brumfield B, Wilson J (2014) 'Miraculous day' as American Ebola patients released. CNN. http://www.cnn.com/2014/08/21/health/ebola-patient-release/index.html?hpt=hp_t1. Accessed 1 Aug 2014

Butty J (2014a) Sierra Leone Ebola death toll doubles. VOA News. http://www.voanews.com/content/sierra-leone-ebola-death-toll-doubles/1933223.html. Accessed 26 Aug 2014

Butty J (2014b) Liberia's Ebola quarantine affecting livelihoods. VOA News. http://www.voanews.com/content/liberias-west-point-residents-say-ebola-quarantine-affecting-their-livelihoods/2424248.html. Accessed 22 Aug 2014

Camara K (2014) Guinea student who brought Ebola to Senegal back home. VOA News. http://www.voanews.com/a/guinea-student-who-brought-ebola-to-senegal-back-home/2463601.html. Accessed 29 Jan 2017

Caulderwood K (2014) Million-dollar fruit bat trade could be spreading Ebola, UN warns. International Business Times. http://www.ibtimes.com/million-dollar-fruit-bat-trade-could-be-spreading-ebola-un-warns-1634630. Accessed 22 Jul 2014

CBC News (2014) Ebola outbreak: Canadians pulled from Sierra Leone as precaution. CBC News. http://www.cbc.ca/news/world/ebola-outbreak-canadians-pulled-from-sierra-leone-as-precaution-1.2746945. Accessed 27 Aug 2014

CBS New York (2014) Area airports on alert to look for passengers with Ebola symptoms. CBS
    News. http://newyork.cbslocal.com/2014/08/01/area-airports-on-alert-to-look-for-passengers-
    with-ebola-symptoms/. Accessed 1 Aug 2014
CBS News (2014a) Nancy Writebol, U.S. Ebola survivor, breaks her silence. CBS News. http://
    www.cbsnews.com/news/nancy-writebol-u-s-ebola-survivor-breaks-her-silence/. Accessed 10
    Jan 2017
CBS News (2014b) Ebola patients soon expected to arrive in United States. CBS News. http://
    www.cbsnews.com/news/experimental-ebola-serum-given-to-stricken-u-s-woman/. Accessed
    14 Jan 2017
Centers for Disease Control and Prevention (2014a) As West Africa Ebola outbreak worsens CDC
    issues Level 3 Travel Warning. 31 Jul 2014
Centers for Disease Control and Prevention (2014b) Guidance for safe handling of human remains
    of Ebola patients in U.S. hospitals and mortuaries. 25 Aug 2014
Centers for Disease Control and Prevention (n.d.-a) Travel health notices. CDC. https://wwwnc.
    cdc.gov/travel/notices#travel-notice-definitions. Accessed 10 Jan 2017
Centers for Disease Control and Prevention (n.d.-b) CDC emergency response activation levels.
    https://www.cdc.gov/media/dpk/2014/images/ebola-outbreak/img29.pdf.   Accessed   15   Jan
    2017
Channels Television (2014) First Consultants Medical Centre explains efforts managing Ebola
    case. Channels Television. http://www.channelstv.com/2014/07/29/first-consultants-medical-
    centre-explains-efforts-managing-ebola-case/. Accessed 16 Aug 2014
Cheng M (2014) Ebola outbreak: health workers battle death, heat, rumours in desperate struggle
    to save patients. The Huffington Post. http://www.huffingtonpost.ca/2014/08/18/ebola-out-
    break-west-africa_n_5686873.html. Accessed 18 Jan 2017
Cheng M, Giles C (2014) Miguel Pajares dies: Spanish missionary was infected with Ebola virus
    In Liberia. The Huffington Post. http://www.huffingtonpost.com/2014/08/12/miguel-pajares-
    dies_n_5670811.html. Accessed 12 Aug 2014
Chiacu D (2014) U.S. allows use of Ebola test overseas as crisis deepens. Reuters. http://www.
    reuters.com/article/2014/08/06/us-health-ebola-testing-idUSKBN0G61YK20140806.
    Accessed 6 Aug 2014
Chiejina A (2014) Ebola containment A rare piece of good news from Nigeria. Business Day.
    http://businessdayonline.com/2014/08/ebola-containment-a-rare-piece-of-good-news-from-
    nigeria/#.U_NIgrd0ziw. Accessed 19 Aug 2014
Cocks T (2014) Nigeria isolates Lagos hospital where Ebola victim died. Reuters. http://www.
    reuters.com/article/2014/07/28/us-health-ebola-nigeria-idUSKBN0FX15420140728.
    Accessed 28 Jul 2014
Cocks T, Payne J (2014) Doctor dies of Ebola in Nigeria's oil hub Port Harcourt. Reuters. http://
    www.reuters.com/article/2014/08/28/us-health-ebola-nigeria-idUSKBN0GS0S120140828.
    Accessed 28 Aug 2014
Collins D (2014) British Ebola victim kept in 'isolation bubble' after landing back in UK. The
    Mirror.   http://www.mirror.co.uk/news/uk-news/british-ebola-victim-kept-isolation-4100802.
    Accessed 22 Jan 2017
Cooper C (2014) Ebola deadly outbreak crosses border as mistrust hampers medical staff. The
    Independent.   http://www.independent.co.uk/news/world/africa/ebola-deadly-outbreak-
    crosses-border-as-mistrust-hampers-medical-staff-9456917.html. Accessed 25 Aug 2014
Copeland L, Stanglin D (2014) 2nd U.S. Ebola patient arrives at hospital in Atlanta. USA Today.
    http://www.usatoday.com/story/news/world/2014/08/05/ebola-world-bank/13611523/.
    Accessed 15 Jan 2017
Cruz M (2014) Officials testing woman for Ebola at UNM Hospital. KOAT. http://www.koat.
    com/news/health-dept-working-with-cdc-to-rule-out-ebola-in-patient/27566304#!bFzT0S.
    Accessed 18 Aug 2014

Davis R (2014) Panic in the parking lot: a hospital sees its first Ebola case. NPR. http://www.npr.
    org/sections/goatsandsoda/2014/10/14/356045068/panic-in-the-parking-lot-a-hospital-sees-
    its-first-ebola-case. Accessed 9 Jan 2017

Dawson S (2014) Exclusive: emergency food drops eyed for quarantined Ebola region of West
    Africa. Reuters. http://www.reuters.com/article/2014/08/14/us-health-ebola-hunger-exclusive-
    idUSKBN0GE2CW20140814. Accessed 15 Aug 2014

Daygbor JN (2014) Dogs feed on Ebola victims. The New Dawn. http://www.thenewdawnli-
    beria.com/index.php?option=com_content&view=article&id=12468:dogs-feed-on-ebola-
    victims&catid=25:politics&Itemid=59. Accessed 26 Aug 2014

Diallo M (2014) 'I was so scared to die' living with the fear of Ebola in West Africa. International
    Federation of the Red Cross and Red Crescent Societies. https://www.ifrc.org/en/news-and-
    media/news-stories/africa/guinea/i-was-so-scared-to-die-living-with-the-fear-of-ebola-in-
    west-africa-66127/. Accessed 22 Aug 2014

Diallo B, Roy-MacCaulay C (2014) 2 new Ebola deaths confirmed in West Africa. The Huffington
    Post.   http://www.huffingtonpost.com/2014/05/27/ebola-deaths-west-africa-guinea-sierra-
    leone_n_5396951.html. Accessed 20 Aug 2014

DiLorenzo S (2014) Doctors without borders: Ebola 'out of control.' http://bigstory.ap.org/article/
    ebola-out-control-doctors-without-borders. Accessed 22 Aug 2014

Dione B (2014) Senegal confirms its 1st case of Ebola. ABC News. http://abcnews.go.com/
    International/wireStory/ebola-cases-past-week-25172474. Accessed 29 Aug 2014

Disease Outbreak News (2014a) Ebola virus disease, West Africa – update. World Health
    Organization. 30 May 2014

Disease Outbreak News (2014b) Ebola virus disease, West Africa – update. World Health
    Organization. 4 June 2014

Disease Outbreak News (2014c) Ebola virus disease, West Africa – update. World Health
    Organization. 18 June 2014

Disease Outbreak News (2014d) Ebola virus disease, West Africa – update. World Health
    Organization. 24 June 2014

Disease Outbreak News (2014e) Ebola virus disease, West Africa – update. World Health
    Organization. 1 Jul 2014

Disease Outbreak News (2014f) Ebola virus disease, West Africa – update. World Health
    Organization. 3 Jul 2014

Disease Outbreak News (2014g) Ebola virus disease, West Africa – update. World Health
    Organization. 8 Jul 2014

Disease Outbreak News (2014h) Ebola virus disease, West Africa – update. World Health
    Organization. 10 Jul 2014

Disease Outbreak News (2014i) Ebola virus disease, West Africa – update. World Health
    Organization. 17 Jul 2014

Disease Outbreak News (2014j) Ebola virus disease, West Africa – update. World Health
    Organization. 19 Jul 2014

Disease Outbreak News (2014k) Ebola virus disease, West Africa – update. World Health
    Organization. 24 Jul 2014

Disease Outbreak News (2014l) Ebola virus disease, West Africa – update. World Health
    Organization. 27 Jul 2014

Disease Outbreak News (2014m) Ebola virus disease, West Africa – update. World Health
    Organization. 31 Jul 2014

Disease Outbreak News (2014n) Ebola virus disease, update – west Africa. World Health
    Organization. 4 Aug 2014

Disease Outbreak News (2014o) Ebola virus disease, update – west Africa. World Health
    Organization. 6 Aug 2014

Disease Outbreak News (2014p) Ebola virus disease, update – west Africa. World Health
    Organization. 8 Aug 2014

Disease Outbreak News (2014q) Ebola virus disease, update – west Africa. World Health
    Organization. 11 Aug 2014
Disease Outbreak News (2014r) Ebola virus disease, update – west Africa. World Health
    Organization. 13 Aug 2014
Disease Outbreak News (2014s) Ebola virus disease, update – west Africa. World Health
    Organization. 15 Aug 2014
Disease Outbreak News (2014t) Ebola virus disease, update – west Africa. World Health
    Organization. 19 Aug 2014
Disease Outbreak News (2014u) Ebola virus disease, update – west Africa. World Health
    Organization. 20 Aug 2014
Disease Outbreak News (2014v) Ebola virus disease, update – west Africa. World Health
    Organization. 22 Aug 2014
Disease Outbreak News (2014w) Ebola virus disease, update – west Africa. World Health
    Organization. 28 Aug 2014
Dixon R (2014) As Ebola virus spreads in West Africa, some blame health workers. LA Times.
    http://www.latimes.com/world/africa/la-fg-africa-ebola-20140703-story.html. Accessed 24
    Aug 2014
Doherty R (2014) Ebola scare at Gatwick as woman dies after flight from Sierra Leone. AOL.
    http://travel.aol.co.uk/2014/08/04/ebola-scare-gatwick-woman-dies-flight-sierra-leone/.
    Accessed 4 Aug 2014
Doloquee F (2014) Liberia Ganta records first Ebola death. The New Dawn. http://allafrica.com/
    stories/201407231033.html. Accessed 23 Jul 2014
Dosso Z (2014) In Liberia village, shunned Ebola victims left to die. Yahoo News. http://news.
    yahoo.com/liberia-village-shunned-ebola-victims-left-die-023813543.html. Accessed 13 Aug
    2014
Dosso Z (2015) World's largest Ebola unit dismantled as outbreak retreats. Yahoo News. https://
    www.yahoo.com/news/worlds-largest-ebola-unit-dismantled-outbreak-retreats-142258740.
    html?ref=gs. Accessed 18 Jan 2017
Doucleff M (2014) Doctors aren't sure how to stop Africa's deadliest Ebola outbreak. NPR. http://
    www.npr.org/blogs/health/2014/06/18/323213138/doctors-aren-t-sure-how-to-stop-africa-s-
    deadliest-ebola-outbreak. Accessed 22 Aug 2014
Duhaime-Ross A (2014) This is the bogus drug that scammers are selling to cure Ebola. The
    Verge. http://www.theverge.com/2014/8/15/6006641/these-are-the-companies-profiting-from-
    the-ebola-crisis. Accessed 15 Aug 2014
Early S (2014) British doctor: Ebola is 'a terrifying disease'. DW. http://www.dw.de/british-doc-
    tor-ebola-is-a-terrifying-disease/a-17857482. Accessed 15 Aug 2014
ECDC (2014) Outbreak of Ebola virus disease in West Africa – second update, 9 June 2014. The
    European Center for Disease Prevention and Control. 9 June 2014
Economist (2014) Ebola in Sierra Leone – which doctor? The Economist. http://www.economist.
    com/blogs/baobab/2014/06/ebola-sierra-leone. Accessed 29 Aug 2014
Edwards A (2014) Ebola patients headed for treatment in US are sparking outbreak fears. Fox
    News, CNN Wire. http://fox13now.com/2014/08/01/ebola-patients-headed-for-treatment-in-
    us-sparking-outbreak-fears/ Accessed 13 Jan 2017
Elbagir N, Berlinger J (2014) Two Liberian medical workers discharged after recovering
    from Ebola. CNN. http://www.cnn.com/2014/08/30/world/africa/ebola-west-africa/index.
    html?hpt=hp_t2. Accessed 31 Aug 2014
Estrada C (2014) Ebola, snakes and witchcraft: stopping the deadly disease in its tracks in West
    Africa.   IFRC.   https://www.ifrc.org/en/news-and-media/news-stories/africa/sierra-leone/
    ebola-snakes-and-witchcraft-stopping-the-deadly-disease-in-its-tracks-in-west-africa-66215/.
    Accessed 22 Aug 2014
Farge E (2014a) Struggling Liberia creates plague villages in Ebola epicenter. Reuters. http://www.
    reuters.com/article/2014/08/17/us-health-ebola-liberia-insight-idUSKBN0GH0EY20140817.
    Accessed 17 Aug 2014

Farge E (2014b) Senegal blocks Liberia aid flight, imposes Ebola travel curbs. Reuters. http://uk.reuters.com/article/2014/08/22/us-health-ebola-senegal-idUKKBN0GM1HV20140822. Accessed 22 Aug 2014

Farge E, Oberstadt A (2014) Senegal tracks route of Guinea student in race to stop Ebola. Reuters. http://www.reuters.com/article/us-health-ebola-senegal-idUSKBN0H414F20140909. Accessed 29 Jan 2017

Fieldstadt E, Snow K, Williams S (2014) Ebola patient Dr. Kent Brantly arrives at U.S. hospital from Liberia. NBC News. http://www.nbcnews.com/storyline/ebola-virus-outbreak/ebola-patient-dr-kent-brantly-arrives-u-s-hospital-liberia-n171241. Accessed 14 Jan 2017

Filou E (2014) Ebola: voices from the epicentre of the epidemic. The Guardian. http://www.theguardian.com/global-development-professionals-network/2014/jul/14/ebola-epidemic-guinea-sierra-leone-liberia-msf-world-health-organisation. Accessed 24 Aug 2014

Fink S (2014a) 3 Liberian health workers with Ebola receive scarce drug after appeals to U.S. New York Times. http://www.nytimes.com/2014/08/17/world/africa/three-liberian-health-workers-get-experimental-ebola-drug.html. Accessed 1 Jan 2017

Fink S (2014b) With aid doctors gone, Ebola fight grows harder. New York Times. http://www.nytimes.com/2014/08/17/world/africa/with-aid-doctors-gone-ebola-fight-grows-harder.html?_r=0. Accessed 16 Aug 2014

Fofana U (2014a) Death toll from Ebola in Sierra Leone more than doubles to 12. Reuters. http://www.reuters.com/article/2014/06/09/us-leone-ebola-idUSKBN0EK1HT20140609. Accessed 22 Aug 2014

Fofana U (2014b) Fear, suspicion undermine West Africa's battle against Ebola. Reuters. http://www.reuters.com/article/2014/06/30/us-health-ebola-leone-idUSKBN0F520F20140630. Accessed 24 Aug 2014

Fofana U (2014c) First Ebola victim in Sierra Leone capital on the run. Reuters. http://www.reuters.com/article/2014/07/25/us-health-ebola-africa-idUSKBN0FU1DB20140725. Accessed 25 Jul 2014

Fofana U (2014d) Runaway Sierra Leone Ebola patient dies in ambulance. Reuters. http://news.yahoo.com/runaway-sierra-leone-ebola-patient-dies-ambulance-115730446.html. Accessed 27 Jul 2014

Fofana U (2014e) Sierra Leone declares emergency as Ebola death toll hits 729. Reuters. http://www.reuters.com/article/2014/07/31/us-health-ebola-leone-idUSKBN0G00TG20140731. Accessed 31 Jul 2014

Fofana U, Coulibaly M (2014) WHO shuts Sierra Leone lab after worker infected with Ebola. Reuters. http://www.reuters.com/article/us-health-ebola-idUSKBN0GQ17920140826. Accessed 25 Jan 2017

Fofana U, Giahyue JH (2014) Health workers strike at major Ebola clinic in Sierra Leone. Reuters, Hartford Courant. http://www.courant.com/nation-world/chi-health-workers-strike-ebola-clinic-20140830,0,7734377.story?page=2. Accessed 31 Aug 2014

Fofana U, MacDougall C (2014a) Troops deploy in Sierra Leone, Liberia to try to stop Ebola spread. Reuters. http://af.reuters.com/article/worldNews/idAFKBN0G41D820140804?pageNumber=3&virtualBrandChannel=0. Accessed 4 Aug 2014

Fofana U, MacDougall C (2014b) Sierra Leone army blockades Ebola areas Liberia declares emergency. Reuters. http://www.reuters.com/article/2014/08/07/us-health-ebola-africa-idUSK-BN0G70WW20140807. Accessed 7 Aug 2014

Fonbuena C (2014) PH pulling out peacekeepers in Liberia, Golan Heights. http://www.rappler.com/nation/67016-philippines-pullout-liberia-golan. Accessed 22 Jan 2017

Foote W (2014) On the front lines of Ebola my interview with an entrepreneur in Liberia. Forbes. http://www.forbes.com/sites/willyfoote/2014/08/25/on-the-front-lines-of-ebola-my-interview-with-an-entrepreneur-in-liberia/. Accessed 25 Aug 2014

Fox M (2014a) Ebola may have been smoldering for years, study says. NBC News. http://www.nbcnews.com/health/health-news/ebola-may-have-been-smoldering-years-study-says-n158641. Accessed 20 Jul 2014

Fox M (2014b) Docs declare Ebola patients Kent Brantly and Nancy Writebol no risk to pub-lic. NBC News. http://www.nbcnews.com/storyline/ebola-virus-outbreak/docs-declare-ebola-patients-kent-brantly-nancy-writebol-no-risk-n185626. Accessed 19 Jan 2017

Fox M, Edwards E (2014) Ebola scare briefly closes Charlotte ER. NBC News. http://www.nbc-news.com/storyline/ebola-virus-outbreak/ebola-scare-briefly-closes-charlotte-er-n168731. Accessed 30 Jul 2014

Frankel TC (2014a) Alarm grows as Ebola outbreak spurs more flight cancellations, border clo-sures. The Washington Post. http://www.washingtonpost.com/world/africa/alarm-grows-as-ebola-outbreak-spurs-more-flight-cancellations-border-closures/2014/08/25/87e6d020-2c66-11e4-994d-202962a9150c_story.html. Accessed 25 Aug 2014

Frankel TC (2014b) It was already the worst Ebola outbreak in history. Now it's mov-ing into Africa's cities. Washington Post. http://www.washingtonpost.com/world/africa/it-was-already-the-worst-ebola-outbreak-in-history-now-its-moving-into-africas-cities/2014/08/30/31816ff2-2ed6-11e4-bb9b-997ae96fad33_story.html. Accessed 31 Aug 2014

Freeman C, Akkoc R (2014) Ebola outbreak BA suspends flights to Sierra Leone and Liberia over virus. The Telegraph. http://www.telegraph.co.uk/news/aviation/11013996/Ebola-outbreak-BA-suspends-flights-to-Sierra-Leone-and-Liberia-over-virus.html. Accessed 5 Aug 2014

Gardner B (2014) Ebola: infected British healthcare worker William 'begged' to treat dying patients. The Telegraph. http://www.telegraph.co.uk/news/worldnews/ebola/11054039/Ebola-Infected-British-healthcare-worker-William-begged-to-treat-dying-patients.html. Accessed 24 Aug 2014

Garloch K, Funk T (2014) Charlotte's Nancy Writebol, other Ebola patient released from Atlanta hospital. Charlotte Observer. http://www.charlotteobserver.com/2014/08/21/5119405/write-bol-doctor-ebola-released.html#.U_dTWLd0ziw. Accessed 21 Aug 2014

Garrett L (2014) You are not nearly scared enough about Ebola. http://www.foreignpolicy.com/articles/2014/08/14/you_are_not_nearly_scared_enough_ebola_vaccine_west_africa_out-break. Accessed 14 Aug 2014

Gbandia S (2014a) Villagers stone workers tracking Ebola in Sierra Leone. Bloomberg. http://www.bloomberg.com/news/2014-05-28/villagers-stone-workers-tracking-ebola-in-sierra-leone.html. Accessed 20 Aug 2014

Gbandia S (2014b) Ebola spreads to Sierra Leone capital of Freetown as deaths rise. Bloomberg. http://www.bloomberg.com/news/2014-07-12/ebola-spreads-to-sierra-leone-capital-of-free-town-as-deaths-rise.html. Accessed 19 Aug 2014

Geisbert TW (2014) Medical research: Ebola therapy protects severely ill monkeys. Nature 514:41–43

Giahyue JH, Samb S (2014) Celebration in Liberia slum as Ebola quarantine lifted. Reuters. http://www.reuters.com/article/2014/08/30/us-health-ebola-idUSKBN0GU0OJ20140830. Accessed 30 Aug 2014

Gire SK, Goba A, Andersen KG et al (2014) Genomic surveillance elucidates Ebola virus origin and transmission during the 2014 outbreak. Science 345:1369–1372

Gladstone R (2014) Death toll from Ebola surges in West Africa, prompting alarm. New York Times. http://www.nytimes.com/2014/07/16/world/africa/death-toll-from-ebola-surges-in-west-africa-prompting-alarm.html?_r=0. Accessed 24 Aug 2014

Godwin AC (2014) Ebola: Arik Air suspends all flights from Liberia, Sierra Leone. http://dailyp-ost.ng/2014/07/28/ebola-arik-air-suspends-flights-liberia-sierra-leone/. Accessed 28 Jul 2014

Govan F (2014) Ebola outbreak Spain to accept Europe's first confirmed case of the virus. The Telegraph. http://www.telegraph.co.uk/news/worldnews/europe/spain/11017332/Ebola-outbreak-Spain-to-accept-Europes-first-confirmed-case-of-the-virus.html. Accessed 15 Jan 2017

Government of Sierra Leone (2014) Address to the nation on the Ebola outbreak by his excellency the President Dr. Ernest Bai Koroma July 30, 2014. ReliefWeb. https://reliefweb.int/report/

sierra-leone/address-nation-ebola-outbreak-his-excellency-president-dr-ernest-bai-koroma-july. Accessed 30 Oct 2017

Grady D (2014a) Short staff tries to cope with Ebola. New York Times. http://www.nytimes.com/2014/07/29/world/africa/short-staff-tries-to-cope-with-ebola.html?_r=0. Accessed 29 Jul 2014

Grady D (2014b). With Ebola cases still few, populous Nigeria has chance to halt its outbreak. New York Times. http://www.nytimes.com/2014/08/16/science/with-ebola-cases-still-few-populous-nigeria-has-chance-to-halt-its-outbreak.html?_r=0. Accessed 16 Aug 2014

Grady D, Fink S (2014) Tracing Ebola's breakout to an African 2-year-old. New York Times. http://www.nytimes.com/2014/08/10/world/africa/tracing-ebolas-breakout-to-an-african-2-year-old.html?_r=0. Accessed 9 Aug 2014

Greenfieldboyce N (2014) How much bigger is the Ebola outbreak than official reports show? NPR. http://www.npr.org/blogs/goatsandsoda/2014/08/21/341992005/how-much-bigger-is-the-ebola-outbreak-than-official-reports. Accessed 21 Aug 2014

Guardian (2014a) Relatives remove Sierra Leone Ebola patients from clinic. The Guardian. http://www.theguardian.com/world/2014/may/28/relatives-sierra-leone-ebola-patients-clinic. Accessed 20 Aug 2014

Guardian (2014b) Ebola crisis: Guinea closes borders with Sierra Leone and Liberia. The Guardian. http://www.theguardian.com/society/2014/aug/09/ebola-guinea-sierra-leone-liberia. Accessed 9 Aug 2014

Gupta S, Dellorto D (2014) Experimental drug likely saved Ebola patients. CNN. http://www.cnn.com/2014/08/04/health/experimental-ebola-serum/. Accessed 13 Jan 2017

Haglage A (2014) Kissing the corpses in Ebola country. The Daily Beast. http://www.thedailybeast.com/articles/2014/08/13/kissing-the-corpses-in-ebola-country.html. Accessed 13 Aug 2014

Hammer J (2015) All of my nurses are dead, and I don't know if I'm already infected. https://medium.com/matter/did-sierra-leones-hero-doctor-have-to-die-1c1de004941e#.cvvxs8kth. Accessed 10 Jan 2017

Harvard T.H. Chan School of Public Health (2014) Poll finds many in U.S. lack knowledge about Ebola and its transmission. 21 Aug 2014

Hasting D, Hutchison B (2014) Emory University Hospital in Georgia is expected to receive Ebola virus patient as American aid workers are evacuated from Liberia. NY Daily News. http://www.nydailynews.com/life-style/health/american-ebola-virus-patient-u-s-article-1.1887776. Accessed 13 Jan 2017

Hille P (2014) Senegalese Ebola patient evacuated to Germany for treatment. Deutsche Welle. http://www.dw.com/en/senegalese-ebola-patient-evacuated-to-germany-for-treatment/a-17881359. Accessed 27 Jan 2017

Hinshaw D, McKay B (2014) Ebola virus crisis worsens for lack of global help. The Wall Street Journal. http://online.wsj.com/articles/ebola-crisis-worsens-for-lack-of-global-help-1409269141. Accessed 29 Aug 2014

Hogan C (2014a) 'There is no such thing as Ebola.' The Washington Post. http://www.washingtonpost.com/news/morning-mix/wp/2014/07/18/there-is-no-such-thing-as-ebola/?tid=hp_mm. Accessed 18 Jul 2014

Hogan C (2014b) Ebola striking women more frequently than men. The Washington Post. http://www.washingtonpost.com/national/health-science/2014/08/14/3e08d0c8-2312-11e4-8593-da634b334390_story.html. Accessed 14 Aug 2014

Huggler J (2014) Ebola Germany accepts infected patient for treatment. The Telegraph. http://www.telegraph.co.uk/news/worldnews/europe/germany/10998367/Ebola-Germany-accepts-infected-patient-for-treatment.html. Accessed 29 Jul 2014

Hussain M (2014a) Red Cross removes staff from Ebola operations after Guinea knife threat. http://news.trust.org//item/20140702083611-3yofq. Accessed 7 Jan 2017

Hussain M (2014b) Liberia adds new Ebola centres as tries to contain virus outbreak. AllAfrica. http://allafrica.com/stories/201408310069.html. Accessed 31 Aug 2014

Hussain M, Samb S (2014) Guinea announces two new cases of Ebola in previously unaf-
    fected area. Reuters. http://www.reuters.com/article/2014/05/23/us-ebola-guinea-idUSK-
    BN0E31Y220140523. Accessed 20 Aug 2014
Ibeh N (2014) Shocking Jonathan sacks 16,000 resident doctors in Nigeria. Premium Times.
    https://www.premiumtimesng.com/news/166732-shocking-jonathan-sacks-16000-resident-
    doctors-in-nigeria.html#sthash.CQruypOe.rSEHPRQw.dpbs. Accessed 16 Aug 2014
Ibekwe N (2014a) Exclusive: how Liberian govt cleared Patrick Sawyer to travel to Nigeria while
    under observation for Ebola. Premium Times. http://www.premiumtimesng.com/foreign/west-
    africa-foreign/166559-exclusive-how-liberian-govt-cleared-patrick-sawyer-to-travel-to-nige-
    ria-while-under-observation-for-ebola-2.html Accessed 9 Jan 2017
Ibekwe N (2014b) Video shows Liberian, Patrick Sawyer, was 'terribly ill' possibly knew he
    had Ebola before traveling to Nigeria. Premium Times. https://www.premiumtimesng.com/
    news/166176-video-shows-liberian-patrick-sawyer-was-terribly-ill-possibly-knew-he-had-
    ebola-before-traveling-to-nigeria.html#sthash.s5CWwSZJ.dpbs. Accessed 16 Aug 2014
Jansen B (2014) WHO urges exit screening in countries with Ebola. USA Today. http://www.
    usatoday.com/story/travel/news/2014/08/18/who-ebola-exit-screening/14230779/.   Accessed
    18 Aug 2014
Johnson RM (2014) 'Miracle' mum-to-be in Sierra Leone tells of Ebola recovery. AFP, The Daily
    Star. http://www.dailystar.com.lb/News/International/2014/Jun-14/260087-miracle-mum-to-
    be-in-sierra-leone-tells-of-ebola-recovery.ashx. Accessed 29 Aug 2017
Jones S (2014) West Africa Ebola epidemic is out of control. The Guardian. http://www.the-
    guardian.com/global-development/2014/jun/23/west-africa-ebola-epidemic-out-of-control.
    Accessed 22 Aug 2014
Joseph J, Karikari-apau, N, Holland L (2014) First WHO worker stricken with Ebola. CNN. http://
    www.cnn.com/2014/08/24/world/africa/ebola-outbreak/index.html?hpt=hp_t2.   Accessed   24
    Aug 2014
Kassam A (2014) Ebola: Spanish missionary infected with virus in Liberia flown to Spain. The
    Guardian.   https://www.theguardian.com/world/2014/aug/07/ebola-spanish-missionary-
    miguel-pajares-virus-liberia-flown-spain. Accessed 15 Jan 2017
Katz A (2014) Harrowing images of Liberia's Ebola outbreak. Time. http://lightbox.time.
    com/2014/08/19/ebola-outbreak-liberia-john-moore-photographs/#1. Accessed 20 Aug 2014
Kay C, Ibukun Y (2014) Nigeria suspects Ebola cases after officials see progress. Bloomberg.
    http://www.bloomberg.com/news/2014-08-20/nigeria-may-be-ebola-free-in-a-week-as-cases-
    fall-minister-says.html. Accessed 20 Aug 2014
Keith B (2014) Ebola concerns will leave three western African athletes barred from Youth
    Olympic   Games.   https://swimswam.com/ebola-concerns-will-leave-three-western-african-
    athletes-youth-olympic-games/. Accessed 17 Jan 2017
Kitamura M, Gbandia S (2014) Ebola cases mix with malaria creating 'slow-motion' disaster.
    Bloomberg.   http://www.bloomberg.com/news/2014-08-06/malaria-cases-mix-with-ebola-
    amid-slow-motion-disaster-.html. Accessed 7 Aug 2014
Kitching C (2014) British Airways halts flights to Ebola-hit Sierra Leone and Liberia for the rest of
    the year amid concerns over worst outbreak ever. The Daily Mail. http://www.dailymail.co.uk/
    travel/travel_news/article-2735875/British-Airways-halts-flights-two-Ebola-hit-nations-rest-
    year-amid-growing-concerns-worst-outbreak-ever.html. Accessed 29 Jan 2017
Kollewe J (2014) GSK to start production of Ebola vaccine as tests on humans begin. The
    Guardian.   http://www.theguardian.com/society/2014/aug/28/gsk-to-testing-ebola-vaccine-
    humans. Accessed 28 Aug 2014
Kollie SD (2014) Liberia: deadly virus victims' bodies left unburied in Johnsonville. AllAfrica,
    Front Page Africa. http://allafrica.com/stories/201408041814.html. Accessed 15 Jan 2017
Kpodo K (2014) Fear, cash shortages hinder fight against Ebola outbreak. Reuters. http://
    www.reuters.com/article/2014/07/02/us-health-ebola-westafrica-redcross-idUSK-
    BN0F714220140702. Accessed 24 Aug 2014

Krever M (2014) Scientist who discovered Ebola: 'This is unprecedented.' CNN. http://amanpour.blogs.cnn.com/2014/07/02/scientist-who-discovered-ebola-this-is-unprecedented/. Accessed 7 Jul 2014

Lancet (2014) Ebola in West Africa: gaining community trust and confidence. Lancet 383(9933):1946

Lazuta J (2014a) Liberia works to contain new Ebola outbreak amid renewed fear. VOA News. http://www.voanews.com/content/liberia-works-to-contain-new-ebola-outbreak-amid-renewed-fear/1939740.html. Accessed 22 Aug 2014

Lazuta J (2014b) Ebola outbreak now most deadly ever in West Africa. USA Today. http://www.usatoday.com/story/news/world/2014/06/28/ebola-west-africa-outbreak/11615045/. Accessed 24 Aug 201

Levine A (2014) One woman walked in and the Ebola nightmare began. CNN. http://www.cnn.com/2014/09/24/health/ebola-epidemic-liberia/index.html. Accessed 27 Sept 2014

Lewis R (2014) Spanish priest infected with Ebola to receive experimental treatment. Aljazeera. http://america.aljazeera.com/articles/2014/8/10/ebola-spain-zmapp.html. Accessed 15 Jan 2017

Live Press (2014) Ebola virus may have made its way into Spain. The Live Press. http://www.theolivepress.es/spain-news/2014/06/27/ebola-may-have-made-its-way-into-spain/. Accessed 24 Aug 2014

Loftus P (2014) Maker of experimental 'ZMapp' Ebola drug says supply is exhausted. The Wall Street Journal. http://online.wsj.com/articles/maker-of-experimental-zmapp-ebola-drug-says-its-supply-is-exhausted-1407799150. Accessed 12 Aug 2014

Look A (2014) Doctors without borders worried about spread of Ebola outbreak. VOA News. http://www.voanews.com/content/doctors-without-borders-worried-about-spread-of-ebola-outbreak/1929425.html. Accessed 20 Aug 2014

Lupkin S (2014a) Ebola-stricken doc gives 'experimental serum' to coworker. ABC News. http://abcnews.go.com/Health/WorldNews/ebola-stricken-american-doctor-turn-worse/story?id=24791024. Accessed 13 Jan 2017

Lupkin S (2014b) Why American Ebola survivor got so many hugs. ABC News. http://abcnews.go.com/Health/american-ebola-survivor-hugs/story?id=25070559. Accessed 21 Aug 2014

Lynch D (2014) Ebola outbreak death toll poised to break record by September 1. International Business Times. http://www.ibtimes.com/ebola-outbreak-death-toll-poised-break-record-september-1-1665798. Accessed 22 Aug 2014

Lyon GM, Mehta AK, Varkey JB et al (2014) Clinical care of two patients with Ebola virus disease in the United States. N Engl J Med 371:2402–2409

MacDougall C (2014a) Consignment of experimental Ebola drug arrives in Liberia. Reuters. http://uk.reuters.com/article/uk-health-ebola-idUKKBN0GD1VQ20140814. Accessed 16 Jan 2017

MacDougall C (2014b) Liberia gives experimental Ebola drug to three African doctors. Reuters. http://www.reuters.com/article/us-health-ebola-liberia-idUSKBN0GG0L020140816. Accessed 17 Jan 2017

MacDougall C (2014c) Chaos and fear overtake Liberia's Ebola response. Aljazeera. http://america.aljazeera.com/articles/2014/8/19/chaos-and-fear-overrunliberiasebolaresponse.html. Accessed 19 Aug 2014

MacDougall C, Flynn D (2014) Update 1-bodies dumped in streets as West Africa struggles to curb Ebola. Reuters. http://in.reuters.com/article/2014/08/05/health-ebola-africa-idINL6N-0QB62Q20140805. Accessed 5 Aug 2014

MacDougall C, Giahyue JH (2014) Update 4-Liberia police fire on protesters as W Africa's Ebola toll hits 1,350. Reuters. http://www.reuters.com/article/2014/08/20/health-ebola-liberia-protests-idUSL5N0QQ2FU20140820. Accessed 20 Aug 2014

MacDougall C, Nebehay S (2014) Liberia fights Ebola in capital, West Africa toll tops 1,200. Reuters. http://uk.reuters.com/article/2014/08/19/uk-health-ebola-idUKKBN0GI1LU20140819. Accessed 19 Aug 2014

Mark M (2014a) Ebola virus causes outbreak of infectious dance tune. The Guardian. https://www. theguardian.com/world/2014/may/27/ebola-virus-outbreak-infectious-dance-tune.   Accessed 19 Aug 2014

Mark M (2014b) Fear and ignorance as Ebola 'out of control' in parts of west Africa. The Guardian.   http://www.theguardian.com/world/2014/jul/02/-sp-ebola-out-of-control-west-africa. Accessed 24 Aug 2014

Mark M (2014c) Ebola outbreak nurse who treated first victim in Nigeria dies. The Guardian. http://www.theguardian.com/world/2014/aug/06/ebola-outbreak-nurse-nigeria-dies. Accessed 6 Aug 2014

Mark M (2014d) Ebola epidemic takes toll on business in quarantine zones and across Africa. The Guardian. http://www.theguardian.com/world/2014/aug/27/ebola-epidemic-business-impact-africa. Accessed 28 Aug 2014

Mazen M (2014) Nigeria acknowledges slow response in Ebola case. ABC News. http://abcnews. go.com/Health/wireStory/nigerian-official-show-ebola-symptoms-24848708. Accessed 5 Aug 2014

McClam E (2014) Nancy Writebol, second American Ebola patient, arrives at Atlanta hospital. NBC News. http://www.nbcnews.com/storyline/ebola-virus-outbreak/nancy-writebol-second-american-ebola-patient-arrives-atlanta-hospital-n173146. Accessed 15 Jan 2017

McCoy T (2014a) Why the escape of numerous Ebola patients in Liberia's worst slum is so terrifying. The Washington Post. http://www.washingtonpost.com/news/morning-mix/wp/2014/08/18/why-the-escape-of-numerous-ebola-patients-in-liberias-worst-slum-is-so-terrifying/?tid=hp_mm. Accessed 18 Aug 2014

McCoy T (2014b) The nightmare of containing Ebola in Liberia's worst slum. The Washington Post. http://www.washingtonpost.com/news/morning-mix/wp/2014/08/21/the-nightmare-of-containing-ebola-in-liberias-worst-slum/. Accessed 21 Aug 2014

McCray V (2014) Family of Ebola victim mourns his loss. The Blade. http://www.toledoblade. com/Medical/2014/08/01/Family-of-Ebola-victim-mourns-his-loss.html.   Accessed 10 Jan 2017

McGregor S, Mokhema T (2014) Country confusion keeps Ebola-fearing tourists out of Africa. Bloomberg.   http://www.bloomberg.com/news/2014-08-28/country-confusion-keeps-ebola-fearing-tourists-away-from-africa.html. Accessed 29 Aug 2014

McKay B (2014) Ebola virus American patient hopes for discharge soon. The Wall Street Journal. http://online.wsj.com/articles/american-ebola-patient-hopes-for-discharge-soon-1408126329. Accessed 16 Aug 2014

Médecins Sans Frontières (2014a) Resurgence of epidemic Ebola in West Africa. Médecins Sans Frontières. http://www.msf.org/article/resurgence-epidemic-ebola-west-africa. Accessed 20 Aug 2014

Médecins Sans Frontières (2014b) West Africa: MSF activities in Ebola outbreak. Médecins Sans Frontières. http://www.msf.org/article/west-africa-msf-activities-ebola-outbreak. Accessed 24 Aug 2014

Médecins Sans Frontières (2014c) Struggling to contain the Ebola epidemic in West Africa. Médecins Sans Frontières. http://www.doctorswithoutborders.org/news-stories/voice-field/struggling-contain-ebola-epidemic-west-africa. Accessed 24 Aug 2014

Médecins Sans Frontières (2014d) Ebola epidemic confirmed in Democratic Republic of Congo: MSF sends specialists and material to the epicentre. Médecins Sans Frontières. http://www. msf.org/en/article/ebola-epidemic-confirmed-democratic-republic-congo-msf-sends-special-ists-and-material. Accessed 27 Jan 2017

Monnier O (2014) Senegal puts 20 people on watch for Ebola after first case. Business Week. http://www.businessweek.com/news/2014-08-30/senegal-puts-20-people-on-watch-for-ebola-virus-after-first-case. Accessed 31 Aug 2014

Moriba S (2014) Sierra Leone News: nurses demand relocation of Ebola centre. Awoko. http:// awoko.org/2014/07/22/sierra-leone-news-nurses-demand-relocation-of-ebola-centre/. Accessed 23 Jul 2014

Mueller K (2014) Burying Ebolas victims in Sierra Leone. IFRC. http://www.ifrc.org/en/news-and-media/news-stories/africa/sierra-leone/burying-ebolas-victims-in-sierra-leone-66528/. Accessed 13 Jan 2017

Muhindo C, Bwambale T (2014) Ugandan doctor dies of Ebola in Liberia. New Vision. http://www.newvision.co.ug/new_vision/ncws/1342263/ugandan-doctor-dies-ebola-liberia. Accessed 8 Jan 2017

Mundasad S (2014) Travel ban to Ebola affected countries, UK officials say. BBC. http://www.bbc.com/news/health-28966419. Accessed 28 Aug 2014

NBC News (2014a) Liberia declares 'state of emergency' amid Ebola outbreak. NBC News. http://www.nbcnews.com/storyline/ebola-virus-outbreak/liberia-declares-state-emergency-amid-ebola-outbreak-n174586. Accessed 15 Jan 2017

NBC News (2014b) Priest Miguel Pajares is flown to Spain for Ebola treatment. NBC News. http://www.nbcnews.com/storyline/ebola-virus-outbreak/priest-miguel-pajares-flown-spain-ebola-treatment-n174786. Accessed 15 Jan 2017

NBC News (2014c) Ontario hospital treating patient with Ebola-like symptoms. NBC News. http://www.nbcnews.com/storyline/ebola-virus-outbreak/ontario-hospital-treating-patient-ebola-symptoms-n176691. Accessed 9 Aug 2014

Nebehay S, MacDougall C (2014) WHO warns of 'shadow zones,' hidden cases in Ebola outbreak. Reuters. http://www.reuters.com/article/2014/08/22/us-health-ebola-who-idUSK-BN0GM0RW20140822. Accessed 22 Aug 2014

Nebehay S, Samb S (2014) West Africa Ebola outbreak still spreading, 'situation serious:' WHO. Reuters. http://www.reuters.com/article/2014/05/28/us-ebola-westafrica-idUSK-BN0E81IQ20140528. Accessed 20 Aug 2014

New Vision (2014) Liberian nurses contract Ebola after death of Ugandan doctor. New Vision. http://www.newvision.co.ug/news/657836-liberian-nurses-contract-ebola-after-death-of-ugandan-doctor.html. Accessed 22 Jul 2014

Newsroom America (2014) WHO identifies countries at risk for spread of Ebola. Newsroom American. http://www.newsroomamerica.com/story/440565.html. Accessed 30 Aug 2014

Nigerian Bulletin (2014) ECOWAS Diplomat who imported Ebola to Port Harcourt to face manslaughter charges? Nigerian Bulletin. http://www.nigerianbulletin.com/threads/ecowas-diplomat-who-imported-ebola-to-port-harcourt-to-face-manslaughter-charges.90315/d increased to 160. Accessed 31 Aug 2014

Nossiter A (2014a) Fear of Ebola breeds a terror of physicians. New York Times. http://www.nytimes.com/2014/07/28/world/africa/ebola-epidemic-west-africa-guinea.html?_r=0. Accessed 28 Jul 2014

Nossiter A (2014b) 'Don't touch the walls': Ebola dears infect an African hospital. New York Times. http://www.nytimes.com/2014/08/08/world/africa/dont-touch-the-walls-ebola-fears-infect-hospital.html?&_r=0. Accessed 8 Aug 2014

Nossiter A (2014c) At heart of Ebola outbreak a village, frozen by fear and death. New York Times. http://www.nytimes.com/2014/08/12/world/africa/at-heart-of-ebola-outbreak-a-village-frozen-by-fear-and-death.html?_r=0. Accessed 12 Aug 2014

Nossiter A (2014d) Sierra Leone again loses a top doctor to Ebola. New York Times. https://www.nytimes.com/2014/08/14/world/africa/ebola-claims-another-sierra-leone-doctor.html?_r=0. Accessed 16 Aug 2014

Nossiter A (2014e) Those who serve Ebola victims soldier on. New York Times. http://www.nytimes.com/2014/08/24/world/africa/sierra-leone-if-they-survive-in-ebola-ward-they-work-on.html?_r=0. Accessed 23 Aug 2014

NPR (2014a) Medical aid group: Liberia's Ebola cases spiral upward. NPR. http://news.stlpublicradio.org/post/medical-aid-group-liberias-ebola-cases-spiral-upward. Accessed 15 Aug 2014

NPR (2014b) Has an Ebola corner been turned? One perspective: 'no, no, no, no'. NPR. http://www.npr.org/blogs/goatsandsoda/2014/08/15/340401916/has-an-ebola-corner-been-turned-one-perspective-no-no-no-no. Accessed 15 Aug 2014

NPR (2014c) Rare good news regarding 5 Ebola patients in Nigeria. NPR. http://www.npr.
org/2014/08/19/341542600/rare-good-news-regarding-5-ebola-patients-in-nigeria. Accessed
19 Jan 2017

Odunsi W (2014) Sawyer: we prevented spread of Ebola in Nigeria – First Consultants Hospital
releases statement. Daily Post. http://dailypost.ng/2014/08/23/prevented-spread-ebola-nigeria-
first-consultants-hospital-releases-statement/. Accessed 23 Aug 2014

Okolie A (2014) Ebola: First Consultant Hospital, victims' families may sue Liberian government. This Day. http://www.thisdaylive.com/articles/ebola-first-consultant-hospital-victims-
families-may-sue-liberian-government/187189/. Accessed 24 Aug 2014

Olu-Mammah J, Fofana U (2014). Ebola causing huge damage to West Africa economies: development bank. Reuters. http://www.reuters.com/article/2014/08/27/us-health-ebola-idUSK-
BN0GQ17920140827. Accessed 27 Aug 2014

Onishi N (2014a) Clashes erupt as Liberia imposes quarantine to curb Ebola. New York Times.
http://www.nytimes.com/2014/08/21/world/africa/ebola-outbreak-liberia-quarantine.html?_
r=0. Accessed 20 Aug 2014

Onishi N (2014b) Liberian boy dies after being shot during clash over Ebola quarantine. New York
Times. http://www.nytimes.com/2014/08/22/world/africa/liberian-boy-dies-after-being-shot-
during-clash-over-ebola-quarantine.html?_r=0. Accessed 21 Aug 2014

Onishi N (2014c) As Ebola grips Liberia's capital, a quarantine sows social chaos. New York
Times. http://www.nytimes.com/2014/08/29/world/africa/in-liberias-capital-an-ebola-out-
break-like-no-other.html. Accessed 28 Aug 2014

Onishi N (2014d) Quarantine for Ebola lifted in Liberia slum. New York Times. http://www.
nytimes.com/2014/08/30/world/africa/quarantine-for-ebola-lifted-in-liberia-slum.html?_r=0.
Accessed 30 Aug 2014

Onuah F, Miles T (2014) Nigeria government confirms Ebola case in megacity of Lagos.
Reuters. http://www.reuters.com/article/2014/07/25/us-heath-ebola-nigeria-idUSKBN-
0FU1LE20140725. Accessed 25 Jul 2014

Paye-Layleh J (2014a) Liberia president declares Ebola curfew. ABC News. http://abcnews.
go.com/Health/wireStory/liberia-missing-quarantined-patients-found-25033856. Accessed 20
Aug 2014

Paye-Layleh J (2014b) Sealed off Liberia slum calm amid Ebola outbreak. Associated Press,
Sacramento Bee. http://www.sacbee.com/2014/08/21/6643867/who-officials-to-visit-liberian.
html. Accessed 21 Aug 2014

Paye-Layleh J (2014c) Liberian ministers who defied Ebola order fired. ABC News. http://abc-
news.go.com/International/wireStory/liberia-doctor-experimental-ebola-drug-dies-25111371.
Accessed 26 Aug 2014

Paye-Layleh J, Larson K (2014) Liberia opens 2nd Ebola treatment center in capital amid fears
of mounting death toll. U.S. News and World Report. http://www.usnews.com/news/world/
articles/2014/08/16/liberia-opens-2nd-ebola-center-in-capital. Accessed 16 Aug 2014

Paye-Layleh J, Williams W (2014) Clashes in Liberia slum sealed off to halt Ebola. The
Washington Post. https://www.washingtonpost.com/world/clashes-in-liberian-slum-sealed-
off-to-halt-spread-of-ebola-virus/2014/08/20/deb45f52-2884-11e4-86ca-6f03cbd15c1a_story.
html?utm_term=.9736daf04a66. Accessed 19 Jan 2017

Pflanz M (2014) Ebola out of control in West Africa as health workers rush to trace 1,500 possible
victims. The Telegraph. http://www.telegraph.co.uk/news/worldnews/africaandindianocean/
guinea/10942598/Ebola-out-of-control-in-West-Africa-as-health-workers-rush-to-trace-1500-
possible-victims.html. Accessed 19 Aug 2014

Pollack A (2014) Opting against Ebola drug for ill African doctor. New York Times. http://www.
nytimes.com/2014/08/13/world/africa/ebola.html?_r=0. Accessed 14 Aug 2014

Poole J (2014) 'Shadow' and 'D-12' sing an infectious song About Ebola. NPR. http://www.npr.
org/blogs/goatsandsoda/2014/08/19/341412011/shadow-and-d-12-sing-an-infectious-song-
about-ebola?utm_medium=RSS&utm_campaign=news. Accessed 19 Aug 2014

Premium Times (2014) Rivers official confirms suspected Ebola death in Port Harcourt. Premium Times. http://www.premiumtimesng.com/news/167383-rivers-official-confirms-suspected-ebola-death-in-port-harcourt.html. Accessed 29 Jan 2017

Qiu X, Wong G, Audet J et al (2014) Reversion of advanced Ebola virus disease in nonhuman primates with ZMapp. Nature 514:47–53

Quist-Arcton O (2014a) In West Africa, officials target ignorance and fear over Ebola. NPR. http://www.npr.org/blogs/parallels/2014/07/10/330390279/in-west-africa-officials-target-ignorance-and-fear-over-ebola. Accessed 24 Aug 2014

Quist-Arcton O (2014b) Skeptics in Sierra Leone doubt Ebola virus exists. NPR. http://www.npr.org/blogs/goatsandsoda/2014/08/06/338234063/skeptics-in-sierra-leone-doubt-ebola-virus-exists. Accessed 15 Jan 2017

Rayner G (2014) British Ebola sufferer William Pooley given experimental drug ZMapp and sitting up in bed. The Telegraph. http://www.telegraph.co.uk/news/worldnews/ebola/11057096/British-Ebola-sufferer-William-Pooley-given-experimental-drug-ZMapp-and-sitting-up-in-bed.html. Accessed 22 Jan 2017

Republic of Liberia (n.d.) Special statement by the president. http://www.emansion.gov.lr/doc/Special%20Statement%20by%20President%20Ellen%20Johnson%20Sirleaf%20-1_1.pdf. Accessed 10 Jan 2017

Reuters (2014a) 5 dead in Sierra Leones first Ebola outbreak as disease continues to spread. Reuters, Fox News. http://www.foxnews.com/health/2014/05/27/5-dead-in-sierra-leone-first-ebola-outbreak-as-disease-continues-to-spread/. Accessed 19 Aug 2014

Reuters (2014b) Ebola patient in Sierra Leone pulled from hospital by family. Reuters, CBC News. http://www.cbc.ca/news/health/ebola-patient-in-sierra-leone-pulled-from-hospital-by-family-1.2655490. Accessed 3 Feb 2016

Reuters (2014c) Ebola: Sierra Leone shuts borders. Reuters, IOL. http://www.iol.co.za/news/africa/ebola-sierra-leone-shuts-borders-1702254#.U5lgovldVOs. Accessed 3 Jan 2017

Reuters (2014d) Ebola-sickened travellers may cross borders, WHO warns. Reuters, CBC News. http://www.cbc.ca/news/health/ebola-sickened-travellers-may-cross-borders-who-warns-1.2689685. Accessed 24 Aug 2014

Reuters (2014e) Sierra Leone's chief Ebola doctor contracts the virus. Reuters. http://af.reuters.com/article/topNews/idAFKBN0FS10V20140723. Accessed 23 Jul 2014

Reuters (2014f) Liberian man in Nigeria's Lagos being tested for Ebola. Reuters. http://af.reuters.com/article/topNews/idAFKBN0FT1Z120140724. Accessed 25 Jul 2014

Reuters (2014g) Protesters march on Ebola center in Sierra Leone. Reuters, Newsweek. http://www.newsweek.com/protesters-march-ebola-center-sierra-leone-261467?piano_t=1. Accessed 26 Jul 2014

Reuters (2014h) Liberia shuts border crossings, restricts gatherings to curb Ebola spreading. Reuters. http://www.reuters.com/article/2014/07/28/us-health-ebola-africa-idUSKBN-0FX00V20140728. Accessed 27 Jul 2014

Reuters (2014i) Bodies of possible Ebola victims found lying in the street of Liberia's capital. Reuters, The Huffington Post. http://www.huffingtonpost.com/2014/08/03/bodies-of-possible-ebola-_n_5645875.html. Accessed 4 Aug 2014

Reuters (2014j) U.S. CDC activates high level emergency operation center for Ebola outbreak. Reuters. http://af.reuters.com/article/commoditiesNews/idAFL2N0QD1Z020140807. Accessed 15 Jan 2017

Reuters (2014k) Lagos overwhelmed: Nigeria asks for Ebola outbreak help. Reuters, DW. http://www.dw.de/lagos-overwhelmed-nigeria-asks-for-ebola-outbreak-help/a-17843552. Accessed 9 Aug 2014

Reuters (2014l) Kenya Airways to suspend flights to Freetown Monrovia due to Ebola. Reuters. http://www.reuters.com/article/2014/08/16/us-health-ebola-kenya-airways-idUSK-BN0GG0F520140816. Accessed 16 Aug 2014

Reuters (2014m) Illness with Ebola-like symptoms kills several in Congo: locals. Reuters. http://news.yahoo.com/illness-ebola-symptoms-kills-several-congo-locals-130456819.html. Accessed 20 Aug 2014

Reuters (2014n) Congo declares Ebola outbreak in northern Equateur province. Reuters. http://www.reuters.com/article/2014/08/24/us-health-ebola-congodemocratic-idUSKBN-0GO0R520140824. Accessed 24 Aug 2014

Reuters (2014o) Swedish hospital investigating possible case of Ebola. Reuters, The Toronto Sun. http://www.torontosun.com/2014/08/31/swedish-hospital-investigating-possible-case-of-ebola. Accessed 31 Aug 2014

Roy-Macaulay C (2014a) New Sierra Leone law makes it illegal to hide Ebola patients. U.S. News & World Report. http://www.usnews.com/news/world/articles/2014/08/23/sierra-leone-makes-hiding-ebola-patients-illegal. Accessed 23 Aug 2014

Roy-Macaulay C (2014b) Nigeria doctors suspend strike over Ebola threat. ABC News. http://abc-news.go.com/Health/wireStory/ebola-spreads-nigeria-liberia-1000-cases-25095840. Accessed 24 Aug 2014

Roy-Macaulay C (2014c) 3rd doctor dies from Ebola in Sierra Leone. ABC News. http://abcnews.go.com/Health/wireStory/ebola-upper-hand-us-official-25130896. Accessed 27 Aug 2014

Roy-Macaulay C, Cheng M (2014) Sierra Leone: another top doctor dies from Ebola. ABC News. http://abcnews.go.com/Health/wireStory/considered-ebola-drug-sierra-leone-doc-tor-24958782. Accessed 16 Aug 2014

RT (2014) Ebola crisis: Air France crews call for flight cancellations. RT. http://rt.com/news/181544-air-france-ebola-petition/. Accessed 20 Aug 2014

Ruble K (2014) Eight now dead from Ebola virus in Liberia's capital. Vice News. https://news.vice.com/article/eight-now-dead-from-ebola-virus-in-liberias-capital. Accessed 22 Aug 2014

Ryall J (2014) Japan ready to offer experimental Ebola drug abroad. The Telegraph. http://www.telegraph.co.uk/news/worldnews/ebola/11054526/Japan-ready-to-offer-experimental-Ebola-drug-abroad.html. Accessed 25 Aug 2014

Sabeti P (2014) A brush with Ebola: the ongoing fight against deadly diseases in West Africa. National Geographic. http://newswatch.nationalgeographic.com/2014/05/31/a-brush-with-ebola-the-ongoing-fight-against-deadly-diseases-in-west-africa/. Accessed 25 Aug 2014

Sahara Reporters (2014a) Ebola survivor stories from Sierra Leone By UNICEF. Sahara Reporters. http://saharareporters.com/2014/08/11/ebola-survivor-stories-sierra-leone-unicef. Accessed 12 Aug 2014

Sahara Reporters (2014b) Wife of doctor who died of Ebola in Port Harcourt moved to Lagos Ebola treatment center. Sahara Reporters. http://saharareporters.com/2014/08/29/wife-doctor-who-died-ebola-port-harcourt-moved-lagos-ebola-treatment-center. Accessed 16 Sep 2017

Samb S, Bailes A (2014) Ebola crisis in West Africa worsened by patients shunning treatment. The Huffington Post. http://www.huffingtonpost.com/2014/07/13/ebola-africa-patients-treatment_n_5582100.html. Accessed 17 Jul 2014

Samba A (2014) Sierra Leone news: as Ebola survivors on the increase… nurse Messie Konneh's husband appears in Daru. Awareness Times. http://news.sl/drwebsite/exec/view.cgi?archive=10&num=25566. Accessed 3 Jan 2017

Satellite (2014a) Important Ebola notice to all employees and contractors. The Satellite, ArcelorMittal Liberia. 11 Jul 2014

Satellite (2014b) Ebola statement. The Satellite, ArcelorMittal Liberia. 25 Jul 2014

Schoepp RJ, Rossi CA, Khan SH et al (2014) Undiagnosed acute viral febrile illnesses, Sierra Leone. Emerg Infect Dis 20:1176–1182

Schram J (2014) NYC hospital patient being tested for Ebola. NY Post. http://nypost.com/2014/08/04/nyc-hospital-testing-patient-for-ebola/. Accessed 4 Aug 2014

Schwartz D (2014) Ebola epidemic unlikely to spread beyond Africa. CBA News. http://www.cbc.ca/news/health/ebola-epidemic-unlikely-to-spread-beyond-africa-1.2695879. Accessed 24 Aug 2014

Shankar S (2014) Ebola outbreak: Guinea declares emergency as overall deaths from Ebola rise to 1,069. International Business Times. http://www.ibtimes.com/ebola-outbreak-guinea-declares-emergency-overall-deaths-ebola-rise-1069-1658220. Accessed 14 Aug 2014

Shinkman PD (2014) UN calls emergency meeting on West Africa Ebola. http://www.usnews.com/news/articles/2014/08/06/crisis-escalates-un-calls-emergency-meeting-on-west-africa-ebola. Accessed 6 Aug 2014

Siddique H (2014) Infected nurse airlifted from Ebola zone speaks of joy at seeing patients recover. The Guardian. https://www.theguardian.com/society/2014/aug/25/will-pooley-ebola-london-hospital-risks-sierra-leone. Accessed 22 Jan 2014

Sierra Leone Ministry of Health & Sanitation (2014) Sierra Leone Health Ministry answers citizens' Ebola questions. Awareness Times. http://news.sl/drwebsite/publish/article_200525509.shtml. Accessed 20 Aug 2014

Sifferlin A (2014) Doctors without borders opens new Ebola ward in Liberia. Time. http://time.com/3145185/ebola-doctors-without-borders-liberia/. Accessed 18 Jul 2017

Silver M (2014a) Panic, pouring rain, a ray of sun: reporting on Ebola in Sierra Leone. NPR. http://www.npr.org/blogs/goatsandsoda/2014/08/11/339302484/panic-pouring-rain-a-ray-of-sun-reporting-on-ebola-in-sierra-leone?utm_medium=RSS&utm_campaign=storiesfromnpr. Accessed 11 Aug 2014

Silver M (2014b) Reporting on Ebola: an abandoned 10-year-old, a nervous neighborhood. NPR. http://www.npr.org/blogs/goatsandsoda/2014/08/20/341705940/reporting-on-ebola-an-abandoned-10-year-old-a-nervous-neighborhood. Accessed 20 Aug 2014

Silver M (2014c) Death, sex and a glimmer of hope: reporting on Ebola from Sierra Leone. NPR. http://www.npr.org/sections/goatsandsoda/2014/07/16/331960686/death-sex-and-a-glimmer-of-hope-reporting-on-ebola-from-sierra-leone. Accessed 24 Aug 2014

Sim D (2014) Ebola outbreak photos: fear and panic as Liberian forces seal West Point slum to contain disease. International Business Times. http://www.ibtimes.co.uk/ebola-outbreak-photos-fear-panic-liberian-forces-seal-west-point-slum-contain-disease-1461985. Accessed 19 Jan 2017

Sirleaf EJ (2014) Nationwide statement by Madam Ellen Johnson Sirleaf President of the Republic of Liberia on the Ebola virus, Saturday, June 28, 2014

Snyder D (2014) Liberia shuts hospital where Spanish priest staff contract Ebola. Business Day. http://www.bdlive.co.za/africa/africannews/2014/08/06/liberia-shuts-hospital-where-spanish-priest-staff-contract-ebola. Accessed 6 Aug 2014

Snyder S (2014) Ebola patient entrance to Emory University Hospital. CNN. http://ireport.cnn.com/docs/DOC-1157861?hpt=hp_c2. Accessed 3 Aug 2014

Sophia M (2014) Saudi Arabia bans Haj pilgrims from Ebola hit countries. Gulf Business. http://gulfbusiness.com/2014/08/saudi-arabia-bans-haj-pilgrims-ebola-hit-countries/. Accessed 4 Aug 2014

South China Morning Post (2014) Nigerian staying at Hong Kong's Chungking Mansions suspected to have Ebola, says Centre for Health Protection. South China Morning Post. http://www.scmp.com/news/hong-kong/article/1570697/nigerian-hong-kong-hospital-suspected-have-ebola-says-centre-health. Accessed 10 Aug 2014

Spain E (2014) Ebola outbreak: NC missionaries evacuating 60 people. WFMY. http://www.wfmynews2.com/story/news/local/2014/07/29/nc-missionaries-ebola-evacuation/13348119/. Accessed 30 Jul 2014

Stanglin D (2014) CDC issues highest-level alert for Ebola. USA Today. https://www.usatoday.com/story/news/world/2014/08/06/ebola-nigeria-saudi-arabia-virus-death-toll/13663973/. Accessed 14 Dec 2017

Sullivan G, Moyer J (2014) In traumatized Liberia Sierra Leone and Guinea Ebola chaos. The Washington Post. http://www.washingtonpost.com/news/morning-mix/wp/2014/08/08/in-traumatized-liberia-and-sierra-leone-ebola-chaos/?tid=hp_mm. Accessed 8 Aug 2014

Sutton J, Yan H (2014) American doctor in Liberia infected with Ebola. CNN. http://www.
    cnn.com/2014/07/27/world/africa/ebola-american-doctor-infected/index.html?hpt=hp_t2.
    Accessed 27 Jul 2014
Szabo L (2014) Ebola outbreak could lead to food crisis, U.N. says. USA Today. http://
    www.usatoday.com/story/news/nation/2014/08/28/ebola-food-crisis/14737281/?utm_
    source=feedblitz&utm_medium=FeedBlitzRss&utm_campaign=usatoday-newstopstories.
    Accessed 28 Aug 2014
Thompson D (2014) Ebola's deadly spread in Africa driven by public health failures, cultural
    beliefs. National Geographic. http://news.nationalgeographic.com/news/2014/07/140702-
    ebola-epidemic-fever-world-health-guinea-sierra-leone-liberia/. Accessed 19 Aug 2014
Times Live (2014) South Africa bans entry for non-citizens from Ebola affected countries. The
    Times Live. http://www.timeslive.co.za/politics/2014/08/21/south-africa-bans-entry-for-non-
    citizens-from-ebola-affected-countries. Accessed 21 Aug 2014
Tommy E (2014) Sierra Leone News: do not scare tourists away! Tourism Minister calls for
    responsible and objective Ebola reporting. Awareness Times. http://news.sl/drwebsite/publish/
    article_200525804.shtml. Accessed 21 Jul 2014
Trenchard T (2014) Ebola: shattering lives in Sierra Leone. Aljazeera. http://www.aljazeera.com/
    indepth/features/2014/07/ebola-shattering-lives-sierra-leone-201472134839888944.html.
    Accessed 24 Aug 2014
U.S. Department of State (2014a) U.S. orders departure of eligible family members from Liberia;
    sending additional disease specialists to assist. 7 Aug 2014
U.S. Department of State (2014b) U.S. Orders Departure of Eligible Family Members from Sierra
    Leone. 14 Aug 2014
UNICEF (2014) Misconceptions fuel Ebola outbreak in West Africa. http://www.unicef.org/
    media/media_74256.html. Accessed 11 Jul 2014
United Nations News Center (2014) Ebola outbreak 'not out of hand', UN health agency says ready-
    ing response. UN. http://www.un.org/apps/news/story.asp?NewsID=48156#.U_oM17d0ziw.
    Accessed 24 Aug 2014
Vanguard (2014) Iyke Enemuo's widow, sixth Ebola victim also has virus. Vanguard. http://www.
    vanguardngr.com/2014/08/iyke-enemuos-widow-sixth-ebola-victim-also-virus/. Accessed 31
    Aug 2014
Vogel G (2014) Genomes reveal start of Ebola outbreak. Science 345(6200):989–990
Voice of America News (2014a) WHO warns West Africa countries of Ebola spread. VOA News.
    http://www.voanews.com/content/who-warns-west-africa-countries-of-ebola-spread/1946558.
    html. Accessed 24 Aug 2014
Voice of America News (2014b) Germany, Guinea-Bissau react to Ebola outbreak. VOA News.
    http://www.voanews.com/content/germany-guinea-bissau-react-to-ebola-outbreak/2411822.
    html. Accessed 13 Aug 2014
Voice of America News (2014c) Guinea declares public health emergency over Ebola. VOA
    News. http://www.voanews.com/content/nigeria-confirms-11th-case-of-ebola/2413025.html.
    Accessed 14 Aug 2014
Walters S, Adams S (2014) UK Ebola alert as infected medic to fly home: desperate bid to save
    first Briton struck by virus. The Daily Mail. http://www.dailymail.co.uk/news/article-2732679/
    BREAKING-NEWS-Briton-living-Sierra-Leone-tests-positive-Ebola-assessed-doctors.html.
    Accessed 23 Aug 2014
Weintraub K (2014) Universities adjust plans in face of Ebola crisis. USA Today. http://www.
    usatoday.com/story/news/nation/2014/08/11/universities-ebola-study-abroad/13900291/.
    Accessed 11 Aug 2014
Weise E (2014) Liberians protest as bodies of Ebola victims left uncollected. USA Today.
    http://www.usatoday.com/story/news/2014/08/09/ebola-liberia-bodies-outbreak-virus-
    africa/13835091/. Accessed 9 Aug 2014

Williams CJ (2014) U.S. doctor treating patients in Liberia tests positive for Ebola. LA Times. http://www.latimes.com/world/africa/la-fg-liberia-us-doctor-ebola-20140726-story.html. Accessed 10 Jan 2017

Wilson J (2014a) Ebola fears hit close to home. CNN. http://edition.cnn.com/2014/07/29/health/ ebola-outbreak-american-dies/. Accessed 9 Jan 2017

Wilson J (2014b) Ebola doctor in Sierra Leone dies. CNN. http://www.cnn.com/2014/07/29/ health/ebola-doctor-dies/index.html?hpt=hp_t2. Accessed 29 Jul 2014

Wilson J (2014c Borders closing over Ebola fears. CNN. http://www.cnn.com/2014/08/22/health/ ebola-outbreak/. Accessed 21 Jan 2014

Wiseman P (2014) Ebola starting to take an economic toll in region. The Miami Herald. http:// www.miamiherald.com/2014/08/09/4280651/ebola-starting-to-take-an-economic.html. Accessed 9 Aug 2014

World Health Organization (2014a) WHO risk assessment – human infections with Zaïre Ebolavirus in West Africa, 24 June 2014

World Health Organization (2014b) Statement on the 1st meeting of the IHR Emergency Committee on the 2014 Ebola outbreak in West Africa. 8 Aug 2014

World Health Organization (2014c) Ebola situation assessment: no early end to the Ebola outbreak. 14 Aug 2014

World Health Organization (2014d) Why the Ebola outbreak has been underestimated. 22 Aug 2014

World Health Organization (2014e) Situation assessment – unprecedented number of medical staff infected with Ebola. 25 Aug 2014

World Health Organization (2014f) Ebola response roadmap. 28 Aug 2014

World Health Organization (2014g) Ebola situation in Port Harcourt, Nigeria. 3 Sep 2014

Yahoo News (2014) Ebola-hit Liberia bans sailors from disembarking. Yahoo News. https:// au.news.yahoo.com/world/a/24856656/ebola-hit-liberia-bans-sailors-from-disembarking/. Accessed 30 Aug 2014

Zaimov S (2014) Deadliest Ebola outbreak continues 'frightening' spread; Samaritan's Purse directing efforts at Liberia isolation center. Christian Post. http://www.christianpost.com/news/ deadliest-ebola-outbreak-continues-frightening-spread-samaritans-purse-directing-efforts-at-liberia-isolation-center-123083/. Accessed 24 Aug 2014

Chapter 4
The Peak in Africa (September 2014)

Abstract By September 2014, the Ebola outbreak had overwhelmed West African healthcare systems. Treatment centers were filled beyond capacity and new centers could not be opened fast enough to deal with the increasing number of cases. Overflowing medical facilities had to turn away newly arriving infected patients. Heartbreaking scenes occurred as sick patients crisscrossed cities looking for space in treatment centers only to find that no space was available. As conditions worsened, Sierra Leone took the unprecedented step of holding a 3-day, nationwide lockdown. During the lockdown, healthcare workers visited every house in the country. They gave residents information about Ebola and looked for new cases. Levels of foreign aid remained relatively low, but efforts were beginning to ramp up. In the middle of September, the United States launched a major Ebola offensive and began to send military personnel to Liberia. On the very last day of the month, news broke that an active Ebola case had been detected in Dallas, Texas. Ebola had left Africa and arrived in a western country.

4.1 Day-by-Day Outbreak Entries (September 2014)

September 1, 2014 (Monday)
Liberia has extended a stay-at-home order for nonessential government workers for another month (News 24 2014). All workers will continue to be paid. Nurses at Monrovia's JFK Hospital have gone on strike (Ghana Voice 2014). They are demanding higher wages and better access to PPE. Liberian schools remain closed (News 24 2014).

Near Monrovia, Liberia, the bodies of some Ebola victims are being secretively buried in unmarked graves on Daka Island (Hinshaw 2014).

In Barkedu Town, Liberia, approximately 200 people out of an original population of 8000 have died. The town is now quarantined (Leposo and Elbagir 2014).

In Nigeria, 72 people remain under surveillance in Lagos and 199 in Port Harcourt (Daily Post 2014).

September 2, 2014 (Tuesday)
As part of a UN special briefing today, International President of MSF, Dr. Joanne Liu, provided a grim description of the current Ebola situation:

© Springer International Publishing AG, part of Springer Nature 2018
S. G. Bullard, *A Day-by-Day Chronicle of the 2013-2016 Ebola Outbreak*,
https://doi.org/10.1007/978-3-319-76565-5_4

It is impossible to keep up with the sheer number of infected people pouring into facilities. In Sierra Leone, infectious bodies are rotting in the streets. Rather than building new Ebola care centres in Liberia, we are forced to build crematoria. (Médecins Sans Frontières 2014a)

She later said:

To curb the epidemic, it is imperative that states immediately deploy civilian and military assets with expertise in biohazard containment. I call upon you to dispatch your disaster response teams, backed by the full weight of your logistical capabilities. This should be done in close collaboration with the affected countries. Without this deployment, we will never get the epidemic under control. (Médecins Sans Frontières 2014a)

Echoing these concerns, Director of the CDC Dr. Thomas Frieden said the outbreak is spiraling out of control, and the window of opportunity to control the outbreak is closing (Mai-Duc 2014).

A third American doctor has tested positive for Ebola (Lupkin 2014a). The 51-year-old doctor [Richard Sacra] has been treating pregnant women at ELWA hospital in Monrovia, Liberia, as part of the group Serving in Mission (Fay 2014; Lupkin 2014a). He was diagnosed with Ebola about 1800 h Monday, September 1, 2014 (UNMEER 2014). Dr. Sacra arrived in Monrovia on August 4, 2014. At that time, medical aid in the city was very limited, and many of the women Dr. Sacra treated were extremely sick with pregnancy complications. There was no way to know if any of the patients had Ebola. He almost certainly became infected while treating them (UNMEER 2014). Dr. Sacra describes his initial symptoms:

It was a Friday night [August 29, 2014] *I had been feeling a little off during the day but.* [sic] *I didn't think anything of it. I thought I was just tired or something. Then in the evening around 10pm I had a chill and knew I was getting a fever. I took a temperature. I had a 100.8 degrees Fahrenheit. It's not high but high enough to let me know I had a fever. From that moment, I isolated myself and I didn't leave the apartment where I was staying. I started checking my temperature basically every hour or two. I didn't have any other symptoms that whole weekend – that was a Friday evening. All day Saturday, all day Sunday – I didn't really have any other symptoms, maybe a slight headache, mild nausea; mild symptoms. I was on the phone with my wife talking about it. I told her that I thought I probably had Ebola because I really felt like this was different than anything I have had because normally when you have a fever, with Malaria or other things, you'll spike a temp and then it will break. And you'll feel chilly, you'll get a temp and then you'll sweat, then it will break. Then it will wait a few hours and you'll have another temp. Like when you get a virus it kind of goes up and down. This one was just up. It just stayed there. Mine didn't get that high. I never broke the whole weekend I had a temperature. Both nights did take Tylenol, one or two nights when I went to bed to help me sleep. It made me feel a little better so I could rest.* (UNMEER 2014)

As the disease progressed:

… Some people have had terrible pain with it. I heard people say I felt like this, I felt like that. Some people had terrible pain with it – horrible headaches with it; really terrible pain. I did not have a lot of pain. I had some achy muscles – nothing more than a normal virus would do, it's just that it lasted longer, was more severe. For me, it wasn't a different category then having a bad stomach bug. When you have a bad stomach bug, you have it for 24 hours and then it's gone. But this kept going and going. (UNMEER 2014)

Patients in Liberian Ebola clinics are reportedly going hungry. At least one patient broke out of ELWA Hospital in Monrovia in search of food. When he reached a nearby market, he was recognized as being a patient. He was chased away from the market and returned to the clinic (Murphy 2014).

The UN warns that food prices are increasing in Ebola-affected areas. For example, the price of cassava has recently risen by 150% in Liberia. Food is a major household expense in West Africa and can account for 80% of family income. Thus, rising food prices can cause extreme hardship for people in the region (Associated Press 2014a).

A 39-year-old woman has been injected with the experimental GlaxoSmithKline Ebola vaccine at the NIH Clinical Center in Bethesda, Maryland. She is the first person to receive the fast-tracked experimental serum. The goal of the trial is to see if the vaccine is safe in humans and if it can illicit an appropriate immune response (Lupkin 2014b).

The WHO reports that 31 people have died from Ebola in the Democratic Republic of the Congo (AFP 2014a). Seven of the dead are healthcare workers (World Health Organization 2014a). The virus responsible for this outbreak is genetically distinct from the strain circulating in West Africa. It is very similar to the 1995 Kikwit strain. Thus, the outbreak in the Democratic Republic of the Congo is a separate disease event from the West Africa outbreak (World Health Organization 2014a). This separate outbreak will no longer be discussed in this book.

September 3, 2014 (Wednesday)
There have been more than 1900 Ebola deaths in West Africa during the current outbreak (Clarke and Samb 2014). This means that more deaths have occurred in the present outbreak than in all previous Ebola outbreaks combined (Bennett 2014).

The UN now estimates it will cost $600 M to contain the Ebola outbreak (Clarke and Samb 2014). This is up from the $490 M figure quoted a week ago in the WHO roadmap (World Health Organization 2014b). Sierra Leone says it has already spent $18.2 M fighting Ebola during the last 6 months (Awoko 2014a).

In Sierra Leone, workers in treatment centers and members of burial parties are given a $113 hazard bonus each week (Awoko 2014a).

The WHO is monitoring over 200 Ebola contacts in Port Harcourt, Nigeria. It also has a 26-bed isolation ward ready to receive Ebola patients (World Health Organization 2014c).

The African Union will meet next week to develop a comprehensive strategy to deal with the Ebola outbreak (The News 2014a).

British Ebola victim, William Pooley, has fully recovered and been discharged from the hospital. He says his passport has been incinerated so he cannot go anywhere. He thinks this will make his mother happy (Gallagher 2014).

Steep budget cuts at the WHO may help explain why the agency did not flood support into Ebola-affected areas as soon as the outbreak started. Since the 2007–2008 global financial crisis, the WHO's budget has decreased by $1 billion to $3.98 billion – roughly a 20% reduction. The outbreak and emergency response section was particularly hard-hit by cuts. The epidemic and pandemic response department was dissolved, and staff levels for an emergency response unit dropped from 94 to 34 individuals. Possibly as a result of this reduced capacity, Dr. Margaret Chan, the current director of the WHO, says the role of the WHO is to provide support and advice. It is up to the affected governments to take care of their people (Fink 2014).

September 4, 2014 (Thursday)

Total cases: 3707 (638 new)   Fatalities: 1848 (296 new)
                                         (Disease Outbreak News 2014)

Dr. Abdulsalami Nasidi, Project Director at the Nigerian CDC, says more than 380 people are now under surveillance in Port Harcourt. The health status of these people is being assessed twice a day (Nebehay 2014).

Dr. Rick Sacra, the most recently infected American doctor, will be flown to the United States for treatment. He will be taken to the Nebraska Medical Center in Omaha Friday morning and will be treated in the center's Biocontainment Patient Care Unit. Dr. Sacra is currently in stable condition (Izadi 2014).

The United States will provide $75 M to help fight Ebola. The funds will be used to buy 130,000 protective suits and to support the deployment of 1000 more treatment beds (Associated Press 2014b).

Researchers have produced a model that combines air traffic patterns with Ebola's epidemiological profile. The model predicts there is an 18% chance that at least one Ebola case will reach the United States by late September 2014 (Knox 2014).

September 5, 2014 (Friday)

Total cases: 3967 (260 new)   Fatalities: 2105 (257 new)
                                         (World Health Organization 2014d)

Ebola transmission in West Africa remains high. Over the last month, about 200 new cases have occurred each week in Liberia, 150 in Sierra Leone, and 100 in Guinea (World Health Organization 2014d).

In West Point, Liberia, the price of goods is starting to fall back to pre-quarantine levels (AllAfrica 2014a).

Nigeria will reopen its schools earlier than initially planned (Mohammed 2014). Schools will reopen on September 22, 2014, instead of October 13, 2014. To help protect students, all schools will have at least two trained staff members on site who can identify and deal with suspected Ebola cases (Mohammed 2014). People in Nigeria are relatively calm, but they avoid shaking hands and often carry disinfectant with them (Maja-Pearce 2014).

Dr. Rick Sacra has arrived in Nebraska (McKay and McWhirter 2014). Soon after he arrived, he was given a transfusion of blood from US Ebola survivor Kent Brantley (Associated Press 2014c).

The WHO recommends using convalescent blood to treat Ebola victims (Butler 2014; Kroll 2014a). During the 1995 Ebola outbreak in Kikwit, Zaire, seven of eight patients who were given convalescent blood survived (Mupapa et al. 1999). It is hoped that convalescent blood will similarly help patients in this outbreak. The WHO also says that preliminary Ebola vaccine safety trials could be completed as early as November 2014 (Kroll 2014a). As soon as the trials are finished, the vaccines can be given to healthcare workers (Batty 2014).

The EU will provide $227 M to help fight Ebola (Reuters 2014a).

September 6, 2014 (Saturday)

Sierra Leone has announced that the country will conduct a 3-day, nationwide lockdown to fight the Ebola outbreak (Batty 2014; O'Carroll 2014a). The lockdown will take place from September 18–21, 2014. During the lockdown, people will be required to stay in their homes. Security patrols will make sure people do not leave. The lockdown will allow healthcare workers to identify and isolate Ebola cases (Batty 2014). International health officials are highly skeptical of the plan (O'Carroll 2014a). They worry that the lockdown might actually increase the spread of Ebola. They also worry that the lockdown could make people more afraid of Ebola and reduce their trust in the government and healthcare workers (O'Carroll 2014a).

Overcrowded Liberian Ebola clinics cannot always accommodate newly arriving patients. In one recent case, six unattended patients – reported to be vomiting and urinating – were left outside the Paynesville Center in Monrovia. Some local residents fled the area in fear (AAP 2014a).

Volunteer militia groups on Senegal's border with Guinea are acting as self-appointed border guards. They prevent people from entering Senegal, detain them, or report their movements to security forces (Rokhy 2014).

September 7, 2014 (Sunday)

President Obama says the US military will likely become involved in controlling the West African Ebola outbreak. If it does, the military will set up isolation units and provide security for healthcare workers (Sun and Eilperin 2014).

The 17,000 residents of Dolo Town, Liberia, have been quarantined since August 20, 2014 (Dosso 2014). At least 30 people in the town have died from Ebola. Food supplies are dwindling. Some lucky residents have family members outside the community who can get food to them through the checkpoints (Dosso 2014). People without this option have to rely on the supplies delivered by agencies like the World Food Programme. Residents are starting to refer to their community as an Ebola jail (Dosso 2014; Epatko 2014a).

In Lagos, Nigeria, workers in the Infectious Diseases Hospital at the Yaba Mainland Hospital are threatening to strike over unpaid wages. Staff were promised $250–400 a shift to work with Ebola patients, but they have not been paid in 2 weeks (Premium Times 2014).

Stanley et al. (2014) assessed the effectiveness of the experimental GlaxoSmithKline Ebola vaccine (Gilblom 2014). The vaccine generally protected macaques from infection. All macaques ($n = 4$) survived exposure to Ebola 5 weeks after they had been injected with the vaccine (Stanley et al. 2014). When they were exposed to the virus 10 months after they had received the vaccine, 50% of the macaques became sick. If they were provided with a booster vaccine 2 months after their initial injection, all of the macaques survived (Stanley et al. 2014). These results are very encouraging, but the sample size is low (four macaques in each test). It is also unclear if the vaccine will be as effective in humans.

A US air marshal was attacked with a syringe in Lagos Airport, Nigeria, today (Associated Press 2014d). Several air marshals were about to pass through security when a group of men approached them. One man stabbed a syringe into an air marshal's arm, and then the group of men ran away (KPRC 2014). It is unclear what was in the syringe. The syringe was recovered and the victim has been transported to a hospital in Houston, Texas, for observation and testing (Associated Press 2014d).

Canadian officials locked down the Hilton Hotel in Saint John, New Brunswick, due to an Ebola scare. The hotel was secured from 1115 to 1700 h today because a woman who had recently been in Cameroon became ill (Canadian Press 2014). The episode highlights the generalized fear western countries have of Ebola. Cameroon is adjacent to Nigeria, but so far the country has not had any Ebola cases.

September 8, 2014 (Monday)

Total cases: 4293 (326 new)   Fatalities: 2296 (191 new)
                                    (World Health Organization 2014e)

The WHO has released a stark report about conditions in Liberia. The agency says the outbreak in Liberia is beyond the scale that local doctors and on-the-ground international aid groups can handle. The WHO warns that in the coming weeks there could be thousands of new Ebola cases in Liberia and says a massive increase in assistance is needed to control the situation (World Health Organization 2014f). The report states:

> In Montserrado county, the team estimated that 1000 beds are urgently needed for the treatment of currently infected Ebola patients. At present only 240 beds are available, with an additional 260 beds either planned or in the process of being put in place. These estimates mean that only half of the urgent and immediate capacity needs could be met within the next few weeks and months.
>
> In Monrovia, taxis filled with entire families, of whom some members are thought to be infected with the Ebola virus, crisscross the city, searching for a treatment bed. There are none. As WHO staff in Liberia confirm, no free beds for Ebola treatment exist anywhere in the country.
>
> ...development partners need to prepare for an 'exponential increase' in Ebola cases in countries currently experiencing intense virus transmission. Many thousands of new cases are expected in Liberia over the coming 3 weeks. (World Health Organization 2014f)

Clarence K. Massaquoi, an official in Lofa County, Liberia, says the number of deaths in his district is underreported (AllAfrica 2014b). He thinks this is because many of the communities in his rural district are off the main road and difficult to reach and assess. He also confirms that the mayor of Kolba City, Mary Ngaima, has died from Ebola. She tested positive for the disease on August 25, 2014 (AllAfrica 2014b; Liberia Peacebuilding Office 2014). Separately, the quarantine of Dolo Town has been lifted (Vanguard 2014).

Liberian body collection units continue their work. One team says it has been collecting about 15 bodies a day. They think all the teams in their area are collecting between 30 and 50 bodies a day. On a recent trip to Banjor, a slum outside of Monrovia, the team recovered the body of a 20-year-old pregnant woman named Fatimah Jakemah. Neighbors were afraid to interact with Jakemah after she became sick. They ignored her cries for food and water. Eventually Jakemah died. On the same trip, the team arrived at a location where they expected to recover two bodies. Instead they found two critically ill, but still living patients. The team told a community leader that they could only take the dead and could not transport the sick. The distraught leader thanked the team for coming and promised to call them again when the patients had died. Disregarding this rather odd statement, the team called an ambulance to come and pick up the patients (AFP 2014b).

During the upcoming nationwide lockdown, Sierra Leone plans to send medical representatives to every home in the country. The government is recruiting 21,400 volunteers for this effort. The volunteers will inform people about Ebola, identify potential Ebola cases, and locate unreported bodies (Johnson 2014a).

Sierra Leone officials say fewer goods are reaching Sierra Leone because of travel restrictions and border closings. This has led to some people eating substandard or expired food (Awareness Times 2014a).

Nigeria has released 319 people from observation (The News 2014b).

Emory University Hospital in Atlanta, Georgia, has announced that a fourth Ebola patient will be flown to the United States for treatment (Associated Press 2014e). The victim [Ian Crozier] is a US doctor who has been working in Kenema, Sierra Leone (Associated Press 2014e; Loftus 2015). He began feeling ill on September 6, 2014 (O'Carroll 2014b). Dr. Crozier requested that his identity remain confidential while he was undergoing treatment, so his name was not publically known until December 2014 (Loftus 2015; Sifferlin 2014). Dr. Crozier was the sickest Ebola patient treated by Emory University Hospital. He had a viral load more than 100 times higher than any other patient at Emory (Loftus 2015).

Ebola is returning to areas thought to have been cleared of the disease. For example, Macenta, Guinea, was affected early in the outbreak. Ebola seemed to have died out in the community, and no cases were seen for some time. Since the beginning of September, however, 45 new cases have been identified in Macenta. This type of reintroduction is likely due to the high mobility of West African people (Diallo and DiLorenzo 2014a).

Aid workers fighting Ebola in West Africa are often frustrated by the lack of coordinated international assistance. Sebastien Vidal of MSF says that conditions are getting progressively worse and seem to be getting out of control. Even so, western countries appear mainly focused on helping themselves. They have been mainly concerned with taking steps to control any imported cases that may enter their borders. He urgently requests that western countries send trained workers to fight the outbreak in West Africa (Quist-Arcton 2014).

The British military will set up a 62-bed Ebola treatment facility near Freetown, Sierra Leone (Independent.ie 2014). Fifty of the beds will be used to treat local victims; 12 will be set aside for international workers (Independent.ie 2014).

Separately, the US military will build a 25-bed facility in Monrovia, Liberia, to treat infected healthcare workers (CBS News 2014). It is hoped that having more dedicated beds available for medical staff will encourage more healthcare workers to volunteer to fight the disease. At present there are a total of 570 Ebola treatment beds in Guinea, Sierra Leone, and Liberia (CBS News 2014).

September 9, 2014 (Tuesday)
Liberia's defense minister, Brownie Samukai, says Ebola is a serious threat to Liberia's national existence (Nichols 2014). Liberian President Ellen Johnson Sirleaf sent an urgent letter to President Obama saying that if the chain of transmission is not broken, the virus will overwhelm the country (Cooper 2014).

Sophie-Jane Madden of MSF says the situation in Monrovia, Liberia, is already chaotic and the outbreak is expected to get larger and worse. People are already being turned away from her treatment facility (Sami 2014).

Contact tracing and surveillance teams are deployed throughout Nigeria. Faisal Shuaib, head of Nigeria's Ebola Emergency Operation Center, is pleased with the effectiveness of the teams and is encouraged by the willingness of citizens to help them. At present, 477 people are under surveillance in Port Harcourt (Hogan 2014). In Kaduna State, the government is providing 10,000 thermometers to schools and is training teachers how to detect Ebola cases (Bella Naija 2014).

Senegal continues to trace the steps of the Guinean student [Mamadou Alimuo Diallo] who brought Ebola to the country. At present, 33 people, including a 2-month-old baby, are under surveillance in a quarantine house. Each person is checked for fevers twice a day (Farge and Oberstadt 2014).

MacIntyre et al. (2014) question the Ebola PPE protocols recommended by the WHO and CDC. Both agencies say medical staff should wear googles and masks when working with Ebola patients, but that they do not need to wear respirators. The authors think these recommendations are inadequate. It is unclear how easily Ebola aerosolizes or if healthcare workers can be infected from aerosolized Ebola particles. MacIntyre et al. (2014) point out that laboratory workers working with Ebola are required to wear full PPE with respirators, even though laboratory settings are generally less hazardous than healthcare settings. They also say the current recommendations are obviously not working given the large number of healthcare workers who have been infected during the outbreak (MacIntyre et al. 2014). An opposing view by Martin-Moreno et al. (2014) supports the current PPE recommendations. These authors emphasize that Ebola is primarily transmitted by contact with bodily fluids. As such, wearing full PPE is generally not needed when working with Ebola patients. Respiratory protection is expensive. The West African countries affected by the disease cannot afford to purchase it in large quantities. Additionally, even if healthcare workers had access to respiratory protection, it would be unavailable to the general population. It could increase the public's fear of Ebola if they saw healthcare workers wearing respirators but knew they did not have access to respirators themselves (Martin-Moreno et al. 2014).

China will build an Ebola laboratory and holding center at the Sierra Leone-China Friendship Hospital in Freetown, Sierra Leone (MCT and Xinhua 2014).

The infected American doctor [Ian Crozier] arrived at Emory University Hospital in Atlanta at 1025 h today (Associated Press 2014f). So far, he has only been identified as a "male US citizen" (Christensen et al. 2014). British Ebola survivor William Pooley says he will return to Sierra Leone to help victims of the disease (O'Carroll 2014c).

September 10, 2014 (Wednesday)

Overcrowded Ebola clinics often have to turn patients away. In Monrovia, Liberia, one obviously ill man who was not admitted said that he had come to the clinic, but no space was available for him. He had a bad headache and fever and was trying to return home (AAP 2014b).

MSF has two treatment centers in Liberia, the ELWA-3 unit in Monrovia, and a treatment center in Foya (AllAfrica 2014c). The ELWA-3 unit has 140 beds and has treated 489 patients since mid-August 2014 (AllAfrica 2014c). Twelve survivors were released from ELWA-3 today (Campbell 2014).

Infectious Ebola particles can remain in the semen of survivors for at least 7 weeks after they have recovered from the disease. In Liberia, a woman died after she was infected through sexual contact with her boyfriend. He was an Ebola survivor who had recently left a treatment center (BBC 2014).

There is much discussion in Nigeria about the reopening of schools (News Ghana 2014a; Nigerian Bulletin 2014). Initially, the government planned to reopen them on October 13, 2014. As the Nigerian outbreak was brought under control, the reopening date was advanced to September 22, 2014. Parents are now concerned that this is too soon (News Ghana 2014a). Teachers in the Rivers State, where Port Harcourt is located, are petitioning the governor to keep schools closed until all of the people under surveillance have been released (Nigerian Bulletin 2014).

The Guinean student [Mamadou Alimuo Diallo] who brought Ebola to Senegal has recovered (Reuters 2014b).

There do not appear to have been any pathogens in the syringe used to attack a US air marshal on September 7, 2014 (Associated Press 2014g).

Home remedies for Ebola continue to emerge in West Africa. One female Nigerian student says students at her school bathe in a mixture of kerosene and salt water to try to ward off the virus (Dike 2014).

The Bill & Melinda Gates Foundation will donate $50 M to help fight Ebola; $10 M of this has already been provided (Bill and Melinda Gates Foundation 2014). The United States donated five ambulances to Sierra Leone today (Roy-Macaulay and Kargbo 2014).

September 11, 2014 (Thursday)

The risk of Ebola has reached the President of Liberia's office. A woman who worked for Liberia's Foreign Minister died from Ebola on Monday, September 8, 2014 (News Ghana 2014b). The woman's husband, who is now quarantined, is a staff member for the country's President (News Ghana 2014b). Separately, the Antoinette Tubman Soccer Stadium in Monrovia will be turned into two large Ebola treatment centers (AFP 2014c).

Pierre Trbovic works at the MSF Ebola center in Monrovia, Liberia. The center is filled well beyond capacity and cannot accept any new patients. As a result, someone has to stand at the gate and turn people away. Trbovic did this job for 1 week. He says the first person he turned away was a father who had brought his sick teenage daughter to the clinic. The man knew his daughter would probably die, but he wanted to get her into the clinic so she would not infect the rest of the family. Some people abandon their sick relatives at the clinic. They seem to think if an ill person is left there, they will have to be admitted. One girl died at the gate. Her body remained where it lay until a corpse removal team collected it. The job was so heart-wrenching that Trbovic occasionally had to go behind one of the tents and cry (Trbovic 2014).

A fourth top Sierra Leone doctor, Dr. Olivet Buck [reported by Ross (2014) as Olivette Busk], has contracted Ebola (Ross 2014). Dr. Buck will be evacuated to another country for treatment, but it is unclear where she will go (Ross 2014). Dr. Buck contracted Ebola while treating an infected boy at the Lumley Government Hospital in Freetown (Sierra Express Media 2014).

German virologist Jonas Schmidt-Chanasit of the Bernhard Nocht Institute for Tropical Medicine believes the West African Ebola outbreak may be past the point where external aid can help. He anticipates the virus will burn itself out in the region, infect everyone who is susceptible, and possibly kill as many as five million people. Officials from various aid agencies strongly reject this assessment (Osterath 2014).

September 12, 2014 (Friday)

Total cases: 4390 (97 new)   Fatalities: 2226 (−70 new)
                             (World Health Organization 2014g)

The WHO is calling for more healthcare workers to assist with the Ebola outbreak (World Bulletin 2014). Director Margaret Chan says 500–600 more doctors and 1000 more healthcare workers are needed (World Bulletin 2014). In response, Cuba has promised to send 165 medical personnel to West Africa (Reuters 2014c).

The WHO says there have been no Ebola cases in Senegal other than the initial case. Several people were suspected of having Ebola, but they have all tested negative (World Health Organization 2014h).

Twenty-three people were admitted to the MSF center in Paynesville, Liberia, today. Twenty-five people had to be turned away due to lack of space. The center only provides supportive care to patients, but this can significantly increase their odds of survival. Untreated patients in the community have a mortality rate of about 90%. Patients in the center have a mortality rate of about 70% (Bernstein 2014a).

At the Kenema center in Sierra Leone, Matron Josephine Sindesellu is 1 of the only 2 nurses remaining from a group of 26 who were working at the facility in May 2014 (Calkin 2014). Nineteen of the nurses have died from Ebola. Five others have had the disease and recovered. Sister Nancy Yoko, who worked side-by-side with British nurse William Pooley, died last week (Calkin 2014). Separately, a new Ebola treatment center will be opened this weekend a few miles from Kenema (Hamer 2014).

A black market for convalescent blood serum is developing in West Africa. Patients who survive Ebola possess antibodies in their blood that help fight the disease. If the blood of a survivor is transfused into a sick victim, it could help the new patient's body fight the infection. The use of convalescent blood is experimental, and improperly performed transfusions can transmit other blood-borne pathogens. The WHO is trying to develop standardize techniques so transfusions can be used on a large scale. At present no official sanction has been given for the use of transfusions (Cortez and Kitamura 2014).

A Liberian woman living in Nigeria has hung herself as a result of the Ebola outbreak. Neighbors say the woman, named Kate, had started to look sick and everyone was avoiding her. Some store owners refused to sell to her. It is believed that this rejection led her to take her own life (Iginla 2014).

Germany, the Netherlands, and Dubai sometimes request travelers coming from West Africa produce an Ebola clearance certificate before they are allowed to enter the country. In one case, a Kenyan was invited to visit Dubai for a conference. In order to come, the invitation letter said the Kenyan needed to obtain a passport-sized photo, a copy of their passport, and an Ebola test. The letter did not explain what an "Ebola test" was (Munuhe 2014).

British nurse William Pooley was flown to Atlanta tonight so he could give a blood transfusion to the current Ebola patient [Ian Crozier] at Emory University Hospital (Randhawa 2014). Pooley has the same blood type as the patient. To get to Atlanta, Pooley had to be quickly issued a new passport because his previous one had been incinerated (Randhawa 2014).

China will donate $32.5 M to fight Ebola (Xinhua 2014a). UNICEF has donated 15 ambulances to Guinea (Xinhua 2014b).

September 13, 2014 (Saturday)
Sierra Leone doctor Dr. Olivet Buck has died. She is the fourth top Sierra Leone doctor to die from Ebola. The government had hoped to evacuate her to Germany for treatment (Roy-Macaulay 2014).

Dr. Mosoka Fallah is credited with helping the residents of West Point, Liberia, coordinate their fight against Ebola. The country's government is overwhelmed, so community action is often needed to combat the disease. Dr. Fallah organized volunteer surveillance teams to locate sick and dead victims. Also, with the help of other community leaders, he divided West Point into zones so food and supplies could be distributed equally (Onishi 2014a).

The Red Cross has opened a new 60-bed Ebola treatment center near Kenema, Sierra Leone. The facility is staffed by 19 international and 80 local healthcare workers. The first Ebola fatality, a male nurse in his 30s from Freetown, has already been buried in the center's cemetery (O'Brien 2014).

The United States has sent some supplies to assist with the West African Ebola outbreak. The items provided include 5629 tons of food, 50,000 bars of soap, 10,000 sets of PPE, 10,000 Ebola test kits, 2400 buckets of chlorine disinfectant, 320 infrared thermometers, 100 rolls of plastic sheeting, 2 water treatment systems, 2 portable water tanks, and an unspecified number of body bags (Brumfiel 2014).

Two Dutch doctors have been exposed to Ebola in Sierra Leone. Drs. Nick Zwinkels and Erdi Huizenga were working at the Lion Heart Medical Centre in

Yele. The center mostly deals with malaria cases. While there, they had contact with three patients who died of Ebola. The doctors will be evacuated to the Netherlands on Sunday, September 14, 2014 (AFP 2014d).

The Paul G. Allen Family Foundation will provide $9 M to the CDC to fight Ebola (Canada Journal 2014).

September 14, 2014 (Sunday)
The Liberian economy is now officially in recession. This is largely due to the Ebola outbreak (Brown A 2014).

There is concern that sex workers, especially those in the border regions of affected countries, are at high risk of contracting Ebola (Zambia Daily Mail 2014).

US researchers at the NIH and DOD predict that the outbreak will last another 12–18 months (Greig 2014).

It was reported that doctors had fled from Achimota Hospital in Accra, Ghana, because a suspected Ebola victim had arrived at the facility (GhanaWeb 2014). The hospital's management, however, denies these accusations (Akweiteh 2014).

September 15, 2014 (Monday)
President Obama has signaled that he will launch a major offensive against the West African Ebola outbreak (Lee and McKay 2014). He will officially announce his plans tomorrow in Atlanta at the CDC. Initial reports suggest the President will deploy up to 3000 personnel to West Africa and establish 17 Ebola treatment centers in the region (Cooper et al. 2014). Separately, and likely unrelated, the US State Department has ordered 160,000 hazmat suits (Brown FP 2014).

Head Nurse Issa French is the most senior medical worker at the Ebola center in Kenema Hospital, Sierra Leone. No senior doctors are present (O'Brien 2014).

Agathe Jacob, a 22-year-old nurse working in Kenema, Sierra Leone, contacted Ebola while helping care for infected children. When she fell ill, she was initially diagnosed with malaria. By the time she found out she had Ebola, she had passed the disease onto her family. Her 22-year-old husband Ibrahim, her 2-year-old son Suare, and her 8-month-old son Papa all died from the disease in July (O'Brien 2014).

The 10-bed, Bong Ebola Treatment Unit opened in Bong County, Liberia, today. The unit was built by Save the Children and will serve the rural population of the region. The next closest treatment centers are in Monrovia and Foya, 4 and 6 h away, respectively (Du Cille and Bernstein 2014).

Guinea will use mobilized medical teams near its borders with Liberia and Sierra Leone to identify and treat Ebola patients trying to enter the country (Xinhua 2014b).

Mumbai, India, will no longer allow passengers to disembark from ships coming from West Africa. Additionally, all crew members from Ebola-affected countries will be screened for Ebola (Sequeira 2014).

US universities are struggling to address the Ebola outbreak. Some are providing recommendations and advice to people associated with the school. For example, administrators at Central Connecticut State University sent an informational email to all staff and students today. The message reads in part:

At the recommendation of the CDC, the University's Student Wellness Services asks any student who has returned from Guinea, Sierra Leone, Liberia, or Nigeria within the past 21 days to contact the office… to schedule an appointment with Dr. Christopher Diamond. Dr. Diamond will provide a confidential risk assessment as well as guidance for monitoring your health.

For faculty and staff who have recently returned from those countries within the past 21 days, Dr. Diamond will hold an information session on Thursday, September 18, 1:30 to 3:00 pm, Student Center, Philbrick. (McLaughlin 2014)

September 16, 2014 (Tuesday)

Total cases: 4985 (595 new)   Fatalities: 2461 (235 new)
(World Health Organization 2014i)

A White House factsheet released this morning confirms that the United States will dramatically increase its effort against the West African Ebola outbreak (White House 2014a). President Obama spoke from the CDC in Atlanta at 1600 h. He said the United States is ready to take a lead role in the Ebola outbreak and outlined the steps the United States will take to fight the disease (White House 2014b). The American plan includes deploying 3000 US troops to the region, having US Africa Command coordinate efforts among international agencies and streamline logistical support in the region, establishing an air-bridge to Senegal and then to the affected countries, constructing additional treatment centers in Liberia, training approximately 500 healthcare workers (presumably locals) each week, and providing protection kits for 400,000 households (White House 2014a, b). President Obama ended his address with an anecdote from the outbreak:

> *Let me just close by saying this: The scenes that we're witnessing in West Africa today are absolutely gut-wrenching. In one account over the weekend, we read about a family in Liberia. The disease had already killed the father. The mother was cradling a sick and listless five-year-old son. Her other son, 10-years-old, was dying, too. They finally reached a treatment center but they couldn't get in. And, said a relative, "We are just sitting."*
>
> These men and women and children are just sitting, waiting to die, right now. And it doesn't have to be this way. (White House 2014b)

The UN now estimates it will cost $1 B to control the Ebola outbreak (AFP and Reuters 2014).

Medical workers in West Africa are beginning to develop alternatives to treating Ebola patients in hospitals. When Ebola patients come to hospitals, they can expose the general hospital population to the virus. As a result, Samaritan's Purse is shifting its focus away from hospitalized care to stand-alone Ebola isolation units (Fox 2014). MSF is developing similar isolation units. Also, to reduce within-family Ebola transmission, Samaritan's Purse will provide PPE directly to family members caring for sick individuals (Fox 2014).

A French woman working with MSF in Liberia has contracted Ebola (Reuters 2014d). The patient began showing symptoms Monday, September 15, 2014 (Landauro 2014). She will be transported to France for treatment (Reuters 2014d).

Small businesses in West Africa are being hurt by the outbreak. For example, Patrice Juah's clothing store in Monrovia, Liberia, remains open, but she has had to lay off six of her seven employees (Epatko 2014b).

Fast-tracked vaccine trials underway at the NIH in Bethesda, Maryland, are showing positive results. Ten people have been injected with the GlaxoSmithKline vaccine. So far no major problems have been detected (Phillip 2014).

The World Bank has approved a \$105 M grant for Ebola-affected countries (World Bank 2014a). Of this, \$52 M will go to Liberia, \$28 M to Sierra Leone, and \$25 M to Guinea (World Bank 2014a). Separately, Japan has donated a variety of goods including tents, sleeping mats, and blankets to Liberia (AllAfrica 2014d).

Ebola survivor, Dr. Kent Brantly, met with President Obama in the oval office today before the President left for Atlanta (Sink 2014). Dr. Brantly then testified before a senate committee about his experiences with Ebola (WOKV 2014).

September 17, 2014 (Wednesday)
Eight, ten-man burial teams are working in Freetown, Sierra Leone (Gbandia 2014). Ebola victims must be specially handled, while non-Ebola cases can be handled normally. Tests are conducted to see if a person has died from Ebola. It takes some time to conduct the tests, so bodies are sometimes left for several days before they are recovered. To speed up testing, 26 motorbike riders transport blood samples to the laboratory. Each burial team member is paid \$116 per week. Sas Kargbo, coordinator for the burial details, says the teams have been burying between 20 and 30 corpses a day (Gbandia 2014). Burial parties can be called through two telephone numbers: +23279557733 and +23299671521 (Sierra Express Media 2014).

US Army Africa Commander, Major General Darryl Williams, arrived in Monrovia, Liberia, today with a 12-person assessment team (Baldor 2014).

The World Bank believes Ebola could deal a crippling blow to West African economies. At the moment, fear seems to be having a greater impact on business than the actual disease (World Bank 2014b).

Ben Kangar, pastor of the Calvary Chapel Red Wing, in Red Wing, Minnesota, has been collecting donations for his native Liberia. He recently learned that his niece gave birth to twins in Liberia, but one of them died because medical care was not available (Brun 2014). Most medical assets in Liberia are directed toward fighting Ebola, so there is little assistance available for non-Ebola medical emergencies. There are persistent stories of infants dying during unaided childbirths and people dying from survivable illnesses and accidents.

Britain has begun safety trials of the GlaxoSmithKline Ebola vaccine. In all, 60 volunteers will be given the vaccine. Ruth Atkins, a 48-year-old former nurse, was the first volunteer. She was injected with the vaccine today (Boseley 2014).

Shurina Rose Wiah, Miss Liberia from 2009 to 2010, has died. Rumors spread that she died from Ebola. However, her mother denies this and says Shurina did not have any Ebola-like symptoms (AllAfrica 2014e).

The United Kingdom will support 700 new treatment beds in Sierra Leone. Australia will donate \$6.4 M to fight Ebola (Associated Press 2014h).

September 18, 2014 (Thursday)

Total cases: 5357 (372 new)   Fatalities: 2630 (169 new)
                               (World Health Organization 2014j)

The UN Security Council unanimously passed a resolution today declaring the Ebola outbreak a threat to world peace and security (Sengupta 2014). The UN will create an international mission to help control the outbreak and coordinate management efforts (Cohen 2014). UN Secretary-General Ban Ki-moon says the mission will be known as the United Nations Mission for Ebola Emergency Response or UNMEER. Its goal will be to stop the outbreak, treat infected victims, make sure essential services are provided, ensure stability in affected areas, and prevent future outbreaks (Cohen 2014).

Sierra Leone is preparing for its 3-day, nationwide Ebola lockdown. The lockdown will begin at midnight tonight. During the lockdown, citizens will be required to remain indoors, and all activities unrelated to Ebola will stop. While the lockdown is underway, 7000, 4-person teams will visit every one of Sierra Leone's 1.5 million homes. The teams will distribute soap and explain Ebola prevention. They will not enter homes or collect bodies, but will contact burial teams if they find corpses. Officials think 15–20% more Ebola cases will be found during the operation. Beds have been prepared in hospitals and schools to accommodate the additional Ebola cases. In anticipation of the lockdown, residents are laying in supplies. A large number of people are in the streets (Johnson 2014b). The use of a nationwide lockdown is a very dramatic step. No similar lockdown has been attempted in the modern era.

An Ebola health team has been killed in Guinea. Eight bodies, including those of three journalists, a medical director, and two senior doctors from a regional hospital, were discovered in a latrine in the village of Womey, Guinea. Three of the victims had their throats slit. The group had been missing since Tuesday, September 16, 2014 (Mark 2014). Many villagers in the area deny the existence of Ebola and are distrustful of foreign workers.

The six burial teams in Monrovia, Liberia, face a tremendous workload. Each team has to deal with 10–15 bodies a day. To help with the work, six additional teams are being trained. As the new teams become operational, it is hoped that each team will manage about five bodies a day (World Health Organization 2014j).

Liberian journalist Yaya Kromah has died from Ebola at JFK Hospital in Monrovia, Liberia (AllAfrica 2014f).

The French nurse who contracted Ebola in Liberia has been flown to France for treatment (Landauro 2014)

The first US military aid has arrived in Liberia. A seven-person US team arrived in the country on a C-17 transport (Associated Press 2014i). Separately, France has announced it will set up a military hospital in Guinea to help with the outbreak (Reuters 2014e).

Travel bans pose a challenge for people in Ebola-affected countries. Hawa Dumboya, a 28-year-old student, from Yellowknife, Northern Territories, Canada, has become stranded in Freetown, Sierra Leone. She traveled to the country in May 2014 to finish her master's thesis. She recently lost her return booking because British Airways stopped flying to the country. She has obtained a new ticket on Brussels Airlines, but her new flight doesn't leave until the end of the month (CBC News 2014a).

September 19, 2014 (Friday)
The 3-day, nationwide lockdown has begun in Sierra Leone. In the Krio language, the campaign is being referred to as the "Ose to Ose Ebola Tok" or house-to-house Ebola talk (Johnson 2014c). People appear to be complying with the lockdown order and the streets are empty. Health teams started making rounds at 0715 h (Johnson 2014c). The teams provide each household with soap and an informational poster (Kelto 2014). The posters inform people about Ebola and mark the houses that have been visited. Supplies were not in place at some meeting sites, so some teams had to wait before they could begin their work. In at least one case, the posters did not arrive. Instead, teams used chalk to mark the houses that had been visited (Kelto 2014). It is unclear how effective the campaign will be, but government officials are optimistic. Social welfare organizations are concerned that the poor will have limited access to food and water during the lockdown (AllAfrica 2014g; Kamanda 2014a). Water is a particular concern. Many houses in Sierra Leone do not have running water and people rely on using communal wells (AllAfrica 2014g). Business leaders worry about the potential economic impact. Food prices increased by 30% immediately before the lockdown (Reuters 2014f). Separately, a new treatment facility, the Hastings Treatment Center, has been established near Freetown (Awareness Times 2014b).

Ebola treatment facilities in Liberia remain filled to capacity and are unable to accept additional patients. Some very ill patients have had to be turned away. Recently in Monrovia, a man who was vomiting blood was turned away, as were three members of one family who were all thought to be infected (Gold 2014).

Six people have been arrested in Guinea in connection with the killings of the Ebola team in Womey (Associated Press 2014j).

Germany and France will begin a joint air-bridge to the Ebola-affected region. Germany will position 100 soldiers in Dakar, Senegal, and use 2 Transall transport planes to carry supplies to Sierra Leone, Liberia, and Guinea. The air-bridge will have an airlift capacity of 100 tons a week (Reuters 2014g).

As the American Ebola effort gets underway, the contents of household Ebola kits has been described. Each kit includes a bucket, a sprayer for disinfectant, bags to collect infected material (such as solid clothing), gloves, gowns, masks, soap, chlorine, and an information pamphlet (Aizenman 2014).

Controversy surrounds Australia's offer of Ebola assistance. The country announced on September 17, 2014, that it would donate ~$6.4 M to help fight the disease (Associated Press 2014h). However, MSF has said it will reject its portion of the aid money ($2.5 M) (Dunlevy 2014). MSF Executive Director Paul McPhun explained that the group strongly believes that money is not needed; rather medical workers are needed in the field. Australia responded by saying that it had evaluated the idea of sending personnel to help with the outbreak, but it did not believe it could evacuate infected people back to Australia. Consequently, the government did not consider it appropriate to send personnel (Dunlevy 2014).

The French MSF worker who contracted Ebola in Liberia is being treated in a hospital in Saint-Mandé on the outskirts of Paris (Landauro 2014). She has been given the influenza medicine Avigan and another experimental drug (Bloomberg 2014). Avigan prevents viruses from replicating, so it is hoped it might help Ebola patients (Bloomberg 2014).

Senior UK medical leaders have written a letter urging UK healthcare workers to volunteer to work at a soon-to-be completed Ebola clinic in Kerrytown, Sierra Leone (Davies et al. 2014).

Muslim pilgrims in Nigeria are being screened for Ebola at Murtala Mohammed International Airport in Lagos. The pilgrims are on their way to Mecca for the Hajj (Donnelley 2014).

Cocoa prices have risen dramatically due to the Ebola outbreak. The Ivory Coast and Ghana produce 60% of the world's cocoa. Both countries are very near the infected region and could be affected by the outbreak. Cocoa prices have risen 6% in the last week. Cocoa currently trades at $3240 a ton (Wexler and Jerving 2014).

September 20, 2014 (Saturday)
The nationwide lockdown continues in Sierra Leone. Teams leave stickers on the front doors of houses after they visit (these are likely the "posters" referred to on September 19, 2014) (DeVries 2014). There are three different stickers, each with different Ebola-fighting tips. It is hoped that people will be curious about the stickers and talk to each other about the stickers they received (DeVries 2014). Thousands of people are evading the lockdown by traveling to neighboring countries, especially Guinea (Euronews 2014). Guinean health officials say people are coming through the forest in waves (Euronews 2014).

A burial team in Waterloo, Sierra Leone, was attacked while trying to bury five bodies. Police arrived to assist the team and the burials proceeded (Associated Press 2014k).

Another Spanish priest, Brother Manuel Garcia Viejo, has contracted Ebola. Brother Viejo is the medical director for the San Juan de Dios Hospital in Lunsar, Sierra Leone. He is being returned to Spain for treatment (Associated Press 2014l).

Regular medical care continues to deteriorate in Liberia. Experts say people are dying from malaria, stroke, heart disease, diabetes, diarrhea, pneumonia, etc. Women in labor are sometimes turned away from clinics (Bernstein 2014b).

An UNMEER advance team will begin deploying to Accra, Ghana, on Monday, September 22, 2014 (United Nations 2014a).

Schools in the Rivers District of Nigeria will open October 6, 2014, instead of September 22 (Onukwugha 2014).

The charity organization Direct Relief has sent 100 tons of Ebola supplies to West Africa on a chartered 747 (Szabo 2014a).

September 21, 2014 (Sunday)

The lockdown in Sierra Leone has entered its final day. Sierra Leone's Health Ministry reports that 75% of the country's households have been visited (Clottey 2014). After the lockdown officially ends, outreach efforts will continue in areas that have not yet been fully reached. It is unclear how effective the lockdown has been. Initial observations suggest it may have had mixed results. On the plus side, important information about Ebola has been provided to many households and a large number of previously unidentified bodies have been discovered. About 70 bodies have been found in Freetown alone (AFP 2014e). On the minus side, the quality of instruction given to households has been variable, and field teams have not always able to deliver information effectively (AFP 2014f). Residents generally welcome the Ebola volunteers, but some are afraid of them. Some worry that the soap being distributed is poisonous (Associated Press 2014m). People also appear to be going hungry. Many people in Sierra Leone live hand to mouth and can only afford to buy food as they need it. Stockpiling food before the lockdown was not an option for many poor individuals. The World Food Program distributed food packages before the lockdown, but not everyone received one (Associated Press 2014m).

Medical staff at the JFK Hospital in Monrovia, Liberia, have a strong record of success with Ebola patients. Mortality in the ward is 43%, much lower than elsewhere. However, the hospital's clinical director, 34-year-old Dr. J. Soka Moses, says that the ward is filled well beyond capacity. It was built to hold 35 patients but currently houses 69. Consequently, some patients lie on the floor and not everyone can be admitted. When reporters visited, many patients were waiting outside the clinic's gates. One was a 15-year-old girl named Faje Kan. She was convulsing and had mucus streaming down her face (Freeman and Wintercross 2014).

Katie Meyler is the founder a Liberian charity called More than Me. The group usually focuses on education but has recently shifted its attention to helping with the Ebola crisis. The agency operates an ambulance that takes patients to Redemption Hospital in Monrovia. Meyler has seen many heart-wrenching scenes. She recently saw a woman in a taxi die from Ebola. She also saw an ambulance arrive with a 3-year-old girl. The girl seemed fine, but her whole family was dead. The ambulance crew did not know what to do with the girl, so they had brought her to the hospital (Jozwiak 2014).

In West Point, Liberia, banners have been erected that proclaim the "10 Commandments of Ebola" (transcribed from a photograph taken by Tim Freccia (VICE News 2014); capitalization and wording as it appears on the banners):

1. *Thou shalt not HIDE ANY SICK person, even a family member or friend;*
2. *Thou shalt not SHAKE HAND or TOUCH someone with high fever who is very sick;*
3. *Thou shalt not TOUCH DEAD BODY even if it is your family member or friend who died;*
4. *Thou shalt not PUT MAT DOWN for dead people not even your family member;*

5. *Thou shalt not EAT or DRINK from the same pan, plate or cup with any family member, friend, or anybody;*
6. *Thou shalt not ALLOW ANYBODY even family friend to spend time;*
7. *Thou shalt not HAVE SEX with strangers; be very careful of the person you have sex with, they could have the EBOLA virus – No sleeping around; stick with the person you know very well;*
8. *Thou shalt not PEE PEE OUTSIDE, use a plastic bottle and wash your hands;*
9. *Thou shalt not TOILET OUTSIDE; use a plastic bag and wash your hands;*
10. *Thou shalt call this TELEPHONE NUMBER 4455 for Response Center #1 right away when you have a sick person or dead body in your house*

Liberia is trying to increase its Ebola treatment capacity to 1000 beds. To help reach this goal, the 120-bed Island Clinic opened in Monrovia today (MacDougall 2014).

The governor of Lagos State, Nigeria, says schools in his region will reopen on October 8, 2014 (Okoro 2014).

About 45 more US personnel have arrived in Liberia (AFP 2014g).

Two lounges have been prepared at King Abdulaziz International Airport in Jeddah, Saudi Arabia, to screen Hajj pilgrims arriving from Africa for Ebola (Saudi Gazette 2014). Presumably one lounge is for men, the other is for women.

September 22, 2014 (Monday)

Total cases: 5864 (507 new)   Fatalities: 2811 (181 new)
(World Health Organization 2014k)

Sierra Leone's nationwide lockdown has ended. Officials think it was successful. By the end of the lockdown, 80% of all households had been visited and 150 new Ebola cases had been discovered (AFP 2014h). Residents are happy the lockdown is over. People started coming into the streets before midnight (when the lockdown officially ended), and the streets have been crowded all day (Leveille 2014).

The number of Ebola fatalities in Sierra Leone appears to be underreported. For example, there have been 110 burials in the King Tom Cemetery in Freetown over the last 8 days. Only a few of these deaths are attributed to Ebola, but strong circumstantial evidence suggests that most of the deaths are from the disease. For example, few of the dead are elderly. Most are children, young adults, or middle-aged people – people who do not usually die unless it is from trauma or sudden illness. The official cemetery list also appears to be inaccurate. In one case, five people in one household are known to have died from Ebola, but only one is recorded on the official cemetery list (Nossiter 2014). This kind of underreporting is probably not intentional. Healthcare workers and burial teams face a monumental task in dealing with the flood of victims and bodies. Given the scale and speed of the disaster, these types of errors can easily occur.

The WHO believes Ebola has been contained in Nigeria and Senegal (Al Jazeera 2014a). This is exceptionally good news. It also demonstrates that Ebola can be contained if effective control methods used.

Infected Spanish priest Brother Manuel Garcia Viejo has arrived in Spain. He has been taken to Carlos III Hospital near Madrid for treatment (Associated Press 2014n).

Countries surrounding the Ebola zone are getting ready for the disease. Senegal, Mali, and the Ivory Coast have all set aside emergency funds to deal with the virus. They are also running public awareness campaigns to inform citizens about Ebola. In Nigeria, a Red Cross worker says it is common to see people having their temperature taken (IRIN 2014).

A male nurse was bitten by an Ebola-infected child while working in West Africa on Saturday, September 20, 2014 (the country was not specified). He is being flown to Switzerland for treatment. Officials do not think he has Ebola, but all precautions are being taken (Associated Press 2014o).

The BBC is starting a nightly Ebola news broadcast. The program will be 9 min long and run at 1950 h GMT on the 9915 and 12,095 kHz shortwave frequencies. The broadcast will feature a news roundup and air local reports from the Ebola-affected region (AFP 2014i).

The German Defense Minister is asking soldiers and civilian employees to volunteer to work at a 50-bed Ebola treatment facility that will be built in West Africa. The Minister promises that any infected worker will be returned to Germany for treatment (Associated Press 2014p).

The UK's NHS is encouraging employees to volunteer to assist with the Ebola outbreak (Davies et al. 2014). To date, 164 healthcare staff have signed up (MacRae 2014).

The emergency department at the Royal Alexandra Hospital in Edmonton, Alberta, Canada, was closed from 0630 to 1100 h today because a patient was thought to have Ebola. When the patient was cleared, the ED reopened (Robb 2014).

September 23, 2014 (Tuesday)
An article published today in the *New England Journal of Medicine* by the WHO's Ebola Response Team details the clinical and epidemiological features of the first 9 months of the outbreak (WHO Ebola Response Team 2014). The overall case fatality rate is 70.8%. The majority of victims (60.8%) are between 15 and 44 years old. The mean incubation period is 11.4 days. The mean time from the onset of symptoms to hospitalization (i.e., the period when a patient can most easily spread the disease) is 5.0 days, but this is high variable (± 4.7 days). As of September 14, 2014, the doubling time of the virus is 15.7 days in Guinea, 23.6 days in Liberia, and 30.2 days in Sierra Leone. During the week of September 8–14, 995 known cases needed hospitalization in Ebola-affected countries, but only about 610 beds were available. These numbers do not take into account the assumed underreporting of cases (WHO Ebola Response Team 2014).

Sierra Leone has sealed its borders with Guinea and Liberia. Troops have been sent to patrol all crossing points (Reuters 2014h). Sierra Leone originally closed its borders with these countries on June 11, 2014. It appears the current action is an attempt to increase security and better seal the boundaries.

A Red Cross burial team was attacked in Forecariah, Guinea, today. The team's vehicles were damaged, and a crowd threw rocks through the windows of a nearby health office. One team member was slightly injured in the neck (Diallo and DiLorenzo 2014b).

Nigeria is almost Ebola-free (Kroll 2014b). The Minister of Health, Dr. Onyebuchi Chukwu, says that there are no known cases in the country. Twenty-five people are still under surveillance in Port Harcourt, Nigeria, but it is hoped that they will soon be released (Kroll 2014b). A country is not officially considered to be Ebola-free until two incubation periods (42-days) have passed without a new case (World Health Organization 2014l).

A growing problem in Ebola-affected countries is the increasing number of children orphaned by the disease. At present, there are an estimated 300 Ebola orphans in Liberia (Styles 2014).

CDC models yield a dramatic range of possible outcomes for the current Ebola outbreak. The worst-case scenario predicts 1.4 million Ebola cases by January 20, 2015. The best-case scenario, which assumes the dead are safely buried and 70% of victims receive treatment, predicts the outbreak will be almost over by January 20, 2015 (Grady 2014).

David Nabarro has been appointed the UN's Special Envoy for Ebola (United Nations 2014b). Anthony Banbury has been appointed Special Representative for UNMEER (United Nations 2014b). An UNMEER advance team has arrived in Accra, Ghana (Xinhua 2014c).

US military commanders say US troops in Ebola-affected countries will have an extremely low risk of infection. Major General Darryl Williams also says anyone who is infected will be well cared for (Montgomery 2014).

Dr. Richard Sacra is being treated with the experimental drug TKM-Ebola. The drug is produced by Tekmira Pharmaceuticals and is supposed to stop the Ebola virus from replicating (Engle 2014).

September 24, 2014 (Wednesday)

Total cases: 6263 (399 new)   Fatalities: 2917 (106 new)
(World Health Organization 2014m)

During Sierra Leone's nationwide lockdown, a total of 358 new Ebola cases were identified and 265 bodies were discovered (O'Carroll 2014d). Kamanda, a 19-year-old blogger, describes his experience during the lockdown (Kamanda 2014b). He says over the 3-day period, his family of 27 listened to the radio, prayed, played cards, and watched movies. Healthcare workers visited on the third day. The workers described the signs and symptoms of Ebola, explained how to prevent the disease, and gave the family soap (Kamanda 2014b).

Space inside Liberian Ebola clinics remains scarce. At the MSF clinic in Monrovia, 20–30 patients are admitted each day, while a similar number are turned away (Freeman 2014). In addition to simply being too crowded, patients cannot be admitted to the clinic after dark. Working with Ebola victims is extremely hazardous and it simply cannot be done at night. Some of the people who are not admitted die near the entrance. A 42-year-old man named Dauda Konneh recently died waiting at the clinic. One of the men who brought him said that Konneh had Ebola-like symptoms and was vomiting. They reached the clinic at night, but Konneh was not admitted. He died near dawn (Freeman 2014). Separately, Dr. Attai Omoruto, head of the new Island Clinic in Monrovia, is requesting that Ebola survivors donate blood to help treat infected patients (Giahyue 2014).

Residents in Liberia often try to hide the fact that Ebola is in their community. Mark Korvayan, the leader of a body collection unit in Monrovia, describes a recent trip where his squad recovered the body of a 75-year-old woman. Community leaders said the woman had died from a stroke, not Ebola. However, during the previous month, the woman's daughter and nephew had also died. Korvayan's team had removed their bodies from the same room where the 75-year-old woman was found (Onishi 2014b).

The people of Liberia face numerous hardships due to the outbreak. In addition to medical concerns, violent crimes, especially robberies, have increased. Some attribute this to the 2100–0600 h curfew. Before the curfew, many areas conducted neighborhood watches. With the curfew, watch groups no longer operate (Park 2014).

Improperly conducted funerals continue to be a source of infection in West Africa. Twenty-four people recently died after becoming infected at a funeral in Moyamba, Sierra Leone. Seventeen people were infected at a funeral in Kenema, Sierra Leone (O'Carroll 2014d).

Guinea has arrested 27 people in connection with the killings of the Ebola team in Womey (AFP 2014j).

The WHO believes it might have enough Ebola vaccine (albeit, untested vaccine) available by the end of the year to have some impact on the outbreak (Belfast Telegraph 2014).

Pope Francis is asking Catholics to pray for Ebola victims (CNA Daily News 2014).

Many agencies and individuals are helping Ebola victims. Even small-scale efforts can provide significant help. For example, the YMCA in Missoula, Montana, is the sister organization of the YMCA in Freetown, Sierra Leone. The Missoula YMCA has been sending supplies and money to the Freetown YMCA. The Freetown YMCA is delivering food to families under quarantine (Whitney 2014).

US nurses attending a convention in Las Vegas staged a protest against the lack of Ebola preparedness in American hospitals. Hundreds of nurses wore red shirts in support of the protest. Some staged a mock "die-in," where participants dropped to the sidewalk and had chalk outlines drawn around them (KTVU 2014).

Sham Ebola cures and preventatives continue to be marketed. The FDA issued warning letters today to three US companies whose websites claim their products can be used to prevent or treat Ebola (Reuters 2014i).

September 25, 2014 (Thursday)

Sierra Leone has quarantined Port Loko, Bombali, and Moyamba Districts. Kenema and Kailahun Districts are already under quarantine. In all, 1.2 million people (about 20% of the country's 6 million) are now under quarantine. Corridors have been established to allow supplies and essential goods to enter the quarantine zones. The corridors will be open from 0900 to 01700 h each day (AFP 2014k).

Medical staff are overstretched throughout Liberia. In Bomi County there are only 2 doctors to care for the county's 85,000 people (Saul 2014).

MSF has started distributing Ebola kits to 50,000 households in Monrovia, Liberia. The kits are similar to US Ebola kits. They include two buckets, chlorine, soap, gloves, a gown, plastic bags, a spray bottle, and masks (Médecins Sans Frontières 2014b).

In the Fassankoni region of Guinea, locals are setting up roadblocks to prevent healthcare workers from entering their communities (Sky News 2014).

Infected Spanish priest, Brother Manuel García Viejo, has died (Reuters 2014j).

American doctor Dr. Rick Sacra is now Ebola-free and has been released from the Nebraska Medical Center. He was treated with the experimental drug TKM-Ebola and received two blood transfusions from Dr. Kent Brantly (Funk 2014).

The UN is holding a high-level meeting about Ebola (Somanader 2014). During the meeting, President Obama encouraged other nations to increase their aid. He warned that speed is critical to stopping the virus. He said:

> Ebola is a horrific disease. It's wiping out whole families. And it has turned simple acts of love and comfort – like holding a sick friend's hand, or embracing a dying child – into potentially fatal acts. If ever there were a public health emergency deserving of an urgent, strong and coordinated international response, this is it. (Somanader 2014)

The US Congress will allow unspent money from the war in Afghanistan to be spent fighting Ebola in West Africa. This means $50 M is immediately available for use (Taylor 2014).

Several drugs are being fast-tracked so clinical trials can start with African Ebola patients (The Pharmaceutical Journal 2014). It is unclear which drugs are involved or when testing will begin.

The World Bank will increase its Ebola funding to $400 M (Webwire 2014).

September 26, 2014 (Friday)

Total cases: 6574 (311 new)   Fatalities: 3091 (174 new)
(World Health Organization 2014n)

The WHO says the Ebola outbreak is the most severe acute public health emergency in modern times. The agency notes that this is the first time a BSL-4 pathogen has infected so many people over such a large area (World Health Organization 2014o).

Dr. Joanne Liu, International President of MSF, stressed the need for additional healthcare workers in West Africa (Kelemen 2014). She commended the international community for agreeing to help with the outbreak but emphasized that the help has been slow in coming. Outside help is urgently needed. This is especially true because it has been getting harder to hire locals to fight the disease (McNeil 2014). Dr. Liu underlined the direness of the situation by describing conditions at the MSF clinic in Monrovia, Liberia:

> Every morning we only open one of our centers for 30 minutes, just to admit people who can fill in the beds of the people who died overnight. This is how bad it is. And the rest of the day, we are turning patients back home to go and infect their neighbors and loved ones. So this is not at all under control. (Kelemen 2014)

MSF says it has 3058 staff on the ground in Guinea, Liberia, Sierra Leone, Nigeria, and Senegal. These personnel are distributed among 6 Ebola centers with a total of 549 treatment beds. So far, MSF has admitted 3299 patients to its centers during the outbreak. Of these, 650 have survived. The youngest survivor is a 3-year-old Liberian boy named James (Médecins Sans Frontières 2014c).

The Ebola holding center in Makeni, Sierra Leone, is located in an empty university building. It does not provide care for patients but holds them until they can be transferred to other facilities. Unfortunately, the nearest treatment center is in Kailahun which takes 16 h to reach by car. Recently, 25 patients were transported to Kailahun during a single night. Four of them died along the way. Axelle Vandoornick of MSF says there are almost always dead bodies in the ambulances when they arrive at Kailahun. As of this morning, there were 100–110 patients at the Makeni Center. Conditions are unpleasant. Beds are uncleaned, trash covers the floor, and numerous infected patients lay in close proximity to one another. Three staff members have died at the center (Bailes 2014).

A 22-year-old Liberian nursing student named Fatu Kekula has developed a form of homemade PPE known as the "trash bag method." Trash bags are placed over the socks and tied with a knot over the calves. A pair of rubber boots is put on and another set of trash bags is placed over the boots. The caregiver's hair is placed in a pair of stockings and covered with a trash bag. A raincoat and four pairs of gloves are worn. Finally, a mask is donned. Using this equipment, Kekula has treated four infected relatives. Three of them have survived. Aid workers are now teaching the technique to others (Cohen 2014a).

Different aid agencies pay international workers different amounts. MSF pays new volunteers $1700 a month. The International Medical Corps pays $4500 a month (McNeil 2014).

The US Ebola-fighting effort is known as Operation *United Assistance* (Newman 2014). Members of the 633rd Medical Group from Joint Base Langley-Eustis, Virginia, deployed today as part of this mission (Newman 2014).

Liberian immigrants who are currently in the United States without a visa will not be returned to Liberia for at least 2 years (Caldwell 2014).

As new Ebola treatment centers are constructed, each 100-bed facility will need to be staffed by about 400 healthcare workers. Each center must contain three separate holding areas: one for confirmed cases, one for probable cases, and one for suspected cases. All of these areas need their own separate restroom facilities. Dressing rooms are needed for staffers. The entire facility has to be enclosed within a double fence, so relatives can talk with patients and staff members without coming into contact with them (McNeil 2014).

Experts are concerned that the Ebola outbreak will cause a dramatic increase in deaths from other infectious diseases, such as malaria. Typically about 100,000 West Africans die from malaria each year. Lack of care due to Ebola outbreak could increase this to 400,000 (Reuters 2014k).

Cuba will send 300 more medical personnel to West Africa to help with the outbreak (Al Jazeera 2014b).

The Ivory Coast plans to resume flights to Ebola-affected countries starting next week. The President of Ivory Coast says that residents of his country are already taking steps to prevent Ebola transmission, and the government is ready to deal with any Ebola cases that may arise. Resuming flights will allow the Ivory Coast to show solidarity with the Ebola-affected countries (Associated Press 2014q).

September 27, 2014 (Saturday)
Lacking other treatment options, Dr. Gobee Logan has treated some Ebola patients in Liberia with the HIV drug lamivudine. He gave the drug to 15 patients within the first 5 days of their illness. Thirteen of them survived. Dr. Logan got the idea after reading a scientific article that said HIV and Ebola replicate in a similar manner (Cohen 2014b).

At the MSF Ebola clinic in Monrovia, Liberia, 30 beds became available this morning. Seven of them were freed because patients had recovered. Twenty-three opened because the patients had died. A 14-year-old boy named D. J. Mulbah was one of the new patients admitted to the clinic. He had been brought to the clinic by his mother and grandmother. They arrived by taxi and had traveled with a bucket to catch his vomit. In addition to space for patients, staffing is also a problem at the clinic. A sign inside the unit tells workers not to insert IV lines until more staff are available (Larson and Cheng 2014).

Dr. Bernice Dahn, one of Liberia's top doctors and Deputy Minister for Health Services, has placed herself in quarantine in Monrovia because her office assistant has died from Ebola (Paye-Layleh 2014).

Monty Jones, special advisor to Sierra Leone's president, says the district quarantines seem to be starting to stabilize the outbreak in the quarantined regions. Fewer cases were seen over the last week in Kailahun and Kenema Districts. Jones also says it is becoming clear that the individual houses of infected people need to be quarantined (Finnan 2014).

The airport at Dakar, Senegal, has started acting as an air-bridge to the Ebola zone. The first aid flight arrived in the city today from Guinea (RFI 2014).

The US Navy's 133rd Mobile Construction Battalion has begun building an Ebola treatment center near the airport in Monrovia, Liberia (Hinshaw and McKay 2014).

An American doctor [Dr. Lewis Rubinson] has been exposed to Ebola while treating patients in Kenema, Sierra Leone (Sellers 2014). He will be transported to the NIH in Bethesda, Maryland, for observation (Levine 2014). Dr. Rubinson accidentally punctured his hand while he was disposing an infected needle (Sellers 2014).

Two medical workers have been fired from the Nebraska Medical Center for inappropriately looking through Dr. Sacra's medical file (Associated Press 2014r).

September 28, 2014 (Sunday)
The Bong County Ebola Treatment Center in Liberia has been open for 13 days. Its cemetery already has seven filled graves. Nineteen pre-dug, empty graves are waiting to receive new Ebola victims (Besser 2014).

Dr. Lewis Rubinson has arrived at the NIH in in Bethesda, Maryland (Sellers 2014).

US military aid continues to arrive in West Africa. Over the weekend, C-17 transport planes brought additional personnel, a deployable 25-bed hospital, and two Ebola testing labs to Monrovia, Liberia (AllAfrica 2014h). Separately, a chartered 747 arrived in Monrovia today with 2016 rolls of plastic sheeting to help construct the new US treatment centers (Hinshaw and McKay 2014).

The WHO thinks that several hundred new doses of ZMapp will be available by the end of 2014 (Reuters 2014l).

September 29, 2014 (Monday)
People in Sierra Leone think the government is underreporting or misrepresenting the number of Ebola cases in the country. The government says there have been 2000 confirmed Ebola cases in Sierra Leone and that there are 432 known survivors and 540 deaths. This leaves 1028 patients unaccounted for. Dr. Sylvia Blyden says the difference in the numbers is not intentional. They are the result of the fast-paced nature of the outbreak. Many confirmed Ebola cases die in their communities and never reach an Ebola treatment center. Only deaths at Ebola treatment centers are reported as confirmed deaths (Awareness Times 2014c). It is hoped that all cases will be reviewed and the official government figures revised.

Inaccurate Ebola data are also a problem in Liberia. In Liberia, factors may lead to overestimates or underestimates in the number of Ebola cases. In Monrovia, all dead bodies are collected and cremated (York 2014). Thus, all bodies are essentially assumed to be Ebola victims. This likely leads to an overestimate in the number of Ebola deaths. For example, 24-year-old Theresa Jacob recently died. She had been fighting liver disease for several years and almost certainly died from liver problems, not Ebola. Even so, her body was collected by a body removal team, and she will probably be considered a possible Ebola victim (York 2014). In contrast, other Ebola deaths are unreported. Jean-Pierre Veyrenche of the WHO thinks many people are burying their dead at home and are not notifying government officials about the death (Bastian 2014).

The use of cremation in West Africa creates major cultural problems. Burial is the norm in most West African countries (York 2014). Without a burial plot to visit, families are unable to properly pay their respects to the dead. For example, Decoration Day is an important Liberian holiday where families visit graveyards to clean and decorate the graves of their relatives (York 2014). Cremated Ebola victims have no grave. Their remains are currently being stored at the crematorium (e.g., Paye-Layleh 2015). Consequently, relatives have no place to commemorate their loved ones.

Phebe Hospital in Liberia has received a large donation from Actalliance Liberia Forum (AllAfrica 2014i).

Lungi Airport in Sierra Leone is struggling to handle the large quantity of incoming Ebola supplies. Little warehouse space is available, so supplies must remain on the runway until they can be removed by handling teams. This can take up to a week. The weather has been very rainy, and some supplies have been damaged while waiting to be collected (Awoko 2014b).

Anthony Banbury, head of UNMEER, arrived in Ghana today (United Nations 2014c).

The Toronto-based Defyrus company is working to commercialize ZMapp. They hope to produce tens of thousands of doses in 2015. In addition to the costs associated with upscaling production, one hurdle to making the drug is that some of the drug's antibodies are cultured in tobacco plants. The plants physically need the time to grow before they can be harvested (CBC News 2014b).

French President Hollande says Air France will continue to fly to Conakry, Guinea, out a sense of solidarity with the Ebola-affected country (AFP 2014l).

September 30, 2014 (Tuesday)
An Ebola case has been confirmed in Dallas, Texas (Breman et al. 2014; Doucleff 2014; Yan 2014). The infected man [Thomas Eric Duncan] arrived in Dallas from Liberia on September 20, 2014. At the time of his flight, he had no symptoms and was not visibly ill (Doucleff 2014). He developed symptoms on September 24 and sought treatment on September 25. On September 28, he was placed in isolation at Texas Health Presbyterian Hospital (Doucleff 2014). CDC director Tom Frieden says the man had contact with a handful of people, including relatives and community members (Breman et al. 2014). However, Dr. Frieden is confident the United States can prevent the spread of the disease. Dr. Frieden says that someone who had contact with the patient might develop Ebola, but if so, the chain of transmission will be rapidly stopped (Breman et al. 2014).

Thomas Duncan was a Liberian with strong ties to the United States. In Liberia, he was the driver for the general manager of Safeway Cargo (Stanglin 2014). Duncan probably became infected in Liberia on September 15, 2014. On this date, he helped transport 19-year-old Marthalene Williams [sometimes reported as Nathaline Williams (e.g., Winter et al. 2014)] to an Ebola treatment center in Monrovia (Beaubien 2014; Winter et al. 2014). Williams was pregnant and very sick. Unfortunately, four separate Ebola centers turned Williams away due to lack of space. Williams and Duncan returned home where Duncan helped carry Williams inside. Williams later died (Beaubien 2014). On September 19, Duncan began traveling to the United States (Winter et al. 2014). On his passenger screening form at Roberts International Airport in Liberia, he checked "no" in the box asking if he had taken care of, or had touched the body fluids of, an Ebola patient (Stanglin 2014). His first flight was from Monrovia to Brussels, Belgium, on Brussels Airlines Flight 1247 (Winter et al. 2014). He next took United Airlines Flight 951 from Brussels to Dulles Airport, Washington D.C. Finally, he took United Flight 822 from Washington to Dallas. He arrived in Dallas on September 20 (Winter et al. 2014). Duncan began developing Ebola symptoms on September 24. At 2237 h on September 25, he went to the emergency department of Texas Health Presbyterian Hospital complaining of abdominal pain, dizziness, nausea, and headache (Energy and Commerce Committee 2014; Winter 2014; Winter et al. 2014). During his initial assessment, Duncan said that he had recently come from Africa. A notation was made in Duncan's medical record about this, but the information was not verbally conveyed to the attending physician. In reviewing Duncan's charts, the physician either missed or did not recognize the importance of Duncan's African connection (Energy and Commerce Committee 2014). Duncan's laboratory tests were more or less normal. He was diagnosed with sinusitis and abdominal pain and was discharged with antibiotics at 0337 h on September 26 (Energy and Commerce Committee 2014; Winter 2014; Winter et al. 2014). Ebola was not suspected. After returning home, his condition continued to worsen. On September 28, Dallas Fire and Rescue transported Duncan back to Texas Health Presbyterian Hospital (Winter et al. 2014). A witness said Duncan was throwing up at the time and his family members were screaming (Reuters 2014m). The Paramedics who transported him were later isolated (Yan 2014). Duncan's Ebola diagnosis was confirmed on September 30.

When news of the first US Ebola case was released, over 50,000 twitter tweets an hour were sent about Ebola (Yan 2014).

Poor communication with the families of Ebola patients is a problem in West Africa. MSF operates three phone lines to update relatives about patient progress. However, most families receive their information secondhand via other patients or hospital guards. Sometimes families do not learn about the death of a loved one until days after it has occurred. Other times, relatives hear that a person has died only to find out later the person is still alive (Larson 2014).

The economy of Liberia is being heavily impacted by the outbreak. Fewer people are farming either because they have contracted Ebola or because they are afraid they may get the disease if they work in the fields. Travel restrictions have reduced the amount of food arriving in the country and have made it difficult to distribute the food that is available. As a result, food prices have increased. About 45% of the Liberian work force is in the service sector, but Ebola has dramatically decreased demand for services. Exports have dropped, especially of rubber and palm oil. Some mining operations have closed. Government revenue has fallen by 20%. This has reduced the government's ability to provide services (Barbash 2014).

Residents of Makeni, Sierra Leone, celebrated in the streets Monday night and Tuesday morning in the mistaken belief that the Ebola outbreak was over. A group of survivors had been released from the Ebola holding center, and residents seem to have interpreted this as meaning the disease was gone. Government officials restored order and issued a statement saying Ebola is still present in the community (AFP 2014m).

The CDC believes the Ebola outbreak in Nigeria and Senegal may be over (Szabo 2014b). No new cases have been reported in Nigeria since August 31, 2014. The only case in Senegal was reported on August 28, 2014.

UNICEF estimates that 3700 children have lost one or both parents to Ebola (Fox News 2014).

The Pentagon will deploy 1400 more US troops to Liberia. About half of the new personnel will be from the headquarters element of the 101st Airborne. The rest will be combat engineers (Carroll 2014).

References

AAP (2014a) Liberia Ebola patients 'lying in street.' AAP. News.com.au. http://www.news.com. au/world/liberia-ebola-patients-lying-in-street/news-story/3bb09bf3ef863d11526cb239cc0e 57c7. Accessed 10 Feb 2017

AAP (2014b) Ebola overwhelming African health services. AAP, Geelong Advertiser. http:// www.geelongadvertiser.com.au/news/world/ebola-cases-number-more-than-4000/story-fnjb-nxoi-1227053292667. Accessed 10 Sept 2014

AFP (2014a) Ebola kills 31 people in DR Congo. WHO, AFP, Z News. http://zeenews.india.com/ news/world/ebola-kills-31-people-in-dr-congo-who_1464021.html. Accessed 2 Sept 2014

AFP (2014b) Liberia's Ebola disposal teams preserve life after death. AFP, The Jakarta Globe. http://www.thejakartaglobe.com/international/liberias-ebola-disposal-teams-preserve-life-death/. Accessed 8 Sept 2014

AFP (2014c) Monrovia soccer stadium to house Ebola centre. FIFA. AFP, Yahoo News. http:// news.yahoo.com/monrovia-soccer-stadium-house-ebola-centre-fifa-195200380--sow.html. Accessed 11 Sept 2014

AFP (2014d) Dutch Ebola doctors 'to be evacuated on Sunday.' AFP, Yahoo News. https://uk.news. yahoo.com/dutch-ebola-doctors-evacuated-sunday-212316365.html#BRFngnw. Accessed 13 Sept 2014

AFP (2014e) Ebola shutdown uncovers 70 dead. AFP, IOL. http://www.iol.co.za/news/africa/ ebola-shutdown-uncovers-70-dead-1.1754072#.VB7g17d0ziw. Accessed 21 Sept 2014

AFP (2014f) Criticism grows as Sierra Leone's Ebola shutdown enters final day. AFP, Times Live. http://www.timeslive.co.za/africa/2014/09/21/Criticism-grows-as-Sierra-Leones-Ebola-shutdown-enters-final-day. Accessed 17 Mar 2017

AFP (2014g) More US troops in Ebola-hit Liberia: airport source. AFP, Yahoo News. http://news. yahoo.com/more-us-troops-ebola-hit-liberia-airport-source-192002446.html. Accessed 22 Sept 2014

AFP (2014h) Sierra Leone Ebola lockdown found at least 200 infected, dead: government. AFP, NDTV. http://www.ndtv.com/world-news/sierra-leone-ebola-lockdown-found-at-least-200-in-fected-dead-government-669234. Accessed 18 Mar 2017

AFP (2014i) BBC begins nightly Ebola service in west Africa. AFP, Modern Ghana. http://www. modernghana.com/thread/267002/570563/1. Accessed 22 Sept 2014

AFP (2014j) Guinea arrests 27 over Ebola health team murders. AFP, Yahoo News. http://news. yahoo.com/guinea-arrests-27-over-ebola-health-team-murders-173455358.html. Accessed 24 Sept 2014

AFP (2014k) Ebola epidemic Sierra Leone quarantines a million people. AFP, The Guardian. http://www.theguardian.com/world/2014/sep/25/ebola-epidemic-sierra-leone-quarantine-un-united-nations. Accessed 25 Sept 2014

AFP (2014l) Air France flies to Ebola-hit Guinea out of solidarity Hollande. AFP, Z News. http:// zeenews.india.com/news/world/air-france-flies-to-ebola-hit-guinea-out-of-solidarity-hol-lande_1477861.html. Accessed 29 Sept 2014

AFP (2014m) Sierra Leone crowds mistakenly celebrate 'end of Ebola'. AFP, The Daily Star. http:// www.dailystar.com.lb/News/World/2014/Sep-30/272517-sierra-leone-crowds-mistakenly-celebrate-end-of-ebola.ashx. Accessed 15 Apr 2017

AFP and Reuters (2014) $US1b needed to fight Ebola: United Nations. AFP, The Sydney Morning Herald. http://www.smh.com.au/world/us1b-needed-to-fight-ebola-united-nations-20140916-10hwfv.html. Accessed 16 Sept 2014

Aizenman N (2014) Inside an Ebola kit: a little chlorine and a lot of hope. NPR. http://www.npr.org/blogs/goatsandsoda/2014/09/19/349908367/inside-an-ebola-kit-a-little-chlorine-and-a-lot-of-hope. Accessed 20 Sept 2014

Akweiteh GA (2014) Ebola hasn't scared doctors away – Achimota Hospital. Citifmonline. http://www.citifmonline.com/2014/09/14/ebola-hasnt-scared-doctors-away-achimota-hospital/. Accessed 14 Sept 2014

Al Jazeera (2014a) WHO: Ebola contained in Nigeria. Aljazeera, Senegal. http://america.aljazeera.com/articles/2014/9/22/ebola-contained-senegalnigeria.html. Accessed 19 Mar 2017

Al Jazeera (2014b) Cuba sends 300 more doctors to fight Ebola. Al Jazeera, Yahoo News. https://uk.news.yahoo.com/cuba-sends-300-more-doctors-fight-ebola-102000129.html#2oPUx1L. Accessed 26 Sept 2014

AllAfrica (2014a) Liberia: 'West Point is heartbeat of Monrovia.' AllAfrica, The News. http://allafrica.com/stories/201409050839.html. Accessed 5 Sept 2014

AllAfrica (2014b) Liberia: 'Ebola deaths, situation in Lofa underreporte' – lawmaker. AllAfrica, Front Page Africa. http://allafrica.com/stories/201409081580.html. Accessed 8 Sept 2014

AllAfrica (2014c) Liberia: MSF 'cannot exceed 400 beds' in Liberia. AllAfrica, The New Republic. http://allafrica.com/stories/201409101008.html. Accessed 10 Sept 2014

AllAfrica (2014d) Liberia: Japan makes huge donation to fight against Ebola in Liberia. AllAfrica, Front Page Africa. http://allafrica.com/stories/201409171253.html. Accessed 17 Sept 2014

AllAfrica (2014e) Liberia: former Miss Liberia 'did not die from Ebola', mom says. AllAfrica, Front Page Africa. http://allafrica.com/stories/201409171310.html. Accessed 17 Sept 2014

AllAfrica (2014f) Liberian journalist succumbs to deadly Ebola virus disease. AllAfrica, Front Page Africa. http://allafrica.com/stories/201409191128.html. Accessed 19 Sept 2014

AllAfrica (2014g) Sierra Leone: poor will not have food or water during lockdown, say Sierra Leoneans. AllAfrica, Reuters. http://allafrica.com/stories/201409191202.html?viewall=1. Accessed 19 Sept 2014

AllAfrica (2014h) Liberia: U.S. military brings mobile Ebola testing labs. AllAfrica, The News. http://allafrica.com/stories/201409301090.html. Accessed 30 Sept 2014

AllAfrica (2014i) Liberia: Phebe hospital gets huge donation. AllAfrica, The News. http://allafrica.com/stories/201409292398.html?page=2. Accessed 29 Sept 2014

Associated Press (2014a) UN warns food prices rising in Ebola-hit countries. Associated Press, Boston.com. http://www.boston.com/health/2014/09/02/warns-food-prices-rising-ebola-hit-countries/1TZD1EzMu9a0bmV2THRjSJ/story.html. Accessed 2 Sept 2014

Associated Press (2014b) US to provide $75M to expand Ebola care centers. Associated Press, The Washington Examiner. http://washingtonexaminer.com/us-to-provide-75m-to-expand-ebola-care-centers/article/feed/2162044. Accessed 4 Sept 2014

Associated Press (2014c) Ebola survivor gives blood to ill American. Associated Press, Business Standard. http://www.business-standard.com/article/pti-stories/ebola-survivor-gives-blood-to-ill-american-114091200051_1.html. Accessed 15 Feb 2017

Associated Press (2014d) Ebola fears after US air marshal attacked with syringe at Lagos airport. Associated Press, The Guardian. http://www.theguardian.com/world/2014/sep/09/us-air-marshal-stabbed-syringe-lagos-airport-nigeria-ebola-fears. Accessed 9 Sept 2014

Associated Press (2014e) 4th Ebola patient to be flown to U.S. for care. Associated Press, WITN. http://www.witn.com/home/headlines/4th-Ebola-Patient-To-Be-Flown-To-US-For-Care-274409901.html. Accessed 8 Sept 2014

Associated Press (2014f) Fourth American aid worker with Ebola arrives at Atlanta hospital. Associated Press, New York Daily News. http://www.nydailynews.com/life-style/health/fourth-u-s-aid-worker-ebola-arrives-atlanta-hospital-article-1.1933276. Accessed 12 Feb 2017

Associated Press (2014g) FBI: air marshal attacked with syringe in Nigeria. Associated Press, First Coast News. http://www.firstcoastnews.com/story/news/health/2014/09/10/air-marshal-attacked-syringe/15404229/. Accessed 10 Sept 2014

Associated Press (2014h) Australia pledges $6.4M to fight Ebola. Associated Press, Fox News. http://www.foxnews.com/health/2014/09/17/australia-pledges-64m-to-fight-ebola/. Accessed 17 Sept 2014

Associated Press (2014i) 1st US anti Ebola military aid arrives in Liberia. Associated Press, Buffalo News. http://www.buffalonews.com/article/20140919/AP/309199830. Accessed 19 Sept 2014

Associated Press (2014j) Arrests made in killings of Guinea Ebola education team. Associated Press, The Wall Street Journal. http://online.wsj.com/articles/arrests-made-in-killings-of-guinea-ebola-education-team-1411144837. Accessed 19 Sept 2014

Associated Press (2014k) Ebola outbreak: burial team attacked in Sierra Leone amid 3-day lockdown. Associated Press, CBC News. http://www.cbc.ca/news/world/ebola-outbreak-burial-team-attacked-in-sierra-leone-amid-3-day-lockdown-1.2772813. Accessed 20 Sept 2014

Associated Press (2014l) Spain repatriates priest with Ebola from Africa. Associated Press, The Charlotte Observer. http://www.charlotteobserver.com/2014/09/20/5187638/spain-repatriates-priest-with.html#.VB3JK7d0ziw. Accessed 20 Sept 2014

Associated Press (2014m) Residents complain of food shortages. Associated Press, The Telegram. http://www.thetelegram.com/News/Canada---World/2014-09-21/article-3877181/Residents-complain-of-food-shortages/1. Accessed 21 Sept 2014

Associated Press (2014n) Spain: Ebola test drug out of supply worldwide. Associated Press, Reading Eagle. http://www.readingeagle.com/ap/article/spain-ebola-test-drug-out-of-supply-worldwide. Accessed 17 Mar 2017

Associated Press (2014o) Nurse bitten by Ebola patient flown to Switzerland as precaution. Associated Press, US News and World Report. https://www.usnews.com/news/world/articles/2014/09/22/man-bitten-by-ebola-patient-flown-to-switzerland. Accessed 19 Mar 2017

Associated Press (2014p) Germany asks soldiers to volunteer to fight Ebola. Associated Press, CNS News. http://www.cnsnews.com/news/article/. Accessed 19 Mar 2017

Associated Press (2014q) Ivory coast to resume flights to countries struck by Ebola virus. Associated Press, The Guardian. https://www.theguardian.com/world/2014/sep/27/ebola-sierra-leone-flights-suspension-lifted. Accessed 20 Mar 2017

Associated Press (2014r) Neb. hospital workers fired for violating Ebola patient's privacy. Associated Press, Modern Healthcare. http://www.modernhealthcare.com/article/20140927/INFO/309279886/neb-hospital-workers-fired-for-violating-ebola-patients-privacy#. Accessed 27 Sept 2014

Awareness Times (2014a) Sierra Leone news: consumer protection alerts the public. Awareness Times. http://news.sl/drwebsite/publish/article_200526166.shtml. Accessed 8 Sept 2014

Awareness Times (2014b) Sierra Leone news: RSLAF opens new Ebola treatment centre. Awareness Times. http://news.sl/drwebsite/publish/article_200526786.shtml. Accessed 2 Dec 2014

Awareness Times (2014c) Sierra Leone news: over 1,000 of 2,000 lab confirmed Ebola cases are not accounted for! Awareness Times. http://news.sl/drwebsite/publish/article_200526287.shtml. Accessed 29 Sept 2014

Awoko (2014a) Sierra Leone news: bonanza for health workers as…Le82.1b dished out to fight Ebola. Awoko. http://awoko.org/2014/09/04/sierra-leone-news-bonanza-for-health-workers-as-le82-1b-dished-out-to-fight-ebola/. Accessed 4 Sept 2014

Awoko (2014b) Sierra Leone news: Ebola exposes Lungi Airport. Awoko. http://awoko.org/2014/09/29/sierra-leone-news-ebola-exposes-lungi-airport/. Accessed 29 Sept 2014

Bailes A (2014) Exclusive: no Ebola treatment at Sierra Leone holding center. VOA News. http://www.voanews.com/content/sierra-leone-treatment-center-ebola-outbreak-patients-find-no-care/2463697.html. Accessed 28 Sept 2014

Baldor LC (2014) US troops heading into Africa soon for Ebola fight. San Diego Union Tribune. http://www.sandiegouniontribune.com/sdut-us-troops-heading-into-africa-soon-for-ebola-fight-2014sep19-story,amp.html. Accessed 26 Feb 2017

Barbash F (2014) Ebola stricken Liberia is descending into economic hell. The Washington Post. http://www.washingtonpost.com/news/morning-mix/wp/2014/09/30/hit-by-ebola-liberia-is-descending-into-economic-hell/. Accessed 30 Sept 2014

Bastian M (2014) Ebola: nobody knows what to do. AFP, IOL. http://www.iol.co.za/news/africa/ebola-nobody-knows-what-to-do-1757508. Accessed 5 Apr 2017

Batty D (2014) Sierra Leone to impose lockdown to halt Ebola spread. The Guardian. http://www.theguardian.com/world/2014/sep/06/sierra-leone-lockdown-ebola-outbreak. Accessed 6 Sept 2014

BBC (2014) Ebola virus: 'Biological war' in Liberia. BBC. http://www.bbc.com/news/world-africa-29147797. Accessed 11 Sept 2014

Beaubien J (2014) Fond memories of Ebola victim Eric Duncan, anger over his death. NPR. http://www.npr.org/sections/goatsandsoda/2014/10/09/354645983/fond-memories-of-ebola-victim-eric-duncan-anger-over-his-death. Accessed 7 Apr 2017

Belfast Telegraph (2014) Hope for Ebola vaccine in months. Belfast Telegraph. http://www.belfasttelegraph.co.uk/news/world-news/hope-for-ebola-vaccine-in-months-30612183.html. Accessed 24 Sept 2014

Bella Naija (2014) Kaduna government allocates N116 million for Ebola detecting equipment in schools. Bella Naija. http://www.bellanaija.com/2014/09/09/kaduna-government-allocates-n116-million-for-ebola-detecting-equipment-in-schools/. Accessed 9 Sept 2014

Bennett S (2014) Ebola milestone: more deaths than past outbreaks combined. Business Week. http://www.businessweek.com/news/2014-09-03/ebola-milestone-more-deaths-than-past-outbreaks-combined. Accessed 3 Sept 2014

Bernstein L (2014a) As Ebola cases accelerate, Liberia's sick must fend for themselves. The Washington Post. http://www.washingtonpost.com/world/africa/as-ebola-cases-accelerate-liberias-sick-must-fend-for-themselves/2014/09/13/6ee71468-3b61-11e4-9c9f-ebb47272e40e_story.html

Bernstein L (2014b) With Ebola crippling the health system, Liberians die of routine medical problems. The Washington Post. http://www.washingtonpost.com/world/africa/with-ebola-crippling-the-health-system-liberians-die-of-routine-medical-problems/2014/09/20/727dcfbe-400b-11e4-b03f-de718edeb92f_story.html. Accessed 21 Sept 2014

Besser R (2014) Burying Ebola victims in Liberia. ABC News, MyCentralOregon.com http://www.mycentraloregon.com/2014/09/28/burying-ebola-victims-in-liberia/. Accessed 28 Sept 2014

Bill & Melinda Gates Foundation (2014) Press release: Bill & Melinda Gates Foundation commits $50 million to support emergency response to Ebola. 10 Sept 2014

Bloomberg (2014) Fujifilm says French Ebola patient is taking its Avigan drug. The Japan Times. http://www.japantimes.co.jp/news/2014/09/27/national/science-health/fujifilm-says-french-ebola-patient-is-taking-its-avigan-drug/#.WMLFPU0zXDc. Accessed 10 Mar 2017

Boseley S (2014) First British volunteer injected with trial Ebola vaccine in Oxford. The Guardian. http://www.theguardian.com/society/2014/sep/17/ruth-atkins-first-british-volunteer-injected-trial-ebola-vaccine-oxford.

Breman M, Dennis B, Izadi E (2014) First U.S. case of Ebola diagnosed in Texas after man who came from Liberia falls ill. The Washington Post. https://www.washingtonpost.com/national/health-science/2014/09/30/2690947e-48f3-11e4-a046-120a8a855cca_story.html?utm_term=.c9d3193fb451. Accessed 15 Apr 2017

Brown A (2014) Liberia in recession due to Ebola economic impact. http://afkinsider.com/72268/liberia-recession-due-ebola-economic-impact/. Accessed 14 Sept 2014

Brown FP (2014) Ebola alarm: U.S. State Department orders 160,000 hazmat suits for the virus. Western Journalism. http://www.westernjournalism.com/ebola-alarm-us-state-department-orders-160000-hazmat-suits-virus/?utm_source=rss&utm_medium=rss&utm_campaign=ebola-alarm-us-state-department-orders-160000-hazmat-suits-virus

Brumfiel G (2014) What the US has given to fight Ebola (and why it's not enough). NPR. http://www.npr.org/blogs/goatsandsoda/2014/09/13/348002838/what-the-u-s-has-given-to-fight-ebola-and-why-its-not-enough. Accessed 13 Sept 2014

Brun M (2014) Ebola pain felt in Red Wing. Republican Eagle. http://www.republican-eagle.com/content/ebola-pain-felt-red-wing. Accessed 17 Sept 2014

Butler D (2014) Blood transfusion called priority Ebola therapy. Nature

Caldwell AA (2014) Government lets Liberians stay in U.S. amid Ebola crisis. The Salt Lake City Tribune, Associated Press. http://www.sltrib.com/sltrib/world/58459783-68/protection-liberians-obama-approved.html.csp. Accessed 22 Mar 2017

Calkin S (2014) Will Pooley nurse colleague dies from Ebola. Nursing Times. http://www.nursingtimes.net/nursing-practice/specialisms/infection-control/will-pooley-nurse-colleague-dies-from-ebola/5074762.article. Accessed 12 Sept 2014

Campbell JF (2014) Liberia: several more patients out from ELWA – pregnant woman gives birth at center. AllAfrica. http://allafrica.com/stories/201409111248.html. Accessed 11 Sept 2014

Canada Journal (2014) Microsoft co-founder Paul Allen to donate $9m for Ebola fight. Can J. http://canadajournal.net/health/microsoft-co-founder-paul-allen-donate-9m-ebola-fight-14694-2014/. Accessed 13 Sept 2014

Canadian Press (2014) Ebola scare locks down New Brunswick hotel. The Chronicle Herald. http://thechronicleherald.ca/canada/1234777-ebola-scare-locks-down-new-brunswick-hotel. Accessed 7 Sept 2014

Carroll C (2014) Kirby: 1,400 troops to deploy to Liberia to fight Ebola, starting in October. Stars and Stripes. http://www.stripes.com/kirby-1-400-troops-to-deploy-to-liberia-to-fight-ebola-starting-in-october-1.305906. Accessed 1 Oct 2014

CBC News (2014a) Yellowknife woman stranded in Ebola stricken Sierra Leone. CBC News. http://www.cbc.ca/news/canada/north/yellowknife-woman-stranded-in-ebola-stricken-sierra-leone-1.2769817. Accessed 18 Sept 2014

CBC News (2014b) Ebola treatment with ZMapp cocktail expected in 2015. CBC News. http://www.cbc.ca/news/health/ebola-treatment-with-zmapp-cocktail-expected-in-2015-1.2781556. Accessed 29 Sept 2014

CBS News (2014) Pentagon deploying assets to Liberia for Ebola outbreak. CBS News. http://www.cbsnews.com/news/pentagon-deploying-mobile-hospital-to-liberia-for-ebola-outbreak/. Accessed 8 Sept 2014

Christensen J, Levs J, Goldschmidt D (2014) American Ebola patient arrives at Emory in Atlanta. CNN. http://www.cnn.com/2014/09/09/health/ebola-patient-emory-atlanta/index.html?hpt=he_c2. Accessed 9 Sept 2014

Clarke T, Samb S (2014) U.N. says $600 million needed to tackle Ebola as deaths top 1,900. Reuters. http://www.reuters.com/article/us-health-ebola-idUSKBN0GY1V320140904. Accessed 5 Feb 2017

Clottey P (2014) Sierra Leone ends Ebola lockdown. VOA News. http://www.voanews.com/a/sierra-leone-official-pleased-with-ebola-containment-measure/2457227.html. Accessed 17 Mar 2017

CNA Daily News (2014) Pope Francis prays issues strong appeal for Ebola victims. CNA, EWTN. http://www.dfwcatholic.org/pope-francis-prays-issues-strong-appeal-for-ebola-victims-82670/.html. Accessed 24 Sept 2014

Cohen J (2014) UN Security Council passes historic resolution to confront Ebola. Science. http://news.sciencemag.org/africa/2014/09/u-n-security-council-passes-historic-resolution-confront-ebola. Accessed 20 Sept 2014

Cohen E (2014a) Woman saves three relatives from Ebola. CNN. http://www.cnn.com/2014/09/25/health/ebola-fatu-family/index.html. Accessed 27 Sept 2014

Cohen E (2014b) Doctor treats Ebola with HIV drug in Liberia – seemingly successfully. CNN. http://www.cnn.com/2014/09/27/health/ebola-hiv-drug/. Accessed 27 Sept 2014

Cooper H (2014) Liberian President pleads with Obama for assistance in combating Ebola. New York Times. http://www.nytimes.com/2014/09/13/world/africa/liberian-president-pleads-with-obama-for-assistance-in-combating-ebola.html?_r=0. Accessed 13 Sept 2014

Cooper H, Shear MD, Grady D (2014) U.S. to commit up to 3,000 troops to fight Ebola in Africa. New York Times. http://www.nytimes.com/2014/09/16/world/africa/obama-to-announce-expanded-effort-against-ebola.html?_r=0. Accessed 15 Sept 2014

Cortez MF, Kitamura M (2014) Black market in blood serum emerging amid Ebola outbreak. Business Week. http://www.businessweek.com/news/2014-09-11/blood-serum-from-recovered-ebola-doctor-used-in-new-case. Accessed 12 Sept 2014

Daily Post (2014) Ebola: minister says 271 people under surveillance in Nigeria. Daily Post. http://dailypost.ng/2014/09/01/ebola-minister-says-271-people-surveillance-nigeria/. Accessed 1 Sept 2014

Davies S, Keogh B, Cosford P, Cummings J (2014) To: NHS Trust Medical and Directors of Nursing, Publications Gateway Ref No. 02266. 19 Sept 2014

DeVries N (2014) Sierra Leone's 3-day Ebola lockdown continues. VOA News. http://www.voanews.com/content/ebola-outbreak-sierra-leone/2456472.html. Accessed 20 Sept 2014

Diallo B, DiLorenzo S (2014a) Ebola is surging in places it had been beaten back. ABC News. http://abcnews.go.com/Health/wireStory/ebola-surging-places-beaten-back-25343632?page=2. Accessed 8 Sept 2014

Diallo B, DiLorenzo S (2014b) Red cross team attacked while burying Ebola dead. ABC News. http://abcnews.go.com/Health/wireStory/ebola-vaccine-ready-year-end-25721068. Accessed 24 Sept 2014

Dike M (2014) Ebola: 'we bathed with kerosene, salt, warm water mixture.' Leadership. http://leadership.ng/news/383551/ebola-bathed-kerosene-salt-warm-water-mixture. Accessed 10 Sept 2014

Disease Outbreak News (2014) Ebola virus disease, outbreak – west Africa. World Health Organization. 4 Sept 2014

Donnelley P (2014) Muslim pilgrims checked for Ebola virus on their way to Mecca as health chiefs announce more than 700 cases emerged in one week as disease sweeps West Africa. The Daily Mail. http://www.dailymail.co.uk/news/article-2761351/Muslim-pilgrims-checked-Ebola-virus-way-Mecca-UN-announces-special-mission-combat-disease-sweeping-West-Africa.html. Accessed 19 Sept 2014

Dosso Z (2014) Resentment simmers in Liberia's 'Ebola jail town'. Yahoo News. http://news.yahoo.com/resentment-simmers-liberias-ebola-jail-town-111547180.html. Accessed 7 Sept 2014

Doucleff M (2014) First U.S. case of Ebola confirmed in Dallas. NPR. http://www.npr.org/sections/health-shots/2014/09/30/352815781/first-u-s-case-of-ebola-confirmed-in-dallas. Accessed 1 Oct 2014

Du Cille M, Bernstein L (2014) Liberian clinic for Ebola gives rural victims hope. The Washington Post, Helsinkitimes. http://www.helsinkitimes.fi/world-int/world-news/international-news/12084-liberian-clinic-for-ebola-gives-rural-victims-hope.html. Accessed 19 Sept 2014

Dunlevy S (2014) Medecins Sans Frontieres slams Australia's Ebola response. News.com.au. http://www.news.com.au/national/medecins-sans-frontieres-slams-australias-ebola-response/story-fncynjr2-1227061379772. Accessed 19 Sept 2014

Energy and Commerce Committee (2014) Committee releases Dallas Ebola timelines. 17 Oct 2014

Engle M (2014) Richard Sacra third American missionary with Ebola being treated with Canadian experimental drug. NY Daily News. http://www.nydailynews.com/life-style/health/american-missionary-ebola-treated-experimental-drug-article-1.1949364. Accessed 23 Sept 2014

Epatko L (2014a) How to help Ebola relief efforts. PBS. http://www.pbs.org/newshour/rundown/help-ebola-relief-efforts/. Accessed 10 Feb 2017

Epatko L (2014b) In Liberia, Ebola takes a toll on small businesses. PBS. http://www.pbs.org/newshour/updates/in-liberia-ebola-takes-toll-on-small-businesses/. Accessed 17 Sept 2014

Euronews (2014) Thousands 'evade' Ebola lockdown in Sierra Leone. Euronews. http://www.euronews.com/2014/09/20/thousands-evade-ebola-lockdown-in-sierra-leone/. Accessed 20 Sept 2014

Farge E, Oberstadt A (2014) Senegal tracks route of Guinea student in race to stop Ebola. Reuters. http://www.reuters.com/article/us-health-ebola-senegal-idUSKBN0H414F20140909. Accessed 9 Sept 2014

Fay A (2014) Doctor from Massachusetts has Ebola virus. WWLP. http://wwlp.com/2014/09/03/doctor-from-massachusetts-has-ebola-virus/. Accessed 3 Sept 2014

Fink S (2014) Cuts at W.H.O. hurt response to Ebola crisis. New York Times. http://www.nytimes.com/2014/09/04/world/africa/cuts-at-who-hurt-response-to-ebola-crisis.html. Accessed 7 Sept 2014

Finnan D (2014) Sierra Leone starting to see 'stabilising' effect of Ebola quarantine, says presidential advisor. http://www.english.rfi.fr/africa/20140928-sierra-leone-starting-see-stabilising-effect-ebola-quarantine-says-presidential-advi. Accessed 27 Sept 2014

Fox M (2014) Are hospitals part of the Ebola problem? Charity wants new strategy. NBC News. http://www.nbcnews.com/storyline/ebola-virus-outbreak/are-hospitals-part-ebola-problem-charity-wants-new-strategy-n202486. Accessed 16 Sept 2014

Fox News (2014) African children orphaned by Ebola shunned, face death, UNICEF says. Fox News. http://www.foxnews.com/world/2014/09/30/thousands-children-orphaned-by-ebola-at-risk-being-shunned-unicef-says/. Accessed 30 Sept 2014

Freeman C (2014) I have never seen this number of bodies before: life at an Ebola clinic in Liberia. The Telegraph. http://www.telegraph.co.uk/news/worldnews/ebola/11118025/I-have-never-seen-this-number-of-bodies-before-Life-at-an-Ebola-clinic-in-Liberia.html. Accessed 24 Sept 2014

Freeman C, Wintercross W (2014) The Ebola prayer that goes unanswered. The Telegraph. http://www.telegraph.co.uk/news/worldnews/ebola/11111573/The-Ebola-prayer-that-goes-unanswered.html. Accessed 21 Sept 2014

Funk J (2014) 3rd US Ebola patient released from hospital. ABC News. http://abcnews.go.com/US/wireStory/nebraska-doctors-give-update-ebola-patient-25751592. Accessed 25 Sept 2014

Gallagher J (2014) British Ebola patient 'discharged'. BBC. http://www.bbc.com/news/health-29045908. Accessed 3 Sept 2014

Gbandia S (2014) Sierra Leones Ebola burial teams struggle as bodies decompose. Business Week. http://www.businessweek.com/news/2014-09-17/sierra-leone-s-ebola-burial-teams-struggle-as-bodies-decompose. Accessed 17 Sept 2014

Ghana Voice (2014) Liberia's nurses go on strike amid Ebola outbreak. Ghana Voice. http://www.ghanavoice.com/2014/09/02/liberias-nurses-go-on-strike-amid-ebola-outbreak/. Accessed 5 Feb 2017

GhanaWeb (2014) Ebola scare: doctors desert patients at Achimota Hospital. GhanaWeb. http://www.ghanaweb.com/GhanaHomePage/NewsArchive/artikel.php?ID=325800. Accessed 14 Sept 2014

Giahyue J (2014) Ebola survivors asked to donate blood to treat victims. Canoe.com, Reuters. http://cnews.canoe.ca/CNEWS/World/2014/09/24/21963026.html. Accessed 24 Sept 2014

Gilblom K (2014) Ebola vaccine fully successful in monkey tests: study. Bloomberg. http://www.bloomberg.com/news/2014-09-07/study-ebola-vaccine-fully-successful-in-monkey-tests.html. Accessed 8 Sept 2014

Gold D (2014) Left to die: Liberia's Ebola victims have nowhere to turn as treatment centers overflow. Vice News. https://news.vice.com/article/left-to-die-liberias-ebola-victims-have-nowhere-to-turn-as-treatment-centers-overflow. Accessed 19 Sept 2014

Grady D (2014) Ebola cases could reach 1.4 million within four months, C.D.C. Estimates. New York Times. https://www.nytimes.com/2014/09/24/health/ebola-cases-could-reach-14-million-in-4-months-cdc-estimates.html?_r=1. Accessed 19 Mar 2017

Greig A (2014) US scientists say Ebola epidemic will rage for another 12 to 18 months. The Daily Mail. http://www.dailymail.co.uk/news/article-2755520/U-S-scientists-say-Ebola-epiodemic-rage-12-18-months.html. Accessed 14 Sept 2014

Hamer A (2014) New clinic key to Sierra Leones Ebola fight. Aljazeera. http://www.aljazeera.com/newś/africa/2014/09/sierra-leone-set-open-major-ebola-clinic-201491271935126793.html

Hinshaw D (2014) In Liberia, burial practices hinder battle against Ebola. Wall Str J. http://online.wsj.com/articles/in-liberia-burial-practices-hinder-battle-against-ebola-1409619832. Accessed 1 Sept 2014

Hinshaw D, McKay B (2014) US troops battling Ebola get off to slow start in Africa. Wall Str J http://online.wsj.com/articles/u-s-troops-battling-ebola-get-off-to-slow-start-in-africa-1411948064. Accessed 29 Sept 2014

Hogan C (2014) More than 400 under surveillance for Ebola in Nigeria's 'oil city.' The Washington Post. http://www.washingtonpost.com/news/morning-mix/wp/2014/09/09/more-than-400-under-surveillance-for-ebola-in-nigeria-oil-city/. Accessed 9 Sept 2014

Iginla A (2014) Wahala de o! Liberian woman hang herself till death in Lagos because of Ebola. O Sun Defender. http://www.osundefender.org/?p=186238&cpage=1. Accessed 12 Sept 2014

Independent.ie (2014) British military to set up 62-bed Ebola treatment centre in Sierra Leone. Independent.ie.   http://www.independent.ie/world-news/europe/british-military-to-set-up-62bed-ebola-treatment-centre-in-sierra-leone-30570541.html. Accessed 8 Sept 2014

IRIN (2014) West Africa gears up to contain Ebola spread. IRIN. http://www.irinnews.org/report/100645/west-africa-gears-up-to-contain-ebola-spread. Accessed 22 Sept 2014

Izadi E (2014) The latest American doctor infected with Ebola is coming to Nebraska for treatment. The Washington Post. http://www.washingtonpost.com/news/national/wp/2014/09/04/the-latest-american-doctor-infected-with-ebola-is-coming-to-nebraska-for-treatment/. Accessed 4 Sept 2014

Johnson RM (2014a) Sierra Leone to visit every home to track down Ebola dead. AFP, Rappler. http://www.rappler.com/world/regions/africa/68546-sierra-leone-home-visits-ebola. Accessed 8 Sept 2014

Johnson RM (2014b) Sierra Leone readies for controversial Ebola lockdown. AFP, Rappler. http://www.rappler.com/world/regions/africa/69502-sierra-leone-ebola-lockdown. Accessed 18 Sept 2014

Johnson RM (2014c) Sierra Leone streets deserted as Ebola shutdown begins. AFP, Rappler. http://www.rappler.com/world/regions/africa/69637-sierra-leone-ebola-lockdown. Accessed 19 Sept 2014

Jozwiak G (2014) Ebola virus outbreak: a first-hand Liberian tragedy – 'We begged, take the baby to hospital… they refused'. The Independent. http://www.independent.co.uk/news/world/africa/ebola-in-liberia-firsthand-tragedy-of-a-teenage-mother-behind-the-quarantine-fence--we-begged-take-the-baby-to-hospital-they-refused-9746387.html. Accessed 21 Sept 2014

Kamanda (2014a) Fear and desperation in Sierra Leone. Plan International, Reuters. http://www.trust.org/item/20140919115949-u0yrs/. Accessed 19 Sept 2014

Kamanda (2014b) Sierra Leone: life after the lockdown in Sierra Leone. AllAfrica. http://allafrica.com/stories/201409241238.html?page=2. Accessed 24 Sept 2014

Kelemen M (2014) Promised help to fight Ebola arriving at 'speed of a turtle'. NPR. http://www.npr.org/sections/goatsandsoda/2014/09/26/351553847/promised-help-to-fight-ebola-arriving-at-speed-of-a-turtle. Accessed 26 Mar 2017

Kelto A (2014) Sierra Leone on lockdown over Ebola. NPR. http://www.npr.org/2014/09/19/349908360/sierra-leone-on-lockdown-over-ebola. Accessed 20 Sept 2014

Knox R (2014) A few Ebola cases likely in U.S., air traffic analysis predicts. NPR. http://www.npr.org/blogs/goatsandsoda/2014/09/04/345767439/a-few-ebola-cases-likely-in-u-s-air-traffic-analysis-shows?utm_medium=RSS&utm_campaign=news. Accessed 4 Sept 2014

KPRC (2014) US air marshal attacked with syringe. Texoma's. http://www.texomashomepage.com/story/d/story/us-air-marshal-attacked-with-syringe/39205/Nnd8I9NCbki8zIhg9vRj8Q. Accessed 9 Sept 2014

Kroll D (2014a) WHO Ebola drug panel: use survivor serum to treat Ebola victims. Forbes. http://www.forbes.com/sites/davidkroll/2014/09/05/who-ebola-drug-panel-use-survivor-serum-to-treat-ebola-victims/. Accessed 7 Sept 2014

Kroll D (2014b) Nigeria free of Ebola, final surveillance contacts released. Forbes. http://www.forbes.com/sites/davidkroll/2014/09/23/nigeria-free-of-ebola-as-final-surveillance-contacts-are-released/. Accessed 23 Sept 2014

KTVU (2014) California nurses stage 'die-in' to protest lack of Ebola preparations. KTVU. http://www.ktvu.com/news/news/local/california-nurses-stage-die-protest-lack-ebola-pre/nhTSS/. Accessed 24 Sept 2014

Landauro I (2014) France's first Ebola patient to get experimental drug. Wall Str J http://online.wsj.com/articles/frances-first-ebola-patient-to-get-experimental-drug-1411113221. Accessed 19 Sept 2014

Larson K (2014) Families wait in agony for word on Ebola patients. AP, The Fresno Bee. http://www.fresnobee.com/2014/09/30/4152198/families-wait-in-agony-for-word.html. Accessed 30 Sept 2014

Larson K, Cheng M (2014) Ebola clinics fill up as Liberia awaits aid. ABC News. http://abcnews.go.com/Health/wireStory/ebola-clinics-fill-liberia-awaits-aid-25801938?singlePage=true. Accessed 27 Sept 2014

Lee CE, McKay B (2014) Obama plans major Ebola offensive. Wall Str J http://online.wsj.com/articles/obama-plans-major-ebola-offensive-1410738096. Accessed 15 Sept 2014

Leposo L, Elbagir N (2014) Funerals, ghost towns and haunted health workers: Life in the Ebola zone. CNN. http://www.cnn.com/2014/09/01/world/africa/ebola-ghost-town/. Accessed 5 Feb 2014

Leveille D (2014) Sierra Leone celebrates the end of its lockdown, but Ebola still looms. PRI. https://www.pri.org/stories/2014-09-22/sierra-leone-celebrates-end-its-lockdown-ebola-still-looms. Accessed 18 Mar 2017

Levine S (2014) American aid worker exposed to Ebola coming to NIH. Politico. http://www.politico.com/story/2014/09/nih-to-treat-american-aid-worker-with-ebola-111374.html. Accessed 27 Sept 2014

Liberia Peacebuilding Office (2014) City mayor of Kolba City, Kolahun District is confirmed Ebola positive. 25 Aug 2014

Loftus M (2015) The long, extraordinary recovery of Ian Crozier. Emory Med Spring 2015:9

Lupkin S (2014a) Another American doctor tests positive for Ebola in west Africa. ABC News. http://abcnews.go.com/Health/american-doctor-tests-positive-ebola-west-africa/story?id=25216376. Accessed 2 Sept 2014

Lupkin S (2014b) Two women receive experimental Ebola vaccine in fast-tracked trial. ABC News. http://abcnews.go.com/Health/women-receive-experimental-ebola-vaccine-fast-tracked-trial/story?id=25236608. Accessed 5 Feb 2017

MacDougall C (2014) 'Everything is with God.' Foreign Policy. http://www.foreignpolicy.com/articles/2014/09/22/ebola_liberia_monrovia_pentagon_obama_redemption. Accessed 22 Sept 2014

MacIntyre CR, Richards GA, Davidson PM (2014) Respiratory protection for healthcare workers treating Ebola virus disease (EVD): are facemasks sufficient to meet occupational health and safety obligations? Int J Nurs Stud 51:1421–1426

MacRae F (2014) 160 NHS Staff volunteer to go to Ebola ravaged West Africa. Daily Mail. http://www.dailymail.co.uk/health/article-2766341/Experimental-Ebola-drugs-tested-West-Africa-time-WHO-predicts-cases-hit-21-000-SIX-weeks.html. Accessed 19 Mar 2017

Mai-Duc C (2014) 'Window of opportunity' to control Ebola is closing, CDC director says. LA Times. http://www.latimes.com/world/africa/la-fg-africa-ebola-cdc-frieden-20140902-story.html. Accessed 2 Sept 2014

Maja-Pearce A (2014) Nigeria in the time of Ebola. New York Times. http://www.nytimes.com/2014/09/06/opinion/adewale-maja-pearce-nigeria-in-the-time-of-ebola.html?_r=0. Accessed 6 Sept 2014

Mark M (2014) Bodies found after Ebola health workers go missing in Guinea. The Guardian. http://www.theguardian.com/society/2014/sep/18/ebola-health-workers-missing-guinea. Accessed 18 Sept 2014

Martin-Moreno JM, Llinás G, Hernández JM (2014) Is respiratory protection appropriate in the Ebola response? Lancet 384:856

McKay B, McWhirter C (2014) Ebola infected doctor arrives in Nebraska for treatment. Wall Str   J   http://online.wsj.com/articles/ebola-infected-doctor-arrives-in-nebraska-for-treat-ment-1409925202. Accessed 5 Sept 2014

McLaughlin MW (2014) Central Connecticut State University, Campus announcement, regarding Ebola virus. 15 Sept 2014

McNeil DG Jr. (2014) Ebola Doctor Shortage Eases as Volunteers Step Forward. New York Times. https://www.nytimes.com/2014/09/27/health/Ebola-Doctor-Shortage-Eases-as-Volunteers-Begin-to-Step-Forward.html?_r=0. Accessed 26 Mar 2017

MCT and Xinhua (2014) China to help Sierra Leone set up Ebola facilities. South China Morning Post.   http://www.scmp.com/news/world/article/1588855/china-help-sierra-leone-set-ebola-facilities. Accessed 10 Sept 2014

Médecins Sans Frontières (2014a) United Nations special briefing on Ebola. 2 Sept 2014

Médecins Sans Frontières (2014b) Liberia: massive distribution of Ebola safety kits. 3 Oct 2014

Médecins Sans Frontières (2014c) Ebola crisis update – Sept 25th. 26 Sept 2014

Mohammed A (2014) Nigeria Govt orders schools to resume September 22. Premium Times. http://www.premiumtimesng.com/news/top-news/167776-nigeria-govt-orders-schools-to-resume-september-22.html. Accessed 6 Feb 2017

Montgomery N (2014) Troops aiding Ebola effort in Africa have minimal chance of infection, USARAF chief says. Stars and Stripes. http://www.stripes.com/news/troops-aiding-ebola-effort-in-africa-have-minimal-chance-of-infection-usaraf-chief-says-1.304726. Accessed 24 Sept 2014

Munuhe M (2014) Travellers told to produce Ebola certificate. The Standard. https://www.stan-dardmedia.co.ke/mobile/?articleID=2000134776&story_title=travellers-told-to-produce-ebola-certificate&pageNo=2. Accessed 12 Sept 2014

Mupapa K, Massamba M, Kibadi K et al (1999) Treatment of Ebola hemorrhagic fever with blood transfusions from convalescent patients. J Infect Dis 179(Suppl 1):S18–S23

Murphy S (2014) Ebola patient flees clinic in search of food. Newstalk. http://www.newstalk.ie/Ebola-patient-flees-clinic-in-search-for-food. Accessed 2 Sept 2014

Nebehay S (2014) Nigeria monitoring 400 contacts of doctor who died of Ebola. Reuters. http://www.reuters.com/article/2014/09/04/us-health-ebola-nigeria-idUSKBN0GZ1EE20140904. Accessed 4 Sept 2014

Newman K (2014) Airmen deploy to deliver Ebola treatment facility with U.S. relief package. http://www.jble.af.mil/News/Article-Display/Article/843828/airmen-deploy-to-deliver-ebola-treatment-facility-with-us-relief-package. Accessed 22 Mar 2017

News 24 (2014) Liberia extends stay at home order. News 24. http://www.news24.com/Africa/News/Ebola-crisis-Liberia-extends-stay-home-order-20140901. Accessed 1 Sep 2014

News Ghana (2014a) October 13 resumption date was to give health officers enough time. News Ghana.   http://www.spyghana.com/october-13-resumption-date-was-to-give-health-officers-enough-time/. Accessed 10 Sept 2014

News Ghana (2014b) Ebola hits hard at Liberian Presidency killing one. News Ghana. http://www.spyghana.com/ebola-hits-hard-at-liberian-presidency-killing-one/. Access 11 Sept 2014

Nichols M (2014) Ebola seriously threatens Liberia's national existence: minister. Reuters. http://af.reuters.com/article/commoditiesNews/idAFL1N0RA1NA20140909?pageNumber=2&virtualBrandChannel=0. Accessed 9 Sept 2014

Nigerian Bulletin (2014) Ebola: teachers urges Gov. Ameachi to reverse decision to reopen schools. Niger Bull http://www.nigerianbulletin.com/threads/ebola-teachers-urges-gov-ame-achi-to-reverse-decision-to-reopen-schools.91605/. Accessed 10 Sept 2014

Nossiter A (2014) Fresh graves point to undercount of Ebola toll. New York Times. http://www.nytimes.com/2014/09/23/world/africa/23ebola.html?action=click&contentCollection=Health&module=RelatedCoverage&region=Marginalia&pgtype=article. Accessed 23 Sept 2014

O'Brien J (2014) Life… and death in the Ebola 'high-risk' zone. Independent.ie. http://www.independent.ie/world-news/africa/life-and-death-in-the-ebola-highrisk-zone-30586734.html#sthash.61OSqIYR.dpuf. Accessed 15 Sept 2014

O'Carroll L (2014a) Sierra Leones planned Ebola lockdown could spread disease further. The Guardian. http://www.theguardian.com/world/2014/sep/06/sierra-leone-lockdown-ebola-outbreak. Accessed 6 Sept 2014

O'Carroll L (2014b) Ebola survivor Ian Crozier: 'Everyone thought he was going to die'. The Guardian. https://www.theguardian.com/world/2014/dec/08/ebola-survivor-ian-crozier-doctor-antibodies-will-pooley. Accessed 12 Feb 2017

O'Carroll L (2014c) William Pooley plans return to the fight against Ebola in Sierra Leone. The Guardian. http://www.theguardian.com/society/2014/sep/09/william-pooley-ebola-sierra-leone-outbreak-epidemic. Accessed 9 Sept 2014

O'Carroll L (2014d) Ebola epidemic house to house search in Sierra Leone reveals 358 new cases. The Guardian. http://www.theguardian.com/world/2014/sep/24/ebola-sierra-leone-curfew. Accessed 24 Sept 2014

Okoro E (2014) Nigeria: Lagos moves schools' resumption to October 8. AllAfrica. http://allafrica.com/stories/201409221945.html. Accessed 22 Sept 2014

Onishi N (2014a) Ebola brings doctor back to Liberia slums he escaped. New York Times, Dallas Morning News. http://www.dallasnews.com/news/news/2014/09/13/ebola-brings-doctor-back-to-liberia-slums-he-escaped. Accessed 19 Feb 2017

Onishi N (2014b) In Liberia, home deaths spread circle of Ebola contagion. New York Times. http://www.nytimes.com/2014/09/25/world/africa/liberia-ebola-victims-treatment-center-cdc.html?_r=0. Accessed 25 Sept 2014

Onukwugha A (2014) Rivers schools to resume October 6. Leadership. http://leadership.ng/news/384638/rivers-schools-resume-october-6. Accessed 21 Sept 2014

Osterath B (2014) Ebola threatens to destroy Sierra Leone and Liberia. DW. http://www.dw.de/virologist-fight-against-ebola-in-sierra-leone-and-liberia-is-lost/a-17915090. Accessed 15 Feb 2017

Park A (2014) Liberians explain why the Ebola crisis is way worse than you think. Mother Jones. http://www.motherjones.com/politics/2014/09/ebola-crisis-liberia-way-worse-you-think. Accessed 24 Sept 2014

Paye-Layleh J (2014) Liberias Chief Medical Officer goes under Ebola quarantine. The Huffington Post. http://www.huffingtonpost.com/2014/09/27/liberia-doctor-ebola-quarantine_n_5892840.html. Accessed 27 Sept 2014

Paye-Layleh J (2015) Liberia removes Ebola crematorium as outbreak is contained. Associated Press, US News & World Report. http://www.usnews.com/news/world/articles/2015/03/08/liberia-removes-ebola-crematorium-as-outbreak-is-contained. Accessed 8 Mar 2015

Phillip A (2014) An Ebola vaccine was given to 10 volunteers, and there are 'no red flags' yet. The Washington Post. http://www.washingtonpost.com/news/to-your-health/wp/2014/09/16/an-ebola-vaccine-was-given-to-10-volunteers-and-there-are-no-red-flags-yet/. Accessed 17 Sept 2014

Premium Times (2014) Lagos Ebola volunteers to go on strike over non-payment of allowances. Niger Bull. http://www.nigerianbulletin.com/threads/lagos-ebola-volunteers-to-go-on-strike-over-non-payment-of-allowances.91184/. Accessed 7 Sept 2014

Quist-Arcton O (2014) In the county where Ebola first struck Liberia, a cry for help. NPR. http://www.npr.org/sections/goatsandsoda/2014/09/08/346735490/in-the-county-where-ebola-first-struck-liberia-a-cry-for-help. Accessed 12 Feb 2017

Randhawa K (2014) Ebola outbreak: survivor William Pooley flown to US to give doctor with virus emergency blood transfusion. The Independent. http://www.independent.co.uk/life-style/

health-and-families/ebola-outbreak-survivor-william-pooley-flown-to-us-to-give-doctor-with-virus-emergency-blood-transfusion-9737888.html. Accessed 17 Sept 2014

Reuters (2014a) EU pledges 227 million in aid to fight Ebola outbreak in West Africa. Reuters. http://www.straitstimes.com/news/world/more-world-stories/story/eu-pledges-4227-million-aid-fight-ebola-outbreak-west-africa-201. Accessed 5 Sept 2014

Reuters (2014b) Guinean who brought Ebola to Senegal recovers from virus. Reuters. http://af.reuters.com/article/worldNews/idAFKBN0H50VV20140910. Accessed 26 Feb 2017

Reuters (2014c) Cuba to send 165 health workers to fight Ebola. Reuters, Eyewitness News. http://ewn.co.za/2014/09/12/Cuba-to-send-165-health-workers-to-fight-Ebola. Accessed 12 Sept 2014

Reuters (2014d) French worker for medical charity MSF contracts Ebola in Liberia. Reuters. http://www.reuters.com/article/2014/09/17/us-health-ebola-france-idUSKBN0HC21B20140917. Accessed 17 Sept 2014

Reuters (2014e) France to set up military hospital to fight Ebola in West Africa. Reuters. http://af.reuters.com/article/topNews/idAFKBN0HD1ZW20140918. Accessed 10 Mar 2017

Reuters (2014f) Sierra Leone's capital at standstill as 3-day Ebola lockdown begins. Reuters, Huffington Post. http://www.huffingtonpost.com/2014/09/19/sierra-leone-ebola-lockdown_n_5848780.html. Accessed 10 Mar 2017

Reuters (2014g) Germany, France to start joint airlift to Ebola-affected countries. Reuters. http://in.reuters.com/article/2014/09/19/us-health-ebola-germany-france-idINKBN-0HE1UA20140919. Accessed 19 Sept 2014

Reuters (2014h) Sierra Leone seals borders with Liberia and Guinea to stop Ebola. Reuters, Global Post. http://www.globalpost.com/dispatch/news/thomson-reuters/140923/sierra-leone-seals-borders-liberia-and-guinea-stop-ebola. Accessed 23 Sept 2014

Reuters (2014i) FDA issues warning letters on Ebola treatment claims. Reuters. http://www.reuters.com/article/2014/09/24/us-health-ebola-fda-idUSKCN0HJ25J20140924. Accessed 24 Sept 2014

Reuters (2014j) Spanish priest suffering from Ebola has died: Madrid health authority. Reuters. http://www.reuters.com/article/2014/09/25/us-ebola-spain-idUSKCN0HK21220140925. Accessed 25 Sept 2014

Reuters (2014k) Collateral death toll expected to soar as Africa deals with Ebola crisis. Reuters, Daily News & Analysis. http://www.dnaindia.com/world/report-collateral-death-toll-expected-to-soar-as-africa-deals-with-ebola-crisis-2021725. Accessed 26 Sept 2014

Reuters (2014l) Trail vaccines for Ebola to be available in January. Reuters, News Ghana. http://www.spyghana.com/trail-vaccines-for-ebola-to-be-available-in-january/. Accessed 28 Sept 2014

Reuters (2014m) Dallas Ebola patient throwing up all over the place on way to hospital. Reuters, The Baltimore Sun. http://www.baltimoresun.com/health/chi-ebola-patient-america-20141002,0,4611727.story. Accessed 2 Oct 2014

RFI (2014) Ebola: le Sénégal ouvre un corridor humanitaire aérien. RFI. http://www.rfi.fr/afrique/20140927-ebola-senegal-ouvre-corridor-humanitaire-aerien-onu-guinee-sierra-leone-liberia-pam-msf. Accessed 26 Mar 2017

Robb T (2014) Edmonton ER reopens after Ebola scare. Toronto Sun. http://www.torontosun.com/2014/09/22/ebola-scare-sparks-edmonton-er-closure. Accessed 19 Mar 2017

Rokhy M (2014) Vigilante 'border guards' keeping Ebola out of Senegal. Yahoo News. http://news.yahoo.com/vigilante-border-guards-keeping-ebola-senegal-115057030.html. Accessed 6 Sept 2014

Ross P (2014) Fourth Sierra Leone doctor contracts Ebola, health workers most at risk in 'war' on disease. International Business Times. http://www.ibtimes.com/fourth-sierra-leone-doctor-contracts-ebola-health-workers-most-risk-war-disease-1686128. Accessed 11 Sept 2014

Roy-Macaulay C (2014) 4th doctor dies of Ebola in Sierra Leone. ABC News. http://abcnews.go.com/Health/wireStory/4th-doctor-dies-ebola-sierra-leone-25489677. Accessed 14 Sept 2014

Roy-Macaulay C, Kargbo K (2014) US gives 5 ambulances to Sierra Leone as country battles Ebola struggles to collect bodies. US News and World Report. https://www.usnews.com/news/world/articles/2014/09/10/us-gives-ambulances-to-sierra-leone-to-fight-ebola. Accessed 26 Feb 2017

Sami M (2014) We're turning Ebola patients away 'every day': MSF. ABC. http://www.abc.net.au/pm/content/2014/s4084249.htm. Accessed 9 Sept 2014

Saudi Gazette (2014) Two lounges at Jeddah airport to check African pilgrims for Ebola. Saudi Gazette. http://www.saudigazette.com.sa/index.cfm?method=home.regcon&contentid=20140922219003. Accessed 21 Sept 2014

Saul H (2014) Ebola virus outbreak: 'just two doctors' available to treat 85,000 people in Liberia county. The Independent. http://www.independent.co.uk/life-style/health-and-families/health-news/ebola-virus-outbreak-just-two-doctors-available-to-treat-85000-people-in-liberia-county-9755580.html. Accessed 25 Sept 2014

Sellers FS (2014) Exposed. After an accidental needle stab, a doctor's Ebola watch begins. The Washington Post. http://www.washingtonpost.com/sf/style/2014/11/03/exposed/. Accessed 3 Nov 2014

Sengupta S (2014) Security council unanimously passes Ebola resolution. http://www.nytimes.com/2014/09/19/world/security-council-unanimously-passes-ebola-resolution.html?_r=0. Accessed 20 Sept 2014

Sequeira R (2014) Ebola alert also at ports: centre. The Times of India. http://timesofindia.indiatimes.com/india/Ebola-alert-also-at-ports-Centre/articleshow/42543145.cms. Accessed 15 Sept 2014

Sierra Express Media (2014) Press briefing – death of Dr. Olivet Buck. Sierra Express Media. http://www.sierraexpressmedia.com/?p=70410. Accessed 18 Sept 2014

Sifferlin A (2014) Emory's 'sickest' Ebola patient, now in recovery, reveals identity. Time. http://time.com/3622735/ebola-emory-university-hospital-ian-crozier/. Accessed 7 Dec 2014

Sink J (2014) Obama, Ebola survivor meet in Oval Office. The Hill. http://thehill.com/blogs/blog-briefing-room/news/217890-obama-ebola-survivor-meet-in-oval-office. Accessed 17 Sept 2014

Sky News (2014) Ebola: roadblocks to stop health workers. Yahoo News, Sky News. https://uk.news.yahoo.com/ebola-roadblocks-stop-health-workers-132157975.html#DyMLelm. Accessed 25 Sept 2014

Somanader T (2014) President Obama to the international community: we must do more to fight Ebola. http://obamawhitehouse.archives.gov/blog/2014/09/25/president-obama-international-community-we-must-do-more-fight-ebola. Accessed 20 Mar 2017

Stanglin D (2014) Liberia says Dallas Ebola patient lied on exit documents. USA Today. http://www.usatoday.com/story/news/nation/2014/10/02/liberia-ebola-patient-thomas-duncan-air-port-screening/16591753/. Initially accessed 2 Oct 2014

Stanley DA, Honko AN, Asiedu C et al (2014) Chimpanzee adenovirus vaccine generates acute and durable protective immunity against ebolavirus challenge. Nat Med 20:1126–1129

Styles R (2014) Abandoned ostracised and left to starve: shocking fate of the hundreds of young children orphaned by Ebola revealed. The Daily Mail. http://www.dailymail.co.uk/femail/article-2766611/Shocking-plight-hundreds-children-orphaned-Ebola-epidemic-revealed.html. Accessed 24 Sept 2014

Sun LH, Eilperin J (2014) Obama: U.S. military to provide equipment, resources to battle Ebola epidemic in Africa. The Washington Post. https://www.washingtonpost.com/world/national-security/obama-us-military-to-provide-equipment-resources-to-battle-ebola-epidemic-in-africa/2014/09/07/e0d8dc26-369a-11e4-9c9f-ebb47272e40e_story.html?utm_term=.63fc99077d74. Accessed 10 Feb 2017

Szabo L (2014a) 100 tons of supplies to fight Ebola sent to West Africa. USA Today. http://www.usatoday.com/story/news/world/2014/09/21/ebola-supplies-airlift/16008215/. Accessed 12 Mar 2017

Szabo L (2014b) CDC: Ebola outbreak in Nigeria and Senegal may be over. USA Today. http://
    www.usatoday.com/story/news/nation/2014/09/30/ebola-over-in-nigeria/16473339/. Accessed
    30 Sept 2014

Taylor A (2014) Congress releases war funds to fight Ebola after Inhofe relents. US News and
    World Report. https://www.usnews.com/news/politics/articles/2014/09/25/congress-releases-
    war-funds-to-fight-ebola. Accessed 20 Mar 2014

The News (2014a) Ebolavirus: AU summons emergency meeting. The News. http://thenewsni-
    geria.com.ng/2014/09/03/ebolavirus-au-summons-emergency-meeting/. Accessed 3 Sept 2014

The News (2014b) Nigeria frees 319 #Ebolavirus suspects. The News. http://thenewsnigeria.com.
    ng/2014/09/08/nigeria-frees-319-ebolavirus-suspects/. Accessed 8 Sept 2014

The Pharmaceutical Journal (2014) Ebola trials fast tracked in Africa. Pharm J http://www.
    pharmaceutical-journal.com/news-and-analysis/news-in-brief/ebola-trials-fast-tracked-in-
    africa/20066628.article. Accessed 25 Sept 2014

Trbovic P (2014) I had to turn people away from an Ebola treatment centre. It's desperate work.
    The Guardian. http://www.theguardian.com/commentisfree/2014/sep/11/ebola-treatment-cen-
    tre-liberia. Accessed 11 Sept 2014

United Nations (2014a) Ban launches UN Ebola response mission; advance teams to arrive in West
    Africa on Monday. 20 Sept 2014

United Nations (2014b) Secretary-General appoints David Nabarro special envoy on Ebola,
    Anthony Banbury special representative, Head of UN Mission for Ebola Emergency Response.
    23 Sept 2014

United Nations (2014c) Head of new UN Ebola emergency response mission arrives in Ghana. 29
    Sept 2014

UNMEER (2014) An interview with Ebola survivor and frontline responder Dr. Rick Sacra.
    http://ebolaresponse.un.org/interview-ebola-survivor-and-frontline-responder-dr-rick-sacra.
    Accessed 5 Feb 2017

Vanguard (2014) Liberia braces for worst as Ebola death toll jumps. Vanguard. http://www.van-
    guardngr.com/2014/09/liberia-braces-worst-ebola-death-toll-jumps/. Accessed 12 Feb 2017

VICE News (2014) In photos: fighting Ebola in the slums of Monrovia. VICE News. https://news.
    vice.com/article/in-photos-fighting-ebola-in-monrovias-west-point-slum. Accessed 21 Sept
    2014

Webwire (2014) World Bank group to nearly double funding in Ebola crisis to $400 Million.
    Webwire.   http://www.webwire.com/ViewPressRel.asp?aId=191149#.VCRMILd0ziw.
    Accessed 25 Sept 2014

Wexler A, Jerving S (2014) Cocoa prices surge on Ebola fears. Wall Str. J http://online.wsj.com/
    articles/cocoa-surges-on-ebola-fears-1411137838. Accessed 19 Sept 2014

White House (2014a) Fact sheet: U.S. response to the Ebola epidemic in West Africa. Office of the
    Press Secretary. 16 Sept 2014

White House (2014b) Remarks by the president on the Ebola outbreak. Office of the Press
    Secretary. 16 Sept 2014

Whitney E (2014) In this year of Ebola, a Montana YMCA is its brother's keeper. KUNC. http://
    www.kunc.org/post/year-ebola-montana-ymca-its-brothers-keeper. Accessed 24 Sept 2014

WHO Ebola Response Team (2014) Ebola virus disease in West Africa – the first 9 months of the
    epidemic and forward projections. N Engl J Med 371:1481–1495

Winter M (2014) Timeline details missteps with Ebola patient who died. USA Today. https://www.
    usatoday.com/story/news/nation/2014/10/17/ebola-duncan-congress-timeline/17456825/.
    Accessed 9 Apr 2017

Winter T, Flynn ML, Dembo R (2014) Timeline: how Ebola made its way to the United States.
    NBC   News.   http://www.nbcnews.com/storyline/ebola-virus-outbreak/timeline-how-ebola-
    made-its-way-united-states-n216831. Accessed 2 Oct 2014

WOKV (2014) Fmr. Ebola patient delivers testimony before Senate committee. WOKV. http://
    www.wokv.com/weblogs/news-cox-washington-bureau/2014/sep/16/fmr-ebola-patient-deliv-
    ers-testimony-senate-commit/. Accessed 17 Sept 2014

World Bank (2014a) Ebola: World Bank group approves US$105 million grant for faster epidemic containment in Guinea, Liberia, and Sierra Leone. 16 Sept 2014

World Bank (2014b) Ebola: economic impact already serious; could be "catastrophic" without swift response. 17 Sept 2014

World Bulletin (2014) WHO asks for more health workers to fight Ebola. World Bulletin. http://www.worldbulletin.net/news/144242/who-asks-for-more-health-workers-to-fight-ebola. Accessed 12 Sept 2014

World Health Organization (2014a) Situation assessment – virological analysis: no link between Ebola outbreaks in west Africa and Democratic Republic of Congo. 2 Sept 2014

World Health Organization (2014b) Ebola response roadmap. 28 Aug 2014

World Health Organization (2014c) Situation assessment – Ebola situation in Port Harcourt, Nigeria. 3 Sept 2014

World Health Organization (2014d) Ebola response roadmap situation report 2. 5 Sept 2014

World Health Organization (2014e) Ebola response roadmap update. 8 Sept 2014

World Health Organization (2014f) Ebola situation in Liberia: non-conventional interventions needed. 8 Sept 2014

World Health Organization (2014g) Ebola response roadmap situation report 3. 12 Sept 2014

World Health Organization (2014h) Situation assessment – Ebola situation in Senegal remains stable. 12 Sept 2014

World Health Organization (2014i) Ebola response roadmap update. 16 Sept 2014

World Health Organization (2014j) Ebola response roadmap situation report. 18 Sept 2014

World Health Organization (2014k) Ebola response roadmap update. 22 Sept 2014

World Health Organization (2014l) Situation assessment – Nigeria is now free of Ebola virus transmission. 20 Oct 2014

World Health Organization (2014m) Ebola response roadmap situation report. 24 Sept 2014

World Health Organization (2014n) Ebola response roadmap update. 26 Sept 2014

World Health Organization (2014o) Experimental therapies: growing interest in the use of whole blood or plasma from recovered Ebola patients (convalescent therapies). 26 Sept 2014

Xinhua (2014a) China offers new aid for combating Ebola. People's Daily. http://english.people-daily.com.cn/n/2014/0912/c90883-8782123.html. Accessed 12 Sept 2014

Xinhua (2014b) Guinea to deploy medical teams along border with Liberia and Sierra Leone. Shanghai Daily. http://www.shanghaidaily.com/article/article_xinhua.aspx?id=240966. Accessed 15 Sept 2014

Xinhua (2014c) UN mission for Ebola emergency response sets up headquarters in Accra. GBC Ghana. http://gbcghana.com/1.1849234. Accessed 23 Sept 2014

Yan H (2014) 1st Ebola diagnosis in the United States: should we worry? CNN. http://www.cnn.com/2014/10/01/health/ebola-us-no-reason-to-panic/. Accessed 7 Apr 2017

York G (2014) Globe in Monrovia: forced cremation a final indignity in Ebola stricken Liberia. The Globe and Mail. http://www.theglobeandmail.com/news/world/ebola-threat-prompts-red-cross-to-remove-all-bodies-infected-or-not/article20852648/. Accessed 30 Sept 2014

Zambia Daily Mail (2014) Ebola sex workers at risk. Zambia Daily Mail. http://www.daily-mail.co.zm/?p=3528. Accessed 14 Sept 2014

Chapter 5
Global Spread (October 2014)

Abstract As the Ebola outbreak continued to rage in West Africa, Western countries began to be directly affected by the disease. On the last day of September 2014, the first active Ebola case was diagnosed in the United States. Officials in Dallas, Texas, scrambled to contain the virus. A few weeks later, tension rose dramatically when two of the nurses who treated the initial US patient developed Ebola. One of the nurses traveled to Ohio and back before becoming sick. She flew by plane and had contact with other travelers. Officials were very worried that Ebola flare-ups would start to occur across the country. On October 6, 2014, a nursing assistant in Spain was diagnosed with Ebola. Like the US nurses, she had helped treat a repatriated Ebola victim. On October 23, 2014, a new US case was identified. A doctor was diagnosed with Ebola in New York City after returning from Guinea. On the same day, an Ebola case was discovered in the West African country of Mali. The Ebola outbreak seemed out of control and poised to start a major international epidemic. In West Africa, however, a corner had been turned. Healthcare efforts had shifted from treating all Ebola patients in medical facilities to providing families with supplies to take care of sick patients at home. Toward the end of October 2014, reports started to surface about there being fewer cases in West Africa, especially in Liberia. These reports were initially treated with caution. As time progressed, however, it became clear that the drop in cases was real.

5.1 Day-by-Day Outbreak Entries (October 2014)

October 1, 2014 (Wednesday)

Total cases: 7178 (604 new)   Fatalities: 3338 (247 new)
(World Health Organization 2014a)

The Texas Ebola patient has been identified as Thomas Eric Duncan (Onishi 2014). NPR reporter Wade Goodwyn provides an in-depth description of Duncan's illness and the events surrounding his diagnosis:

WADE GOODWYN, BYLINE: The story begins on September 19, when a man in Liberia boarded a plane for Texas. He was tested for fever at the airport and showed none. That's important because this strain of Ebola is not contagious until symptoms of the illness begin

© Springer International Publishing AG, part of Springer Nature 2018
S. G. Bullard, *A Day-by-Day Chronicle of the 2013-2016 Ebola Outbreak*,
https://doi.org/10.1007/978-3-319-76565-5_5

to present in the patient. For three days after he arrived in Dallas on the 20th, all was well. But last Wednesday, the man became sick. By Friday, he was so ill he went to the emergency room at Presbyterian Hospital. Dr. Edward Goodman, the top infectious disease specialist at Presbyterian, describes what happened next.

(SOUNDBITE OF ARCHIVED RECORDING)

EDWARD GOODMAN: I think he was evaluated for his illness, which was very nondescript. He had some laboratory tests, which were not very impressive. And he was dismissed on some antibiotic because he was like the majority of people who come in the emergency room.

GOODWYN: If Dr. Goodman sounds the tiniest bit defensive, it's because of what happened next. Although the ER staff didn't realize it, Presby released an infected, contagious Ebola patient back into the general population. It will be this span of time, from when the Ebola symptoms first presented themselves up until when the man was admitted to the hospital, that the Centers for Disease Control and Prevention will focus its tracking effort. As for the man who came from Liberia, as the weekend came to a close, he'd grown so seriously ill with Ebola he returned to Presbyterian. Dr. Goodman says this go-around, the ER staff figured out what they were looking at pretty quickly.

(SOUNDBITE OF ARCHIVED RECORDING)

GOODWYN: I think those caring for him were suspicious of that almost immediately. The emergency room people identified that as a concern and consulted infection prevention department, which is my department, and consulted the infectious disease clinician. And that was on the top of everyone's list.

GOODWYN: Ebola - it had quietly slipped into Dallas through the eighth-busiest airport in the world. Though the diagnosis would not be confirmed by the CDC for another two days, the patient was nevertheless whisked away into the hospital's isolation unit in intensive care. (Goodwyn 2014)

Four members of Thomas Duncan's family have been ordered to stay in their home until October 19, 2014 (Altman 2014; Szabo 2014a). They have also been ordered to submit to health tests, provide blood samples, and report any Ebola-like symptoms to Dallas County Health and Human Services. The written orders were hand-delivered to the family this evening (Altman 2014; Szabo 2014a).

Currently, 12–18 people who had contact with Duncan are being monitored (NBC News 2014a). Healthcare workers who interacted with him have all tested negative for Ebola. They will continue to be monitored for the next 21 days. The Dallas mayor's office says the three-person EMS crew who transported Duncan to the hospital has been quarantined (Whitely 2014). Similarly, the ambulance that carried him, ambulance No. 37, has been isolated and sealed with biohazard tape (Whitely 2014; Yan 2014a). Five students from four different schools, including two elementary schools, a middle school, and a high school, had contact with Duncan (Perez 2014). None of the children have symptoms of Ebola, but they are all being monitored at home. Dallas schools remain open (NBC News 2014a).

Duncan had been staying at the Ivy Apartments in Northeast Dallas (CBS DFW 2014a; Lopez 2014). Residents of the complex are worried that they may have been exposed to Ebola. They are also bothered by the lack of information officials have given them. The city activated a reverse 911 system to notify residents in the area, but people say it did little to remove their fears (Lopez 2014). The level of concern among other Dallas residents varies (Business Journals 2014; Hylton 2014). Some people are exceptionally worried. Others are unconcerned. A few think the dangers of the disease are overstated. Overall, most Dallas residents do not seem overly alarmed by the appearance of Ebola in their community (Business Journals 2014; Hylton 2014).

Stock prices fell on the news of the first US Ebola case. Airline stocks were especially hard-hit. Delta is down to 3.5%. Southwest is down to 2.8%. In contrast, stocks of companies working on Ebola treatments rose. Tekmira Pharmaceuticals is up 17% (Reuters 2014a).

Conditions in the Ebola holding center of Makeni, Sierra Leone, remain grim. During a recent visit, a reporter found a 4-year-old girl lying on the floor. She was in a puddle of urine and had blood coming from her mouth. In the corner was the body of a dead young woman. When a body recovery team arrived, they collected the body and sprayed the living little girl with chlorine (Nossiter 2014a).

Ambulance crews in Liberia do not have the authority to force patients to go for treatment. In Monrovia, an obviously sick man recently refused to board an ambulance. He said that he hadn't been near anyone who had died. Neighbors contradicted this and said that one of the man's family members had recently died. On further questioning, the man said if he left, no one would take care of his children (Larson 2014).

Mauritius will not allow foreign nationals to enter the country if they have visited an Ebola-affected country within 2 months of their arrival (Warner 2014).

October 2, 2014 (Thursday)
Four relatives of Thomas Duncan are quarantined in the apartment where Duncan became sick. They are his partner Louise Troh, her 13-year-old son, and two nephews in their 20s (Associated Press 2014a; Szabo 2014a). Troh is very worried that the apartment is contaminated. The sheets and towels used by Duncan are still in the residence (Martinez 2014).

As of this morning, 80 people had been identified who were known to have had contact with Duncan (Reuters 2014b). By noon, the number had risen to 100 (Altman 2014).

Attendance in Dallas area schools is down (Fernandez et al. 2014). Frightened parents are keeping their children home. School attendance was about 86% today. It is normally around 95% at this time of year (Fernandez et al. 2014). A high school student in Frisco, Texas, has been arrested for posting a false Twitter message saying that Ebola was infecting people in Frisco (Margason 2014).

When Thomas Duncan left Liberia, he answered "no" to questions about whether he had contact with Ebola victims. As a result, Liberia says it will prosecute him if he returns to the country (Stanglin 2014a).

Ashoka Mukpo, a 33-year-old American freelance cameraman working for NBC in Liberia, has contracted Ebola (Barbash 2014; NBC News 2014b). Mukpo had a fever during a routine check on Wednesday, October 1, 2014. Tests confirmed he has Ebola. He will be returned to the United States for treatment. The rest of his news team, including NBC News Chief Medical Editor and Correspondent Dr. Nancy Snyderman, will return with him and be isolated for 21 days (Barbash 2014). Currently, no one else on the team has Ebola symptoms (NBC News 2014b).

It is unclear how to deal with the hazardous waste generated by US Ebola patients. The waste should be incinerated or autoclaved, but few US hospitals are equipped to handle large amounts of infected material (NBC News 2014c).

Save the Children estimates that five people in Sierra Leone are being infected with Ebola every hour (BBC 2014a). The agency also says that last week, only 327 treatment beds were available for 765 new cases (BBC 2014a). Sierra Leone's Ministry of Health and Sanitation says 8478 households have been quarantined since May 2014 (Tommy 2014).

Due to border closures associated with the Ebola outbreak, less food is available in West Africa. Indigenous food production is also down, and food prices have increased. For example, in some areas of Sierra Leone, 40% of farms have been abandoned. The cost of palm oil has increased by 40% in 4 weeks. Overall, trade in West African food markets is down to 50% (Hussain and Arsenault 2014).

Up to 500 troops from the 1st Armored Division will deploy to West Africa in the next few weeks. The troops are currently stationed at Fort Bliss, Texas. They will provide logistic and air support for US Ebola efforts (Kocherga 2014).

Australia has increased its financial support for Ebola-fighting efforts to $16 M. It is still unwilling to send personnel to West Africa (McGuirk 2014).

October 3, 2014 (Friday)

Total cases: 7492 (314 new)   Fatalities: 3439 (101 new)
                               (World Health Organization 2014b)

Five members of the Dallas County Sheriff's Department who entered Thomas Duncan's apartment have been placed on leave (Eiserer 2014). They include three deputies, a sergeant, and a lieutenant. The officers visited Duncan's apartment the night of October 1, 2014, to deliver a court order. The head of Dallas County Health and Human Services Department and a doctor were also present (Eiserer 2014). Late today, Duncan's family was moved to a new location (CBS DFW 2014b). They remain under quarantine but are now in a donated four-bedroom home in an unspecified gated community (CBS DFW 2014b). The number of contacts under surveillance in Dallas has been lowered to about 50. Ten of these are thought to be at high risk of exposure (Dallas News 2014; Ghebremedhin et al. 2014).

Brett Adamson, an Australian aid worker in Monrovia, Liberia, describes the development of the local crematorium. Workers initially cremated about 20 bodies a day at the site. This was not enough, so an additional altar was built to increase the capacity to 60 bodies a day. More recently, a road has been built leading to the crematorium and a large incinerator has been delivered. Now about 100 bodies a day can be cremated (Newcastle Herald 2014).

The Reverend Father Peter Konteh of Sierra Leone describes some of his experiences with the Ebola outbreak. Father Konteh knew the late Dr. Modupeh Cole. Cole worked for Connaught Hospital in Freetown. One day, a patient walked into the hospital and collapsed. Dr. Cole instinctively ran to catch him. After taking care of the patient, Cole realized the patient could be infected with Ebola, so he quarantined himself in a room in his house. Two days later he developed a fever. Dr. Cole died on August 13, 2014. Father Konteh's home is near King Tom Cemetery. He can see the funerals of Ebola victims from his house. He thinks the government is underreporting the number of fatalities. For example, one day the government said three people had died. However, Father Konteh personally witnessed ten burials (Dribben 2014).

Hospitals in Sierra Leone are running out of basic supplies. Standard equipment like body bags, alcohol gel, and gloves are being consumed at a tremendous rate. Adam Goguen, director of academic affairs at the University of Makeni, says the staff has almost no PPE and medicine is becoming scarce (O'Carroll 2014a).

An infected Ugandan doctor, Dr. Michael Mawanda, has arrived at University Hospital in Frankfurt, Germany, for treatment. Dr. Mawanda had been working in Sierra Leone (ABC News 2014a; Agaba 2014). This is the second time an infected person has been transferred to Germany for treatment.

Infected NBC cameraman Ashoka Mukpo will be transported to the Nebraska Medical Center for treatment (Freyer 2014).

UNMEER released a statement saying there is no evidence that Ebola has become airborne (UNMEER 2014a).

About 120 soldiers from Fort Bragg will deploy to West Africa later this month (Associated Press 2014b). The troops will come from the 86th Combat Support Hospital, the 44th Medical Brigade, and the 16th Military Police Brigade (Associated Press 2014b). Fort Carson will send about 160 soldiers from the 615th Engineer Company, 52nd Engineer Battalion, to West Africa (Associated Press 2014c).

The US military says it is continually assessing the situation in West Africa and could request an additional 1000 troops to help with the Ebola outbreak (Vanden Brook and Jackson 2014).

October 4, 2014 (Saturday)
Thomas Duncan is now in critical condition at Texas Health Presbyterian Hospital in Dallas (Karimi and Sutton 2014). He is being treated with the experimental antiviral drug brincidofovir (Keneally and Battiste 2014). The CDC says 114 people in Texas have been tested for Ebola (Zwirko 2014). None of them, including nine people who are considered to be at high risk of exposure, are showing symptoms of the disease (Zwirko 2014).

Workers at the Ebola treatment center in Bong County, Liberia, have walked off the job. They say that the International Medical Corps has not fully paid them and has not provided them with the food it promised. They also lack appropriate PPE (Lomax 2014).

A MSF volunteer nurse has been released from a French hospital after recovering from Ebola. The patient arrived in France on September 18, 2014 (Reuters 2014c).

Canada is sending a second mobile medical lab and two scientists to Sierra Leone to help with the Ebola outbreak (Reuters 2014d).

In Newark, New Jersey, a father and daughter were removed from a United Airlines flight and taken to the hospital. The father had been exhibiting Ebola-like symptoms. The flight was coming from Brussels, and the passengers are thought to be from Liberia (7 Online 2014).

October 5, 2014 (Sunday)
Sierra Leone says there were 121 new Ebola deaths on Saturday October 4, 2014. This is the highest 1-day fatality total to date (Reuters 2014e).

Another high-level doctor, Dr. John Taban Dada, has died from Ebola in Liberia (Agaba 2014).

Politics and bureaucracy are hampering the distribution of Ebola supplies in West Africa. In one case, a shipping container with supplies and PPE has been waiting on the docks of Freetown, Sierra Leone, since August 9, 2014. It is there because a $6500 shipping fee has not been paid (Nossiter 2014b).

The CDC is handling 800 calls a day about Ebola (Villacorta 2014).

Scientists estimate there is a 75% chance Ebola will arrive in France by October 24, 2014. There is a 50% chance it will arrive in Britain by October 24, 2014 (Reuters 2014f).

Israel will send three mobile medical units to West Africa (JTA 2014).

October 6, 2014 (Monday)
A Spanish nursing assistant [María Teresa Romero Ramos] has contracted Ebola in Spain (Brumfield and Levs 2014; Minder and Grady 2014). The nursing assistant helped treat infected priest Brother Manuel Garcia Viejo in Spain's Carlos III Hospital. She developed symptoms on Tuesday, September 30, 2014, and was hospitalized today. Officials are now trying to determine who she had contact with before she was isolated. This is the first documented case of Ebola transmission outside of Africa during the outbreak (Brumfield and Levs 2014; Minder and Grady 2014).

Numerous reporting agencies described María Teresa Romero Ramos's Ebola infection and her efforts to contact medical authorities about her initial symptoms. Taken as a whole, these reports are convoluted and often contradictory. For example, the media usually refers to Ramos as a nurse, though she appears to have been a nursing assistant (e.g., Wheaton 2014). The following represents the best effort to provide an accurate description and timeline of Ramos's activities. Ramos entered Brother Viejo's room twice, once to change his undergarments and once to collect his personal belongings after his death (Alexander H 2014; Phillip and Ferdman 2014). She may have become infected when she touched her face with a gloved hand while removing her PPE (Independent.ie 2014). However, the use of substandard equipment and poor operating procedures may have contributed to her infection. Hospital staff told the investigators that the PPE they were issued did not meet WHO standards (Kassam 2014a; Phillip and Ferdman 2014). For example, gloves were simply sealed with adhesive tape. There were other problems with the care of Ebola patients at the hospital as well. For example, medical waste from Ebola patients was transported out of the hospital via the staff elevator (Kassam 2014a). Ramos left for vacation on the Spanish coast soon after Brother Viejo died (Morris 2014). On September 30, 2014, she developed a fever. She contacted occupational risk personnel at Carlos III Hospital about her condition. Because her fever was below 101.5 °F, she was advised to go to her local clinic (Kassam 2014b). During the early stages of her illness, Ramos used public transportation, visited restaurants and shops, and spent time with friends (Nadeau 2014). On October 2, 2014, she called Carlos III Hospital again to report that she still had a fever. She was directed [presumably meaning her call was routed] to a department of Madrid's regional health service (Botelho et al. 2014). It is unclear what she was told, but no significant action was advised (Kassam 2014b). She called the hospital again today to say she was severely ill (Kassam 2014b). She was advised to go to the nearest emergency facility, which was Alcorcón. She was transported to the hospital by paramedics. At Alcorcón, she told the staff she thought she had Ebola, but she was kept in the general emergency ward (Kassam 2014b).

Infected NBC cameraman Ashoka Mukpo has arrived in Nebraska for treatment. Mukpo may have become infected when he was splashed with disinfectant while cleaning a car in which an Ebola victim had died (Keneally 2014a).

MSF says a Norwegian worker in Sierra Leone [Dr. Silje Michalsen] has contracted Ebola (Médecins Sans Frontières 2014). The patient will be transported to Oslo, Norway, for treatment (Reuters 2014g). The 30-year-old Michalsen developed a fever on October 2, 2014, and tested positive for Ebola on October 3 (The Health Site 2014).

Liberian healthcare workers plan a work slowdown. The workers are trying to get the government to issue their Ebola hazard pay (Reuters 2014h).

US troops have begun constructing the main hospital tent for a new 25-bed facility in Monrovia, Liberia (Associated Press 2014d). Heavy rains are slowing the work.

A US C-130J loaded with Ebola-fighting supplies has been sent from Ramstein Air Base, Germany, to Monrovia (Svan and DeMotts 2014). This is the first time a European-based air unit has been sent to the Ebola zone.

Representative Frank Wolf (R-Virginia) and Senator Jerry Moran (R-Kansas) have sent a letter to President Obama requesting that he appoint an overall US Ebola coordinator (Marcos 2014).

A US airline trade group will meet with government officials to review screening procedures for passengers from Ebola-infected areas (Dastin 2014).

October 7, 2014 (Tuesday)
The infected Spanish nurse [María Teresa Romero Ramos] is being given injections of antibodies from Ebola survivors (Sharkov 2014). The nurse's husband has been quarantined, as has a second nurse who helped treat Brother Viejo (Associated Press 2014e, Morris 2014). The second nurse has diarrhea, but does not have a fever (Associated Press 2014e). Thirty other healthcare workers at Carlos III Hospital have been placed under observation. Twenty-two people at Alcorcón hospital have been contacted by health officials (Bennett 2014). Officials plan to euthanize and cremate the infected nurse's dog, named "Excalibur" (Hatton and Giles 2014).

A group of Spanish healthcare workers protested the poor management of Ebola patients in Spain (Hatton and Giles 2014).

Thomas Duncan remains in critical condition in Dallas. He is now on a ventilator and is receiving kidney dialysis (Garza and Valdmanis 2014). Ashoka Mukpo is being treated with brincidofovir (Herriman 2014).

In Freetown, Sierra Leone, the cemetery at Connaught Hospital is filling rapidly. There are hundreds of recent graves. Most of the graves are unmarked, but some have a cross or a few toys scattered on them. About 400 bodies have been interred in the cemetery in the last few weeks (Mazumdar 2014).

An obviously infected man was recently turned away from an Italian NGO clinic near Freetown, Sierra Leone. He had red eyes and hiccups. A doctor inside the clinic explained that the facility was at capacity and simply could not accept any more patients. If they did, it would put the staff and current patients at risk. The sick man died the next day at an isolation center (Mazumdar 2014).

Burial workers have gone on strike in two of Sierra Leone's districts. They have not been paid in 2 weeks. Each 12-man burial team has been burying between 17 and 35 bodies a day (Reuters 2014i).

The EU has activated its Early Warning and Response System (Román 2014). The network allows EU members to share information about disease outbreaks and coordinate responses (Román 2014). The EU will also increase its aid to Ebola-affected countries. The EU's Emergency Response Coordination Center will begin airlifting supplies to the region starting Friday, October 10, 2014 (UNMEER 2014b).

News of the infected Spanish nurse has led to a drop in tourism-related stocks (Martin 2014). In contrast, shares of Lakeland Industries, a maker of hazmat suits, have risen 40% since Thomas Duncan was diagnosed with Ebola (Udland 2014).

Four major hospitals in the United Kingdom have been placed on standby to receive any future UK Ebola cases. The hospitals are Royal Free Hospital in North London, Royal Liverpool University Hospital Foundation Trust, Newcastle upon Tyne Hospital Foundation Trust, and Sheffield Teaching Hospital NHS Foundation Trust (Donnelly and Knapton 2014).

The Atlanta airport is giving CDC fliers to passengers arriving from Ebola-affected countries. The fliers describe Ebola and encourage readers to seek medical assistance if they have had contact with Ebola victims or develop symptoms (Associated Press 2014f).

Gambia Bird Airlines will resume flights to Freetown, Sierra Leone, starting October 17, 2014 (Awoko 2014).

October 8, 2014 (Wednesday)

Total cases: 8033 (541 new)   Fatalities: 3865 (426 new)
                                    (World Health Organization 2014c)

Thomas Duncan died in Dallas at 0751 h today. His remains were handled according to CDC guidelines. His body was placed inside two sealed body bags, disinfected, and cremated. A service was held for Duncan today at the Wilshire Baptist Church at 4316 Abrams Road in Dallas (Wiley 2014).

Michael Monnig, a Dallas County Sheriff's Deputy who entered Duncan's home, has fallen ill and been isolated (Rahmanzadeh and Mohney 2014). Monnig helped deliver the quarantine order to Duncan's family. He was in the residence for about 30 min, but was not wearing any PPE (CBS DFW 2014c). It is unclear if he has Ebola.

The infected Spanish nurse has been identified as María Teresa Romero Ramos (Wheaton 2014). Her name was revealed when her husband posted an online letter appealing for their dog "Excalibur" to be spared from euthanasia (Wheaton 2014). Unfortunately, the dog was put down today (Minder and Belluck 2014).

Sierra Leone burial teams have returned to work. A government official says their strike has been resolved. During the short strike, there were reports of unattended bodies lying in the streets (Kamara 2014).

A UN medical worker has contracted Ebola in Liberia (Reuters 2014j).

The cost to care for an Ebola patient in the United States is exceptionally high. It is estimated that Thomas Duncan's treatment cost between $18,000 and 24,000 per day (Wayne 2014). Total cost for his care may reach $0.5 M (Wayne 2014). The World Bank estimates that Ebola could cost the global economy up to $32 B, depending on how severe the outbreak becomes (CBS News 2014a).

Dr. Kent Brantly has donated blood for infected NBC cameraman Ashoka Mukpo (NBC News 2014d). Separately, the doctor [Dr. Lewis Rubinson] who had been under observation at the NIH in Maryland after a needlestick has been released (Schnirring 2014). He has not developed symptoms, but will remain at home for another 21-day observation period.

Five US airports (JFK, Newark Liberty, Dulles, O'Hare, and Hartsfield-Jackson) will begin screening passengers from Ebola-affected countries for fevers and will observe passengers for signs of Ebola (Centers for Disease Control and Prevention 2014a). About 150 people arrive in the United States each day from Sierra Leone, Liberia, and Guinea. Of these, 94% arrive at these five major airports (Kelto 2014; Centers for Disease Control and Prevention 2014a). Canada will also screen passengers arriving from West Africa (Hume 2014).

The United Kingdom will deploy 750 troops, three helicopters, and a naval vessel to help fight Ebola in West Africa (Cooper et al. 2014).

October 9, 2014 (Thursday)
María Teresa Romero Ramos's condition has worsened. She is now intubated (Kassam 2014c).

Dr. Juan Manuel Parra helped treat Ramos in the Alcorcón emergency room. He published an open letter describing his interactions with Ramos and raising concerns about the care of Ebola patients in Spain (Ohlheiser and Phillip 2014; Penty and Munoz 2014). Dr. Parra says he worked with Ramos for 16 h during which time she vomited and had diarrhea. The PPE he was issued, however, was inadequate, and the sleeves were too short (Penty and Munoz 2014). Dr. Parra and a second Spanish doctor who treated Ramos have both been placed under observation (Ohlheiser and Phillip 2014). A total of seven people were isolated in Spain today, including two hairdressers who had worked on Ramos (Dowsett 2014).

Dallas Deputy Michael Monnig has tested negative for Ebola (Houston Chronicle 2014).

Because of the Ebola outbreak, the Liberia government will postpone senate elections that were originally scheduled for October 14, 2014 (Sputnik International 2014). A new date for the elections has not been set.

Schools remain closed in Sierra Leone. To make sure children receive some education, the country has started broadcasting educational lessons. Parents are encouraged to have their kids listen to the 4-h programs (Ohlheiser 2014).

Ships sailing directly from West Africa to ports in Brazil and Argentina will have to wait 10 days before they will be allowed to dock. It takes about 10 days for ships to reach South America from Africa. This 10-day travel time, plus the additional 10-day waiting period, will approximate the 21-day Ebola incubation period (Hellenic Shipping News 2014).

A British man who died at the Clinic of Infectious Disease in Skopje, Macedonia, may have had Ebola. The man had Ebola-like symptoms and died soon after he was admitted (Casule 2014; MINA 2014). However, his travel history is unclear, and it is not certain if he had been in an area with Ebola.

In New York, about 200 airline cabin cleaners staged a protest. This was partly due to their concern about possible on-the-job exposure to Ebola. The cleaners say they frequently find hypodermic needles, vomit, and blood as they clean the planes (ABC News 2014b).

One hundred additional US marines have landed in Monrovia, Liberia. This brings the total number of US troops in the country to about 300 (Paye-Layleh and Giles 2014).

Britain will start screening passengers for Ebola at Heathrow and Gatwick airports and at the Eurostar rail terminal (Reuters 2014k).

October 10, 2014 (Friday)

Total cases: 8399 (366 new)   Fatalities: 4033 (168 new)
                               (World Health Organization 2014d)

A total of 14 people are now under observation in Spain (Dowsett 2014). At Carlos III Hospital, some staff are making excuses to avoid work (Kassam 2014d). When Spanish Prime Minister Mariano Rajoy visited the hospital today, angry protestors threw surgical gloves at his car (Reuters 2014l).

Officials in Sierra Leone have begun shifting the focus away from caring for Ebola patients at medical facilities to helping families care for sick individuals at home (Nossiter 2014c). Sierra Leone has realized that it does not have, and will not have, enough beds to care for all of its infected citizens. Currently, there are 304 Ebola treatment beds in the country, but 1148 are needed. Instead of trying to find additional space for victims in hospitals, healthcare workers will now distribute painkillers, rehydrating solution, and gloves to the families of Ebola victims (Nossiter 2014c). There were 140 Ebola deaths in Sierra Leone today, the highest 1-day fatality count to date (Douglas 2014).

Liberia's healthcare system is overwhelmed by the Ebola outbreak. Clinics remain completely full. Non-Ebola cases are often turned away no matter how sick the patient is. In one recent case, a 21-year-old named Nikita Forh died from complications of an asthma attack. Before they would treat her, the doctors at JFK hospital in Monrovia wanted her to provide a certificate proving she did not have Ebola (Reuters 2014m).

Liberian President Ellen Johnson Sirleaf has requested additional governmental powers to combat Ebola. Among other things, Sirleaf is asking for the power to restrict movement, prevent public gatherings, and appropriate property. Some lawmakers worry that Liberia will turn into a police state if the President is given these rights (Paye-Layleh 2014a).

An infected UN Sudanese doctor has been evacuated from Liberia to Leipzig, Germany, for treatment (Health Site 2014). In Liberia, the UN has isolated 41 workers, including 20 military personnel, who had contact with an infected staff member [most likely the Sudanese doctor]. The infected staffer developed Ebola symptoms on October 5, 2014, and tested positive for the disease several days later (AFP 2014a).

Trials of the GlaxoSmithKline Ebola vaccine have begun in Mali. Healthcare workers have been inoculated with the vaccine to assess the vaccine's safety and see if recipients develop Ebola antibodies (Boseley 2014a).

October 11, 2014 (Saturday)
Liberia has banned journalists from Ebola clinics. It is thought that this is to keep reporters from revealing the scope of the outbreak and to prevent them from reporting on protests by healthcare workers. MSF will petition the government to exclude its clinics from the ban (Charlton 2014).

Thirteen-year-old Bintu Sannoh describes her experience with Ebola in Sierra Leone. The disease began in her community when a pharmacist died. He had said that he had a septic ulcer, not Ebola, so he was given a traditional burial. About 2 weeks after his funeral, people who had washed his corpse began to get sick. Soon many people in the community were affected, including Sannoh's aunt. In less than 2 weeks, 26 people developed Ebola. Seventeen of them died. Healthcare workers in full PPE came to the community. They disinfected homes and burned infected bedding. This probably helped control the outbreak, but it terrified the residents and made them even more frightened (Sannoh 2014).

Ebola training for Spanish healthcare workers continues to be substandard. For example, medical experts say it takes 10–14 days to become fully proficient in donning, using, and removing PPE. In contrast, one Spanish doctor says his training consisted of a 10-min briefing followed by being shown some photographs about how to care for Ebola patients (Govan 2014).

Health officials in New Jersey have imposed a mandatory quarantine on Nancy Snyderman's NBC News team (Wagner 2014). The team had returned to the United States after cameraman Ashoka Mukpo contacted Ebola in Liberia. They were in voluntary isolation when at least one team member broke quarantine. This forced officials to legally order the group to remain isolated (Wagner 2014). It was later learned that on October 9, 2014, Nancy Snyderman and several team members were seen outside the Peasant Grill restaurant in Hopewell, New Jersey (Day 2014).

Ebola screening has begun at New York's JFK airport (Malo 2014).

October 12, 2014 (Sunday)
A healthcare worker [Nina Pham] who assisted Thomas Duncan at Texas Health Presbyterian Hospital has tested positive for Ebola (Du Lac et al. 2014; Rainone 2014). This is the first known case of person-to-person Ebola transmission in the

United States. Texas Health Presbyterian Hospital's ER has been put on "diversion," which means no new patients will be admitted (du Lac et al. 2014). The healthcare worker lives on the 3700 block of Marquita Avenue in Dallas (Rainone 2014). The area around the apartment has been decontaminated and secured by police (Rainone 2014). Neighbors have been notified about the case (Fox News 2014a). All telephone lines within a four-block radius of the worker's apartment received a reverse 911 call:

> *THIS IS AN IMPORANT MESSAGE FROM THE CITY OF DALLAS*
>
> *Please be advised that a heath care worker who lives in your area has tested positive for Ebola. This individual is in the hospital and isolated. Precautions are already in process to clean all known potential areas of contact to ensure public health.*
>
> *While this may be concerning, there is no ongoing danger to your health. The virus does not spread through casual contact.*
>
> *The City of Dallas is working closely with the Centers for Disease Control and Prevention, Dallas County, Dallas Independent School District, and Community Leaders to protect your health.*
>
> *For more information please call 311 or Dallas County Health and Human Services at 214-819-2004.* (ABC 13 Eyewitness News 2014)

Nina Pham developed a fever on Friday October 10, 2014, and was isolated late on Saturday (Du Lac et al. 2014; Rainone 2014). Only 90 min elapsed from time Pham realized she had symptoms until she was isolated (Rainone 2014). Pham helped Duncan several times during his second trip to the ER, but she always wore full PPE. As a result, the CDC did not consider her at high risk of exposure (du Lac et al. 2014).

In Liberia, members of the National Health Workers Association are threatening to strike over reduced hazard pay. At the start of the outbreak, Liberia authorized nurses working with Ebola patients to receive $700 a month hazard pay. As the scale of the outbreak increased, this sum was deemed a financial burden to the state. The payment was reduced to $435 a month. The nurses want their pay returned to the initial levels. They will begin striking at midnight Monday October 13, 2014, unless an agreement is reached. It is thought that the government is speeding up the licensing student nurses so they can take the place of striking nurses (Associated Press 2014g).

NPR correspondent Jason Beaubien was in Morovia, Liberia, in August 2014 and has recently returned to the city (Silver 2014). He compares the mood in the city today with his last visit:

> *There's a bit of a sense of Ebola is becoming the new normal. The streets are supercrowded and busy. Despite government declarations that people aren't supposed to gather in large crowds [to prevent the spread of Ebola], the markets look like any street scene. Traffic was fairly light in August but it's once again terrible. There are traffic jams. It feels like, in many ways, life has gone back to normal.*
>
> *On the radio everybody is still talking about Ebola, and there are lots of Ebola songs, some old ones, some new ones, and signs everywhere about Ebola. All schools remain closed.* (Silver 2014)

Operators for Britain's NHS non-emergency 111 number will try to identify possible Ebola cases. If a caller reports Ebola-like symptoms, the operators will ask about their travel history. If Ebola is possible, emergency services will be contacted (BBC 2014b).

Budget and personnel cuts may have weakened the ability of the United States to respond the Ebola crisis. The CDC's Public Health Emergency Preparedness budget declined from $1.1 B in 2006 to $585 M in 2013. Between 2008 and 2013, local health departments shed 48,300 jobs – a 15% reduction in personnel (Begley and Abutaleb 2014).

October 13, 2014 (Monday)
The infected Dallas nurse has been identified as 26-year-old Nina Pham (Associated Press 2014h). She received a blood transfusion from Ebola survivor Kent Brantly today (Associated Press 2014h). Nina Pham's dog, a Cavalier King Charles spaniel named "Bentley," is under surveillance at an undisclosed location (CBS News 2014b; Douglas and Owens 2014). It is unclear if pets can catch or transmit Ebola (CBS News 2014b). To be safe, Spain euthanized María Teresa Romero Ramos's dog. Officials in the United States have been very clear that they plan to save and care for Pham's dog (Douglas and Owens 2014).

While speaking about the Ebola outbreak, WHO Director Dr. Margaret Chan said she had never seen a disease with such a strong potential to cause societal failure within a country (World Health Organization 2014e).

Despite the threat of a strike, healthcare workers in Liberia generally reported for work today (Associated Press 2014i). It is unclear if the issues associated with the planned strike have been resolved or if the strike has been postponed.

Friends of infected cameraman Ashoka Mukpo are raising money to help pay for his medical treatment. It is thought that the total cost for his medical care will be about $500,000. His flight from Liberia to the United States alone cost $150,000. Mukpo had travelers insurance, but it does not cover evacuations caused by disease outbreaks (Associated Press 2014j).

A survey of US nurses finds that 76% have not been provided with an official policy about how to admit Ebola patients to their hospitals. Eighty-five percent say that they have not been provided with interactive Ebola training (Chuck 2014).

The British government has ordered 500,000 hazmat suits from Arco (Cutlack 2014). Germany says it currently has 50 beds available to treat Ebola patients (The Local 2014).

October 14, 2014 (Tuesday)
Police in the Aberdeen community of Freetown, Sierra Leone, used tear gas and live rounds (presumably fired into the air) to disperse angry residents. The residents were protesting the fact that the body of a young woman had been in the streets for 2 days. She is thought to have died from Ebola (Olu-Mammah and Giahyue 2014).

A battalion of 800 Sierra Leone peacekeepers bound for Somalia has been quarantined because a Sierra Leone soldier has tested positive for Ebola (Shankar 2014). The infected soldier is not part of the quarantine unit (Associated Press 2014k). However, the battalion will be quarantined for 21 days before they are deployed (Shankar 2014).

President of Guinea Alpha Condé issued an urgent appeal to retired doctors. He is asking them return to work to help with the Ebola outbreak (Associated Press 2014l).

The CDC is developing specialized Ebola response teams. They will be immediately sent to any US hospital that identifies an Ebola case (Fox 2014).

WHO Assistant Director-General Bruce Aylward warned that by December, 2014, there could be 5000–10,000 new Ebola cases each week in West Africa (Boseley 2014b). However, he also said that the rates of infection have been relatively stable for the past few weeks and this could indicate that the outbreak is slowing down (Achenbach 2014). A press statement released by the WHO today described an unexpected pattern seen in the outbreak. Infected areas often experience a slow decline in cases and then experience a sudden flare-up (World Health Organization 2014f).

The UN worker being treated for Ebola in Leipzig, Germany, has died. He was 56 years old and tested positive for Ebola on October 6, 2014 (Associated Press 2014m).

The *RFA Argus*, a British naval medical vessel, is preparing to sail to West Africa to help with the outbreak (BBC 2014c).

Facebook CEO Mark Zuckerberg and his wife have donated $25 M to help the CDC fight Ebola (Guynn 2014).

October 15, 2014 (Wednesday)

Total cases: 8997 (598 new)   Fatalities: 4493 (460 new)
(World Health Organization 2014g)

A second Dallas nurse who worked with Thomas Duncan has tested positive for Ebola. The new patient is 29-year-old Amber Joy Vinson (Fox News 2014b; Yan 2014b). Unlike Nina Pham who had only been in Dallas before she was diagnosed with Ebola, Vinson had traveled to and from Tallmadge, Ohio (about 30 miles south of Cleveland), before being diagnosed (Berman 2014). Vinson flew to Cleveland on October 10, 2014, and returned October 13 (Berman 2014; Shoichet et al. 2014). She developed a 99.5 °F fever before boarding the return plane (NBC DFW 2014). There were 132 other passengers on her return flight, Frontier Airlines flight 1143 (WKYC 2014). The CDC is asking passengers to contact the agency, so they can determine who might have been exposed to Vinson (Berman 2014; WKYC 2014). Vinson's apartment, located in the Village Apartments in Dallas, is being decontaminated (Associated Press 2014n; Zeeble 2014). Her stepfather's home in the Stonegate Reserve neighborhood in Tallmadge, Ohio, has been cordoned off by police (Harper 2014). Around midday today, health officials decided to move Vinson to Emory University Hospital for treatment. She arrived in Atlanta this evening (NBC News 2014e).

CDC Director Thomas Frieden said he was upset that Vinson had flown even though she had treated an Ebola patient and developed a fever (Shoichet et al. 2014). It was later revealed, however, that Vinson had sought CDC approval before her flight (NBC DFW 2014; WKYC 2014). Vinson called the CDC on Monday. She explained her situation, and said she had a 99.5 °F fever. The person she talked with checked the CDC website for guidance. It said that it was ok for a person with uncertain risk to fly if their temperature was below 100.4 °F (NBC DFW 2014). Dr. Frieden was not aware of these facts when he made his initial statements. In the future, however, the CDC vows that anyone who has had contact with infected patients will not be allowed to travel on commercial airlines (Shoichet et al. 2014). It is unclear how this travel ban will be enforced, but it has been suggested that people under Ebola surveillance might be placed on the Transportation Security Administration's no-fly list (Sheets 2014).

National Nurses United, a US nursing union, has released a highly critical assessment of Texas Health Presbyterian Hospital's handling of Ebola patient Thomas Duncan. Citing unnamed nurses at the hospital, the report describes numerous failings of the facility. Specifically, the report says:

1. Protocols were constantly changing.
2. Duncan was not immediately isolated when he returned to the hospital the second time.
3. The PPE nurses were issued did not cover their necks; instead nurses were instructed to wrap medical tape around their necks.
4. Hazardous waste was not collected in a timely fashion and piled up.
5. Nurses were given no hands-on Ebola training (Shoichet 2014).

The CDC is currently monitoring 125 people in the United States for Ebola symptoms, including 76 who had contact with Thomas Duncan (Washington Examiner 2014).

President Obama canceled a trip to New England and convened an emergency Ebola meeting at the White House. Officials from the CDC, HHS, and DOD attended (Dwyer 2014).

The WHO says there are currently 620 Ebola treatment beds in Liberia, 346 in Sierra Leone, and 160 in Guinea. These represent only 21–50% of the planned number of beds for these countries. Through October 12, 2014, 427 healthcare workers have contracted Ebola. Of these, 236 have died (World Health Organization 2014g).

Several Ebola cases have been confirmed in Koinadugu District, Sierra Leone. Koinadugu was the last unaffected district in the country. Ebola has now reached all 14 of Sierra Leone's districts (Gbandia and Gale 2014).

Liberia is desperately short of Ebola-fighting supplies. According to the Liberian Ministry of Health and Social Welfare, there is too little of almost all essential equipment. Only 4901 body bags are on hand, but 84,841 are expected to be needed within the next 6 months. Only 2199 pairs of rubber boots are available, but 176,304 are needed. Only 309,206 face masks on hand, but 1.7 M are needed (Tharoor 2014).

Two Nigerian students have been rejected from Navarro College in Texas. The school did not want to accept them because they come from a country that has Ebola cases. One of the prospective students, Idris Bello, said that this was rather ironic given the ongoing Ebola outbreak in Dallas, Texas (Mangan 2014).

Three house democrats are requesting that US troops be allowed to directly aid Ebola patients in West Africa. US forces currently act in supporting roles. They are not allowed to have direct contact with Ebola patients (Sullivan 2014).

British Ebola survivor, William Pooley, will return to Sierra Leone to help with the outbreak (O'Carroll 2014b). Doctors think he is now immune to Ebola because he successfully fought off the virus.

There have been a variety of incidents in the United States where people have claimed to have Ebola either as a joke or threat. This evening, a 60-year-old man was arrested at his home in Cleveland, Ohio. While he was at the Horseshoe Casino in Cleveland, he said his wife had Ebola. He had been losing and it is thought that this was meant as a threat (Pinckard 2014).

October 16, 2014 (Thursday)

Amber Vinson may have had Ebola symptoms as early as October 10, 2014, the day she flew from Dallas to Cleveland (Livingston and Powell 2014). The CDC is asking passengers on Vinson's October 10 flight, Frontier Airlines flight 1142, to contact the agency (Centers for Disease Control and Prevention 2014b). Vinson had flown home to plan her wedding. Five of her bridesmaids are now quarantined (Associated Press 2014o; Livingston and Powell 2014). In addition, Coming Attractions Bridal & Formal, a bridal shop that Vinson visited in Akron on October 11, has been closed (Associated Press 2014o). Health officials are asking patrons who visited the shop between 1200 and 1530 h on October 11 to contact them (Livingston and Powell 2014).

Frontier Airlines has placed the six crewmembers from Amber Vinson's October 13 flight on paid leave (NBC News 2014f). The jet that Vinson flew on, registration number N220FR, has been taken out of service. It has been cleaned and the seat covers and carpets near Vinson's seat have been removed. Before being taken out of service, the jet made five additional flights to Cleveland, Fort Lauderdale, and Atlanta (NBC News 2014f). Two Ohio schools, Solon Middle School and Parkside Elementary School, were closed today because a staff member flew on the same plane, but not on the same flight, as Amber Vinson (Szabo 2014b). The schools will be disinfected. The Ohio Department of Health issued the following quarantine protocols for people exposed to Ebola victims:

> For individuals with any direct physical contact with the index case (including brief contact such as a handshake without personal protective equipment), ODH recommends quarantine for 21 days after the last contact in conjunction with public health officials.
>
> For individuals without direct contact, but within a three foot radius of the index case (such as adjacent passengers in an airplane or car) for a prolonged period of time, ODH recommends twice-daily temperature-taking and symptom check (one observed by a public health official) for 21 days after the last contact with the index case.
>
> For individuals without direct contact but in the vicinity of the index case as indicated by a public health official, notification and self-monitoring is recommended. (Ohio Department of Health 2014)

Texas Health Presbyterian Hospital has apologized for mistakes it made in handling Ebola patients (Yan and Shoichet 2014). The hospital is offering to provide hospital rooms to any of its healthcare workers who are under surveillance. Staying at the hospital will ensure that workers do not infect their families or community if they are infected. The use of a room is entirely at the workers' discretion (Yan and Shoichet 2014). Late in the day, all of the healthcare workers who had contact with Thomas Duncan were asked to sign a document legally requiring them to self-quarantine, avoid public places, and not use mass transit (Associated Press 2014p). Dallas is considering asking Governor Rick Perry to declare the county's Ebola outbreak a disaster (NBC News 2014g).

Nina Pham has been transferred to an NIH facility in Maryland for treatment (CBS DFW 2014d).

In Spain, a person who had contact with María Teresa Romero Ramos has developed a fever and been isolated (Associated Press 2014q).

A nurse who treated the French Ebola patient in September has developed Ebola-like symptoms. She has a high, long-lasting fever. The nurse has been taken to the Begin Hospital in Saint-Mande, France, and been isolated (AFP 2014b).

President Obama issued an executive order that allows the Pentagon to call up reservists to help fight Ebola (Korte and Vanden Brook 2014).

A doctoral student at the Yale University School of Public Health has been isolated in the Yale-New Haven Hospital with Ebola-like symptoms (New Haven Register 2014). The student returned from Liberia on Saturday, October 11, 2014, and developed a fever Wednesday night (Donahue and Tensa 2014).

Ebola screening has started at airports in Atlanta, Chicago, New Jersey, and Washington, D.C. (ABC News 2014c).

Ninety-two British medics from the 22 Field Hospital have arrived in Sierra Leone to help with the outbreak (Robinson 2014).

October 17, 2014 (Friday)

Total cases: 9216 (219 new)   Fatalities: 4555 (62 new)
                                 (World Health Organization 2014h)

The Ebola outbreak in Senegal is officially over (World Health Organization 2014i). The only reported case in the country occurred on August 29, 2014. Two, 21-day incubation periods have now passed without any other cases developing. Ebola is no longer considered to be in the country (World Health Organization 2014i). The WHO has congratulated Senegal for its handling of the outbreak (World Health Organization 2014j).

A laboratory supervisor who had contact with Thomas Duncan's medical specimens is on the cruise ship *Carnival Magic* off the coast of Belize (Keneally 2014b). She is considered a low risk of exposure but has agreed to isolate herself in her cabin and the ship is returning to port (Cowell 2014; Keneally 2014b). In Dallas, 75 healthcare workers who assisted Duncan have been placed on the US no-fly list (CBS DC and Associated Press 2014a).

Dealing with the waste generated by Ebola patients is difficult for US hospitals. Texas Health Presbyterian Hospital has been shipping 55 gallon waste drums to Port

Arthur, Texas, for incineration. The waste includes body fluids, contaminated bedding, and used PPE (Wines 2014).

President Obama has appointed Ron Klain as Ebola response coordinator (Tapper 2014). The media is referring to Klain as the Ebola Czar.

Major Alfred Palo Conteh has been appointed Sierra Leone's Ebola Czar (Awareness Times 2014)

Ebola survivors in West Africa are being trained to help care for Ebola orphans (United Nations 2014).

Food prices in Liberia, Sierra Leone, and Guinea are up an average of 24% since the start of the outbreak (Brinded 2014).

A 63-year-old Nigerian man vomited profusely and then died in his seat on an Arik Air flight from Lagos, Nigeria, to New York City (Aminu 2014). This caused tremendous concern about Ebola among the passengers and crew. However, the CDC has determined the deceased passenger did not have Ebola (Aminu 2014). In a separate incident, a woman on a tour of the Pentagon began vomiting in the parking lot and said she had recently been in Sierra Leone (CBS DC and Associated Press 2014b). She later tested negative for Ebola (Morozova 2014).

Benowitz et al. (2014) warn that New York City is especially vulnerable to the arrival of Ebola. New York is a significant transit hub and a major port of entry into the United States. It is also home to many West Africans who travel back and forth to their home countries (Benowitz et al. 2014).

GlaxoSmithKline says safety and efficacy trials of its Ebola vaccine will not be completed until the end of 2015 (Grogan 2014).

Financial contributions to fight Ebola are falling short. The UN has requested $1 B to fight the disease, but so far, only 38% of these funds have been delivered (AFP 2014c).

Burundi, Kenya, Rwanda, Tanzania, and Uganda are sending 619 medical workers to West Africa to fight Ebola (AFP 2014d).

Belize will not issue visas to travelers from West African countries (Associated Press 2014r).

Illinois has opened an Ebola hotline. People can call 800-889-3931 for information about the disease (Nelson 2014).

October 18, 2014 (Saturday)
The number of Ebola cases in Liberia is believed to be underreported. This is partly due to the confusion that normally surrounds large-scale, fast-moving events. But it also appears the government may be trying to downplay the scale of epidemic. Also, when families bury their dead privately, these victims are not recorded on official casualty lists (Townsend 2014).

In Dallas, people who had contact with Thomas Duncan are beginning to come out of their 21-day quarantines. One of the first people released was a man who visited Duncan's apartment in late September (Tsiaperas 2014).

The Transportation Security Administration says one of its agents gave Amber Vinson a routine pat down in Cleveland on October 13, 2014 (Kent 2014). The agent is now on paid leave and is self-monitoring for symptoms (Kent 2014). Separately,

Ohio will not allow people who are being monitored for Ebola in the state to travel internationally (Kesling 2014).

Oxfam says the Ebola outbreak could become the defining humanitarian disaster of the current generation. The agency also calls for more troops to be sent to West Africa to help with the outbreak (Ritchie 2014).

A highly critical internal WHO memo has been leaked to the press. The memo cites numerous flaws in the WHO's initial handling of the outbreak. The WHO is not commenting on the contents of the report (Alexander 2014a, b).

France has begun screening airline passengers arriving from Guinea for Ebola (Chazan 2014).

October 19, 2014 (Sunday)

Spanish nursing assistant María Teresa Romero Ramos has tested negative for Ebola. A second test must also be negative before she can be declared Ebola-free (BBC 2014d).

Dr. Fred Hartman with Management Sciences for Health says the initial panic about Ebola in Monrovia, Liberia, has died down and there are no longer bodies lying in the streets. Even so, the disease is well entrenched in the population and many people are still dying (Kalter 2014).

Infected American doctor Ian Crozier has been released from Emory University Hospital (Loftus 2015; Reuters 2014n). Crozier was exceptionally sick during his illness. He spent 12 days on a ventilator and 24 days on dialysis (Sifferlin 2014).

Ebola survivor William Pooley has returned to Sierra Leone. He will begin working in Freetown on Monday (Gallagher 2014).

The Pentagon will train a 30-member Ebola response team to assist US hospitals with future Ebola cases (Leitsinger 2014).

Rwanda has begun screening passengers from the United States and Spain for Ebola (Stanglin 2014b).

October 20, 2014 (Monday)

The Ebola outbreak in Nigeria is officially over. Two, 21-day incubation periods have passed without any additional cases developing in the country. Ebola is no longer considered to be in Nigeria. The WHO is optimistic about this success and says it shows Ebola can be contained (World Health Organization 2014k).

In Dallas, the observation period for 48 people who had contact with Thomas Duncan, including his fiancée Louise Troh, ended at midnight October 19–20, 2014 (Leitsinger and Jamieson 2014; Sickles 2014). It has been revealed that Troh and her family had been staying at the Catholic Diocese Conference Center in Oak Cliff, Texas (Schechter 2014). About 120 people are still under observation in Texas (Sickles 2014).

Hectic conditions make it difficult to track Ebola patients in Liberia. Relatives have a hard time finding loved ones and often do not know if a person is alive or dead. In one case, Linda Wilson visited Ebola wards in Monrovia for almost a month trying to find her friend, Barbara Bai. Wilson left Bai at Redemption Hospital in mid-September 2014. Patients are often transferred among facilities, and Bai was quickly lost in the system. There was no record of Bai at any medical center.

Eventually, Wilson located a nurse at the Island Clinic who knew about Bai. The nurse said Bai had died and been cremated. The communication problem is often exacerbated because healthcare workers do not want to give families bad news. Sometimes healthcare workers will reassure a family and say a person is ok, even though they know the person has died (Sieff 2014).

Food rations are being distributed to quarantined houses in the Waterloo community near Freetown, Sierra Leone. Ebola is rampant in the area, and at least 350 houses are under quarantine. Ration deliveries started Friday, October 17, 2014. Food packets contain enough food for 30 days (Associated Press 2014s).

The CDC has issued new PPE protocols for healthcare workers working with Ebola patients. The agency recommends all workers receive rigorous PPE training before they work with patients. The PPE needs to cover the entire body and no skin should be exposed. A designated monitor should also watch workers don and doff their PPE to help prevent errors and record any mistakes that do occur (Centers for Disease Control and Prevention 2014c).

The fear of Ebola is causing disruptions around the world. There are daily reports of suspected cases across the globe. There are also reports of people irrationally panicking when confronted with the threat of Ebola. In one recent incident in Zimbabwe, an ambulance crew ran away when they discovered that the woman they had been called to assist had been to Nigeria (AllAfrica 2014a).

Travelers arriving in Canada who do not disclose they have been in West Africa or have had contact with Ebola victims will face a $300,000 fine and jail time (Wolter 2014). Separately, Air Canada will allow flight attendants to wear disposable gloves to help protect them from the virus (Marowits 2014).

The EU is trying to raise $1.27 B to fight Ebola (Associated Press 2014t).

October 21, 2014 (Tuesday)
Ebola cases are increasing rapidly in western Sierra Leone. On Monday, October 20, 2014, 49 new cases were reported in and around Freetown. In contrast, cases appear to be declining in other parts of the country. There were no new cases on Monday in Kenema or Kailahun (Associated Press 2014u).

At least two people were killed in an Ebola-sparked riot in Koindu, Sierra Leone. Healthcare workers tried to collect blood samples from the body of a 90-year-old woman who was thought to have died from Ebola. The woman's son is a youth leader in the community, and a gang of youths prevented the workers from approaching the body. When police arrived to help the healthcare workers, a riot started. During the violence, youths shouted "No more Ebola!" A curfew has been imposed on the town (AFP 2014e).

Decontamination crews filled 53 waste drums with potentially infected material from Amber Vinson's Dallas apartment (Saavedra 2014). Texas is preparing two Ebola biocontainment centers to handle future Texas Ebola cases. One is in Richardson, Texas, the other is at the University of Texas Medical Branch at Galveston (Schluz 2014).

Infected Norwegian doctor Silje Michalsen is now Ebola-free and has been released from Ulleval Hospital in Oslo (The Health Site 2014).

Bogoch et al. (2015) estimate that 2.8 Ebola-infected passengers may travel out of West Africa on commercial airlines each month. Most of these travelers will go to low- or middle-income countries (Bogoch et al. 2015).

There has been a significant drop in the number of air passengers traveling out of the Ebola-affected countries. Compared to last year, 51% fewer air passengers are flying out of Liberia, 66% less from Guinea, and 85% less from Sierra Leone (Bogoch et al. 2015).

The Department of Homeland Security says all travelers, even US citizens, coming to the United States from Guinea, Sierra Leone, or Liberia must enter the United States through one of the five airports screening for Ebola (Reuters 2014o). This regulation will begin Wednesday, October 22, 2014.

Ebola screening has begun at Britain's Gatwick airport (Guardian 2014a).

October 22, 2014 (Wednesday)

Total cases: 9937 (721 new)   Fatalities: 4877 (322 new)
(World Health Organization 2014l)

Forty-five Ebola survivors were released from the Hastings Treatment Center near Freetown, Sierra Leone, today. This is the third mass release of patients from the site. Survivors proudly displayed their health certificates as they left the facility (Associated Press 2014v).

Placards are placed on quarantined West African houses. One such sign in Port Loko, Sierra Leone, reads [(transcribed from photograph credited to AP Photo/ Michael Duff (DiLorenzo 2014)]:

Police Order
Quarantined Home
Unauthorised [sic] *should keep off*

NBC cameraman, Ashoka Mukpo, is now Ebola-free (Szabo 2014c). He has left the Nebraska treatment center and is on his way home to Rhode Island (Associated Press 2014w; Szabo 2014c). Amber Joy Vinson is also Ebola-free. She is still at Emory University Hospital (Winter 2014).

US Ebola Czar Ron Klain started working today (Associated Press 2014w).

Johnson & Johnson hopes to have a million doses of a two-step Ebola vaccine ready by next year. Johnson & Johnson is also in discussions with GlaxoSmithKline to see if the two companies can collaborate on vaccine development (Hirschler 2014).

Travelers arriving in the United States from West Africa are now required to monitor themselves for Ebola symptoms for 21 days and report their morning and evening temperatures to state or local health departments (McNeil and Shear 2014). Nine people in Connecticut have placed themselves in voluntary isolation and are being monitored for Ebola (Hartocollis 2014). They had all traveled to West Africa or had contact with people who had been in the region (Hartocollis 2014).

Insurance companies in the United States and Britain have begun to exclude Ebola from new insurance policies, especially from business policies that involve travel to West Africa (Reuters 2014p).

Rwanda has canceled its Ebola screenings for US and Spanish travelers (Associated Press 2014x).

October 23, 2014 (Thursday)
There is a confirmed Ebola case in New York City. American doctor, Dr. Craig Spencer, has tested positive for Ebola in the city (Santora 2014a). The 33-year-old Spencer had been working with MSF in Guinea. He finished work on October 12, 2014, and returned to New York on October 17 (Santora 2014a; Wulfhorst and Malo 2014). Since his return, he has been self-monitoring for Ebola symptoms. Around 1100 h today, he developed a 100.3 °F fever, nausea, pain, and fatigue (Hartmann 2014; Karimi 2014). He was taken to Bellevue Hospital and quarantined (NYC Health + Hospitals 2014). Three additional people, including his fiancée, have also been isolated in Bellevue Hospital (Santora 2014a). On Wednesday, Spencer traveled in the city (Karimi 2014). He went jogging and bowling. He rode the subway (A, L, and 1 trains), took an Uber ride, and visited *The Gutter* bowling alley (Killough 2014; Santora 2014a). The bowling alley has closed for the night. Dr. Spencer's apartment on West 147th Street has also been quarantined (Hartmann 2014: Karimi 2014).

A 2-year-old girl [Fanta Condé] has tested positive for Ebola in the West African country of Mali (Guardian 2014b). The girl recently came to Mali from Guinea. She is currently in Fousseyni Dao hospital in Kayes, Mali (Höije 2014). Her symptoms include a 102.2° fever, cough, nose bleed, and bloody stools (World Health Organization 2014m). People who had contact with the girl have been isolated. Condé's grand aunt brought Condé to Mali on October 19, 2014. Her father, a healthcare worker, had died in Guinea, almost certainly of Ebola (World Health Organization 2014m; n). Condé and her aunt traveled extensively through Mali. They covered 700 miles, used at least one bus and three taxis, and visited Mali's capital, Bamako (World Health Organization 2014n). They eventually reached Kayes, Mali. On October 21, Condé was admitted to the hospital (World Health Organization 2014n). Given her extensive travel, there is significant concern that Condé may have exposed many people to Ebola.

Forty-three people in the town of Jenewonda, Liberia, are threatening to break quarantine because they have not been provided with food. The UN World Food Programme says provisions are on their way (Paye-Layleh and Roy-Macaulay 2014).

The EU has appointed Christos Stylianides as EU Ebola coordinator (Bendavid 2014).

Texas Health Presbyterian Hospital has suffered a 25% loss in revenue since it treated Thomas Duncan. ER visits are down 53%, and hospital occupancy has fallen from 428 to 337 patients (Murray 2014).

Workers at the two new Texas Ebola containment units are using Tabasco sauce to help learn how to treat patients. Mock patients are sprayed with Tabasco sauce, and workers treat them in full PPE. Any exposure is detected by a tingling sensation on the skin (Lupkin 2014).

Nigeria will send 506 healthcare workers to West Africa to fight Ebola (Akingbule and Hinshaw 2014).

October 24, 2014 (Friday)
CDC experts are working to track Dr. Craig Spencer's movement in New York City and identify potential contacts (James 2014). To help dispel the fear of Ebola in the city, New York Governor Andrew Cuomo says he will ride one of the subway lines taken by Dr. Spencer today (Killough 2014). Ebola survivor, Nancy Writebol, has donated plasma for Dr. Spencer (WSOCTV 2014).

Independent of the federal government, New York and New Jersey have implemented their own enhanced Ebola containment protocols for travelers arriving from West Africa (CBS New York and Associated Press 2014). Officials will assess incoming travelers and determine their risk of Ebola exposure. Those with the highest risk, such as people who had contact with an infected person, will be automatically quarantined for 21 days at a government-regulated facility (CBS New York and Associated Press 2014). Those with lower risk will be monitored. The protocols are new and controversial, but they have already been put into practice. A female healthcare worker [Kaci Hickox] arrived at Newark Liberty International Airport today after treating Ebola patients in West Africa [Sierra Leone] (CBS New York and Associated Press 2014). A legal order was issued to place her in quarantine. At a press conference, the governors of the two states said that the new rules were needed because voluntary quarantines have proven to be ineffective (CBS New York and Associated Press 2014).

Fanta Condé, the 2-year-old Ebola victim in Mali, has died (McNeil 2014; World Health Organization 2014n). The WHO is treating the Mali outbreak as a significant emergency (World Health Organization 2014m). It is sending additional experts to the country (Neuman 2014). Forty-three people in Mali have been identified as potential contacts and are being monitored (Berlinger et al. 2014). The bus that Condé traveled in was located and disinfected; the disinfection was carried out as soon as the bus was found, apparently right in the middle of the street (Höije 2014). The bus had a passenger list, complete with phone numbers, which is being used to search for additional contacts (Höije 2014).

Concerns about burial customs appear to be making Liberians less willing to go to Ebola clinics. Cremation violates the cultural norms of Liberia, but all Ebola victims in Monrovia are cremated. As a result, many Ebola patients are kept at home so they can be secretly buried if they die. At facilities outside of Monrovia, the bodies of Ebola victims are generally buried. But the burials occur away from relatives and often in unmarked graves. Thus, the dead cannot be visited and honored. Recently, only 351 of Liberia's 742 Ebola treatment beds were filled. The empty slots are thought to be caused by people avoiding clinics (Paye-Layleh 2014b).

Nina Pham is now Ebola-free and has been released from isolation (Associated Press 2014y). Soon after her release, she traveled to the White House and met with President Obama. The President hugged her (Worland 2014).

The 101st Airborne will take command of Operation *United Assistance* in Monrovia, Liberia, on Saturday, October 25, 2014 (Levy 2014).

Ethiopia will send 200 healthcare workers to West Africa to fight Ebola (Africa Report 2014).

China will donate $81.7 M to fight Ebola (Liping 2014).

October 25, 2014 (Saturday)

Illinois and Florida are following New York and New Jersey's lead and are implementing enhanced Ebola quarantine protocols (Chicago Tribune 2014; Flegenheimer et al. 2014). Any high-risk traveler who enters the states will be isolated for 21 days. Washington D.C., Maryland, and Virginia (all associated with Dulles International Airport) will not quarantine returning healthcare workers (Hsu and Henderson 2014). Aid groups are very concerned that imposing mandatory quarantines will deter healthcare workers from volunteering to work in the Ebola zone (Hsu and Henderson 2014).

The nurse quarantined in New Jersey has identified herself as Kaci Hickox. She was detained at Newark Liberty International Airport after returning from Sierra Leone. She had been treating Ebola patients in Sierra Leone with MSF. In a letter to the *Dallas Morning News*, Hickox described her arrival in the United States and her subsequent quarantine. She says she arrived at the airport about 1300 h on October 24, 2014. The trip from Sierra Leone had taken 2 days. When she told immigration she had come from Sierra Leone, she was taken to a quarantine office. She was there for 6 h. During this time, many people questioned her. At least one of the questioners was from the CDC. After 4 h, her temperature was taken with a forehead scanner. The reading was 101 °F. Hickox told the officer who took the temperature that she was very upset and the forehead reading was probably inaccurate. However, a more accurate oral temperature was not taken. Around 1900 h, she was told she would have to go to a hospital. Once there, her temperature was taken again, this time both orally and from the forehead. The oral reading was 98.6 °F, and the forehead reading was 101 °F. A blood test for Ebola came back negative (Hickox 2014).

Morgan Dixon, Dr. Spencer's fiancée, has been released from the hospital and has returned to the apartment she shares with Dr. Spencer. She will remain quarantined in the apartment until November 14, 2014. Medical workers will monitor her for symptoms (Rudra 2014).

Different aid groups in West Africa use different PPE. WHO workers use a gown, gloves, a partial hood, a surgical mask, and goggles. The eyes, nose, and mouth are fully covered, but a tiny amount of skin is exposed. MSF workers use much heavier gear that leaves no skin uncovered. The MSF gear provides greater protection but is very hot. Workers can only work in the MSF gear for 45–60 min. The partial skin exposure of the WHO gear is a significant weakness, but the PPE is relatively cheap, quicker to don and doff, and relatively cool (Beaubien 2014a).

Major General Gary J. Volesky, commander of the 101st Airborne, has assumed command of US operations in Liberia (CBS News 2014c).

Mauritania has closed its border with Mali due to the Ebola outbreak (Diarra and Diagana 2014).

October 26, 2014 (Sunday)

There were more than 400 new Ebola cases in Liberia last week (NPR 2014). However, some parts of Liberia are experiencing dramatic drops in case numbers. NPR correspondent, John Hamilton, describes the current conditions in Foya, Liberia:

Earlier today I toured the treatment area, and they showed me the areas where, at one time, they had well over 100 patients with Ebola. Today there are three. So it is just a dramatic, dramatic change. And part of it is that there has been, since they set up the unit here, a place to take people who are very sick. That has meant that they are not at home where they're at risk of infecting other people. But they say the biggest change is probably that they have sent health workers out into the community, people from the community who know the people here, and they have told them that the people at Medecins Sans Frontieres are not the people bringing Ebola but the people who are here to help them with that. And they've taught them about hand washing about how not to have contact with bodies. And it has made just an enormous difference. (NPR 2014)

Residents of Kayes, Mali, are worried about Ebola but are unclear how to avoid catching the disease. Some people are wearing gloves. Others are avoiding handshakes (Ahmed 2014).

Kaci Hickox, the quarantined US nurse, is planning to file a lawsuit questioning the constitutionality of her confinement (Al Jazeera 2014). She is currently in an isolation tent behind Newark University Hospital in New Jersey (Schwartz 2014).

Some healthcare workers at Bellevue Hospital in New York, where Dr. Spencer is being treated, are calling in sick to avoid coming to work (Djuric 2014).

US Ambassador to the UN, Samantha Power, has traveled to Guinea to try to increase international support for Ebola-fighting efforts (Jansing 2014).

The Pentagon is developing plane-portable isolation units that can transport infected personnel. The units will be mounted in C-17 or C-130 transport planes. They will carry 12 walking patients or 8 patients on stretchers (Zoroya 2014).

October 27, 2014 (Monday)

Blackmailers are threatening to spread Ebola in the Czech Republic unless they are given $1.27 M in bitcoins. The blackmailers say that they possess "biological material" from an infected Liberian. Officials say the blackmailers are sophisticated in their use of communication technology, but doubt they have the scientific know-how to collect, transport, and disseminate Ebola (AFP 2014f).

Quarantined nurse Kaci Hickox will be allowed to return home to Maine (Barbaro and Santora 2014). Officials in New Jersey say once she reaches Maine, it will be up to Maine to monitor her. It is unclear if Maine is interested in doing so (Barbaro and Santora 2014). New York has modified its quarantine protocols for medical workers arriving from West Africa (Fox News 2014c). Instead of being isolated at a state facility, workers will be quarantined at home and receive twice-a-day monitoring. The state will reimburse quarantined individuals for any lost pay (Fox News 2014c).

In response to increased concern about Ebola in the United States, the CDC has released new recommendations for monitoring people who may have been exposed to the virus. The agency only recommends restricting the movements of high-risk individuals. High-risk people are those who (1) had an infected needlestick, (2) had direct contact with infected body fluids without PPE, (3) processed infected body fluids without PPE, (4) had direct contact with an infected corpse without PPE, or (5) lived in the same house and provided care to an infected person. People at lower risk may have their movements controlled if it is recommended by public health authorities (Centers for Disease Control and Prevention 2014d). These recommendations are in sharp contrast to, and are far more lenient than, the mandatory 21-day quarantines being imposed by some states on anyone who worked with infected patients.

Due to the intense effort needed to care for Ebola patients, Bellevue Hospital in New York City is transferring some of its other ICU patients to New York University Langone Medical Center (Evans and Karni 2014). Bellevue is currently treating Dr. Craig Spencer. It also ran tests today on a 5-year-old boy with Ebola-like symptoms who had recently traveled to Guinea (Evans et al. 2014). The boy later tested negative for Ebola (Evans et al. 2014).

Mali has identified 111 people who had contact with Fanta Condé. At least 40 of the people have not been located (Monnier and Rihouay 2014).

Ten people in Spain, including María Teresa Romero Ramos's husband, have ended their 21-day observation periods and been released from Carlos III Hospital (Giles 2014).

The Bong County Ebola Treatment Unit in Liberia recently hosted a movie night for its Ebola patients. *The Lion King* was shown to the great delight of the patients. This is the first time a movie has been shown at the facility. 90% of the staff at the Bong County Treatment Unit are Liberian workers, 10% are international workers. The international workers include personnel from Canada, Chad, Ethiopia, France, Germany, Guinea, Iraq, Kenya, Spain, Uganda, and the United States (Sia 2014)

US troops returning from Liberia spend their 21-day quarantines in Vicenza, Italy. Eleven troops, including Major General Darryl Williams, are currently quarantined in Vicenza. Thirty more troops are expected to arrive today (CBS News 2014c).

EU Ebola Coordinator Christos Stylianides would like the number of treatment beds in West Africa to increase to 5000 as soon as possible (Casert 2014).

The University of Nebraska Medical Center and Nebraska Medicine are putting two free Ebola courses online. One is about Ebola in general, and the other describes Ebola treatment techniques (Infection Control Today 2014).

Murray State University in Kentucky announced today that it will defer West African applications. West Africa students may still apply to the school, but they will not be admitted until at least the fall of 2015 (Associated Press 2014z).

Australia will no longer issue visas to travelers from Ebola-affected countries (AFP 2014g).

October 28, 2014 (Tuesday)

Some West African observers think the WHO and CDC assessments of the Ebola situation are overly pessimistic (AllAfrica 2014b). In Liberia, for example, the number of Ebola cases seems to be falling and many treatment centers have large numbers of open beds (AllAfrica 2014b; Fink 2014). The Liberian Red Cross also reports it is collecting fewer bodies than before (AFP 2014h).

Local nurses treating Ebola patients in West Africa are often shunned by their communities. Many end up living at their hospitals. Nurse Joya Koroma, a health-care worker at the Hastings Treatment Center in Sierra Leone, says when landlords find out that their tenants were nurses, they were are longer willing to rent to them (Styles 2014).

Amber Vinson has been released from Emory University Hospital (Achenbach and Dennis 2014).

After her visit to Sierra Leone, US Ambassador Samantha Power tweeted that safe burials in Freetown have gone from 30% to nearly 100% (Power 2014).

The United States says it will allow some infected foreign aid workers into the United States for treatment if needed. Officials say that it would be logical for the United States to treat foreign aid workers who cannot be medivacked back to their own country (Dinan 2014).

October 29, 2014 (Wednesday)

Total cases: 13,703 (3766 new)   Fatalities: 4922 (45 new)
(World Health Organization 2014o)

The WHO has updated its Ebola data. This makes it look like there was a massive rise in Ebola cases over the last week. However, most of the 3766 "new" cases were earlier cases that had not been included in the database (World Health Organization 2014o).

The Ebola outbreak appears to be slowing in Liberia (Sun et al. 2014; World Health Organization 2014o). The number of new cases in Liberia is stabilizing or falling (World Health Organization 2014o).

Liberians have begun 3 days of fasting and prayer aimed at ending the Ebola outbreak (Reuters 2014q).

Schieffelin et al. (2014) describe the clinical features of Ebola during the current outbreak. They examined the records of 106 Ebola patients treated at Kenema Government Hospital in Sierra Leone. Younger people had a higher survival rate than older people. The mortality rate for patients under 21 was 57%, compared to 94% for patients over 45. Patients with fatal outcomes had higher temperatures on admission than patients who survived. Patients with higher viral loads ($>10^7$ ml^{-1}) had higher mortality than patients with lower viral loads ($<10^5$ ml^{-1}) (Schieffelin et al. 2014).

The Disasters Emergency Committee, a group composed of the United Kingdom's 13 top charity organizations, has launched an appeal for help with the Ebola outbreak. This is the first time the committee has requested help for a disease outbreak (Pudelek 2014).

Kaci Hickox is now at her home in Fort Kent, Maine (Mathis-Lilley 2014). She says she will stop staying in isolation as of Thursday, October 30, 2014 (Alman

2014). The governor of Maine Paul LePage is trying to obtain the legal authority to keep her isolated. He says he will use the state police to enforce the quarantine (Alman 2014). Separately, California has ordered a 21-day quarantine for people returning from West Africa who had contact with infected patients (Serna 2014).

Defense Secretary Chuck Hagel has announced that all US troops returning from West Africa will be required to undergo a 21-day quarantine (Burns 2014).

October 30, 2014 (Thursday)

Staff at an Ebola call center in Freetown, Sierra Leone, often field heartbreaking phone calls. One staff member received a call from a woman whose mother, father, and cousin had all died from Ebola. She was calling because their bodies had not been collected by burial teams. The next day the woman called back. She was crying and said that the bodies had still not been collected. Another worker got a call about an abandoned 2-year-old child. The child's mother and father were both dead, and the child was infected. The toddler kept knocking on a neighbor's door and crying for his father (O'Carroll 2014c).

All ambulance drivers in Kailahun, Sierra Leone, wear full PPE. They started doing this in June 2014 after two drivers died from Ebola. Because of the long distances, some ambulances have to travel 4 h or more and there are concerns that ambulance rides may be overly stressful for Ebola patients. Indeed, many patients die on their way to treatment centers (Wonacott 2014).

The state of New York is promising to provide employee protection and to pay and provide healthcare benefits to healthcare workers who are quarantined after returning from West Africa (Santora 2014b). It is hoped this will make workers more willing to comply with quarantine orders.

Researchers who have recently worked in West Africa will not be allowed to attend the American Society of Tropical Medicine and Hygiene's conference in New Orleans. The ban was imposed by the Louisiana Department of Health and Hospitals. The agency says anyone who has been in Guinea, Sierra Leone, or Liberia during the past 21 days should not travel to New Orleans. If they do, they could be quarantined (Beaubien 2014b).

China is sending an elite military unit to Liberia to build a 100-bed treatment facility. The unit has experience from the SARS outbreak (Rajagopalan 2014).

October 31, 2014 (Friday)

Total cases: 13,567 (−136 new)   Fatalities: 4951 (29 new)
                                   (World Health Organization 2014p)

The WHO continues to adjust its Ebola figures. This has led to a drop in official case numbers.

Fanta Condé, the 2-year-old Ebola victim in Mali, is believed to have had contact with 141 people. Fifty-seven of these people have not yet been located. Two known contacts have developed Ebola-like symptoms and are being tested (Miles 2014).

A new 200-bed treatment center has opened in the Congo Town community of Monrovia, Liberia. With its opening, the JFK Medical Center treatment center has closed (Paye-Layleh 2014c).

The WHO has updated its PPE recommendations. The agency says PPE should cover the mouth, nose, eyes, and hands. Face cover, protective foot wear, gowns or coveralls, and head cover are essential (World Health Organization 2014q).

A Maine judge has ruled against a strict quarantine for Kaci Hickox. The judge says the current fear of Ebola in the United States is not entirely rational. Hickox is, however, required to continue monitoring herself for symptoms, report any symptoms that occur, and coordinate travel plans with health officials (Page 2014).

Canada will no longer process the visa applications for residents of countries with widespread and intense Ebola transmission (Associated Press 2014aa). "Widespread and intense transmission" is a category designated by the WHO. At present, these are the countries of Guinea, Sierra Leone, and Liberia (World Health Organization 2014p).

References

7 Online (2014) CDC remove 2 from Newark flight after possible Ebola scare. 7 Online. http://7online.com/health/cdc-investigating-possible-ebola-scare-on-newark-flight-/336774/. Accessed 4 Oct 2014

ABC 13 Eyewitness News (2014) Text of reverse 911 call neighbors of Ebola patient received. ABC 13 Eyewitness News. http://abc13.com/news/text-of-reverse-911-call-neighbors-of-ebola-patient-received/347260/. Accessed 20 May 2014

ABC News (2014a) Ugandan doctor with Ebola treated in Germany. ABC News. http://abcnews.go.com/Health/wireStory/ugandan-doctor-ebola-treated-germany-25937422. Accessed 3 Oct 2014

ABC News (2014b) Airline cabin cleaners strike over Ebola exposure fears. ABC News. http://abc-news.go.com/Health/airline-cabin-cleaners-strike-ebola-exposure-fears/story?id=26066160. Accessed 9 Oct 2014

ABC News (2014c) Nurse who contracted Ebola called CDC before flight, official says. ABC News. http://abcnews.go.com/Health/nurse-contracted-ebola-called-cdc-flight-official/story?id=26232809. Accessed 28 May 2017

Achenbach J (2014) WHO: Ebola spreading in W. Africa, threatens Ivory Coast; some areas see fewer cases. The Washington Post. https://www.washingtonpost.com/news/to-your-health/wp/2014/10/14/who-ebola-spreading-in-w-africa-threatens-ivory-coast-some-areas-see-fewer-cases/?tid=a_inl&utm_term=.3973041f84fd. Accessed 28 May 2017

Achenbach J, Dennis B (2014) Amber Vinson Dallas nurse leaves hospital after Ebola cure. The Washington Post. http://www.washingtonpost.com/national/health-science/amber-vinson-dallas-nurse-leaving-hospital-after-ebola-cure/2014/10/28/d37e7fae-5e95-11e4-8b9e-2ccdac31a031_story.html. Accessed 28 Oct 2014

AFP (2014a) UN quarantines 41 personnel in Ebola-hit Liberia. AFP, News 18. http://ibnlive.in.com/news/un-quarantines-41-personnel-in-ebolahit-liberia/505348-17.html. Accessed 10 Oct 2014

AFP (2014b) Nurse who treated French Ebola patient 'in hospital with fever'. AFP, NDTV. http://www.ndtv.com/world-news/nurse-who-treated-french-ebola-patient-in-hospital-with-fever-680359. Accessed 10 Mar 2017

AFP (2014c) UN Ebola appeal gets just 38% of cash needed. AFP, The Daily Star. http://www.dai-lystar.com.lb/News/World/2014/Oct-17/274454-un-ebola-appeal-gets-just-38-of-cash-needed.ashx#axzz3GPOlx5rR. Accessed 17 Oct 2014

AFP (2014d) East Africa to send 600 health workers for Ebola fight. AFP, Yahoo News UK. https://uk.news.yahoo.com/east-africa-send-600-health-workers-ebola-fight-094254871.html#7bKPmaE. Accessed 17 Oct 2014

AFP (2014e) Two killed after Ebola tests spark riot in Sierra Leone. AFP, The Malay Mail. http://www.themalaymailonline.com/world/article/two-killed-after-ebola-tests-spark-riot-in-sierra-leone. Accessed 22 Oct 2014

AFP (2014f) Blackmailers threaten Czechs with Ebola outbreak. AFP, Yahoo News. https://uk.news.yahoo.com/blackmailers-threaten-czechs-ebola-outbreak-174554858.html#HOe7z7V. Accessed 7 Jun 2017

AFP (2014g) Australia: no immigration from Ebola nations. AFP, Al Jazeera. http://www.aljazeera.com/news/asia-pacific/2014/10/australia-no-immigration-from-ebola-nations-2014102783935140258.html. Accessed 7 Jun 2017

AFP (2014h) Red Cross: fewer bodies in Liberian capital signals Ebola waning. AFP, News Max. http://www.newsmax.com/Newsfront/Health-Ebola-Liberia/2014/10/28/id/603516/. Accessed 8 Jun 2017

Africa Report (2014) 200 Ethiopian volunteers to join West Africa Ebola fight. The Africa Report. http://www.theafricareport.com/East-Horn-Africa/200-ethiopian-volunteers-to-join-west-africa-ebola-fight.html. Accessed 24 Oct 2014

Agaba J (2014) Another Ugandan doctor dies of Ebola. New Vision. http://www.newvision.co.ug/new_vision/news/1311979/ugandan-doctor-dies-ebola. Accessed 16 May 2017

Ahmed B (2014) Mali rushes to track contacts after toddler becomes 1st Ebola death after long journey. Associated Press, Greenfield Reporter. http://www.greenfieldreporter.com/view/story/f2157299bb3b4156be426fe291bff8b0/AF--Mali-Ebola. Accessed 26 Oct 2014

Akingbule G, Hinshaw D (2014) Nigeria to send medics to West African neighbors stricken with Ebola. Wall Str J. http://online.wsj.com/articles/nigeria-to-send-medics-to-west-african-neigh-bors-stricken-with-ebola-1414065052. Accessed 23 Oct 2014

Al Jazeera (2014) Nurse quarantined over Ebola fears plans to file lawsuit. Al Jazeera. http://america.aljazeera.com/articles/2014/10/26/ebola-power-fauci.html. Accessed 27 Oct 2014

Alexander B (2014) WHO not commenting on critical leaked Ebola report. USA Today. http://www.usatoday.com/story/news/world/2014/10/18/ebola-report-world-health-organization-leaked/17502135/. Accessed 18 Oct 2014

Alexander H (2014) Spanish nurse: 'I have no idea how I contracted Ebola'. The Telegraph. http://www.telegraph.co.uk/news/worldnews/ebola/11147947/Spanish-nurse-I-have-no-idea-how-I-contracted-Ebola.html. Accessed 12 Mar 2017

AllAfrica (2014a) Zimbabwe: Ebola – ambulance crew flees Kwekwe scare. AllAfrica, New Zimbabwe. http://allafrica.com/stories/201410210131.html. Accessed 20 Oct 2014

AllAfrica (2014b) Liberia: with all our might Liberians, Guineans and Sierra Leoneans must fight WHO and CDC pessimism! AllAfrica, Daily Observer. http://allafrica.com/stories/201410290989.html. Accessed 28 Oct 2014

Alman A (2014) Maine Gov. Paul LePage sends state police to enforce Ebola quarantine. The Huffington Post. http://www.huffingtonpost.com/2014/10/29/paul-lepage-ebola-quarantine_n_6069740.html. Accessed 29 Oct 2014

Altman A (2014) 4 people quarantined over Ebola fears about 100 being monitored. Time. http://time.com/3456050/ebola-texas/. Accessed 2 Oct 2014

Aminu A (2014) Ebola panic as Nigerian dies in a US bound flight. Daily Times. http://www.dailytimes.com.ng/article/ebola-panic-nigerian-dies-us-bound-flight. Accessed 17 Oct 2014

Associated Press (2014a) Quarantined woman says she's tired of being "locked up". CBS DFW. http://dfw.cbslocal.com/2014/10/02/quarantined-woman-says-shes-tired-of-being-locked-up/. Accessed 2 Oct 2014

Associated Press (2014b) Fort Bragg to send 120 soldiers to fight Ebola. Fox Carolina, AP. http://www.foxcarolina.com/story/26701058/fort-bragg-to-send-120-soldiers-to-fight-ebola. Accessed 3 Oct 2014

Associated Press (2014c) Colorado soldiers going to Africa to combat Ebola. 9News, AP. http://www.9news.com/story/news/local/2014/10/03/colorado-soldiers-going-to-africa-to-combat-ebola/16696617/. Accessed 3 Oct 2014

Associated Press (2014d) U.S. military to put up tent at Liberia Ebola clinic. Associated Press, The Mining Journal. http://www.miningjournal.net/page/content.detail/id/627702/US-military-to-put-up-tent-at-Liberia-Ebola-clinic.html?isap=1&nav=5016. Accessed 6 Oct 2014

Associated Press (2014e) 3 people quarantined after nurse gets Ebola in Spain. Associated Press, New York Post. http://nypost.com/2014/10/07/3-people-quarantined-after-nurse-gets-ebola-in-spain/. Accessed 15 May 2017

Associated Press (2014f) Atlanta airport gives Ebola info to some travelers. Associated Press, The Gazette. http://gazette.com/atlanta-airport-gives-ebola-info-to-some-travelers/article/feed/165226. Accessed 15 May 2017

Associated Press (2014g) Liberian nurses threaten strike amid Ebola epidemic. Associated Press, CBS News. http://www.cbsnews.com/news/ebola-outbreak-liberian-health-care-workers-threaten-strike/. Accessed 12 Oct 2014

Associated Press (2014h) Dallas nurse caught Ebola despite safety gear, can't pinpoint breach. Associated Press, NPR. http://www.npr.org/2014/10/13/355970885/dallas-nurse-caught-ebola-despite-safety-gear-cant-pinpoint-breach. Accessed 13 Oct 2014

Associated Press (2014i) Liberia avoids mass hospital strike amid Ebola. Associated Press, Star Advertiser. http://www.staradvertiser.com/news/apnews/international/article/?ID=7867231. Accessed 14 Oct 2014

Associated Press (2014j) Friends raising money for journalist with Ebola. Associated Press, Times Union. http://www.timesunion.com/news/article/Friends-raising-money-for-journalist-with-Ebola-5819210.php. Accessed 13 Oct 2014

Associated Press (2014k) Soldier gets Ebola but is not among peacekeepers. Associated Press, WSOC. http://www.wsoctv.com/news/ap/top-news/doctors-without-borders-loses-9-medics-to-ebola/nhh5M/. Accessed 14 Oct 2014

Associated Press (2014l) Guinea calls on retired doctors to fight Ebola. Associated Press, My San Antonio. http://www.mysanantonio.com/news/world/article/Guinea-calls-on-retired-doctors-to-fight-Ebola-5824450.php. Accessed 14 Oct 2014

Associated Press (2014m) German hospital: UN worker dies of Ebola. Associated Press, Yahoo News. http://news.yahoo.com/german-hospital-un-worker-dies-ebola-082155030.html. Accessed 14 Oct 2014

Associated Press (2014n) Crews decontaminate Dallas hospital workers apartment, 2nd employee contracted Ebola. Associated Press, The Republic. http://www.therepublic.com/view/story/868683011eaa4c8ea3c048bb66bd70de/TX--Ebola-Apartment. Accessed 15 Oct 2014

Associated Press (2014o) Ohio bridesmaids of nurse with Ebola quarantined, shop closes. Associated Press, Daily Herald. http://www.dailyherald.com/article/20141017/news/141018398/. Accessed 17 Oct 2014

Associated Press (2014p) Officials move to keep Dallas health workers home. Associated Press, WHEC. http://www.whec.com/article/stories/S3592970.shtml?cat=10039. Accessed 16 Oct 2014

Associated Press (2014q) Spain tests 3 with fever for Ebola isolates jet. Associated Press, Townhall. http://townhall.com/news/world/2014/10/16/spain-ebola-patient-improving-1--to-be-tested-n1905923. Accessed 16 Oct 2014

Associated Press (2014r) Ebola travel restrictions vary from country to country. Associated Press, Fox News. http://www.foxnews.com/health/2014/10/18/ebola-travel-restrictions-vary-from-country-to-country.html. Accessed 31 May 2017

Associated Press (2014s) Liberia president says Ebola has brought country to 'a standstill.' Associated Press, Fox News. http://www.foxnews.com/world/2014/10/20/liberia-president-says-ebola-has-brought-country-to-standstill.html. Accessed 31 May 2017

Associated Press (2014t) EU seeks $1.27 billion in Ebola aid for W. Africa. Associated Press, KTVN. http://www.ktvn.com/story/26827485/eu-seeks-127-billion-in-ebola-aid-for-w-africa. Accessed 20 Oct 2014

Associated Press (2014u) Ebola cases rising sharply in western Sierra Leone. Associated Press, Fox News. http://www.foxnews.com/world/2014/10/21/ebola-cases-rising-sharply-in-western-sierra-leone.html. Accessed 2 Jun 2017

Associated Press (2014v) Dozens released Ebola free from Sierra Leone site. Associated Press, McDowell News. http://www.mcdowellnews.com/news/world/ap/dozens-released-ebola-free-from-sierra-leone-site/article_8fb56bb7-f8ef-538b-b009-7a699224e4b0.html. Accessed 22 Oct 2014

Associated Press (2014w) US journalist recovers; Ebola 'czar' gets to work. Associated Press, Midland Daily News. http://www.ourmidland.com/news/world/us-journalist-recovers-ebola-czar-gets-to-work/article_ec69b617-c004-5c67-b913-28b00dd68a2e.html. Accessed 22 Oct 2014

Associated Press (2014x) Rwanda cancels Ebola screenings for people coming from the US. Associate Press, The Daily Mail. http://www.dailymail.co.uk/news/article-2804600/Rwanda-cancels-Ebola-screenings-US-Spain.html. Accessed 23 Oct 2014

Associated Press (2014y) Dallas nurse Ebola free leaving hospital Friday. Associated Press, KOIN. http://koin.com/2014/10/24/dallas-nurse-ebola-free-leaving-hospital-friday/. Accessed 24 Oct 2014

Associated Press (2014z) Murray State deferring applications from Africa. Associated Press, Courier Press. http://www.courierpress.com/gleaner/news/murray-state-deferring-applications-from-africa_32058331. Accessed 27 Oct 2014

Associated Press (2014aa) Canada restricts visas amid Ebola scare. Associated Press, USA Today. https://www.usatoday.com/story/news/world/2014/10/31/canada-visas-ebola/18273133/. Accessed 14 Jun 2017

Awareness Times (2014) Defence Minister Major (rtd) Alfred Palo Conteh takes over from Health Minister Dr. Abu-Bakarr Fofanah in briefing the President on the progress being made in fighting Ebola disease. Awareness Times. http://news.sl/drwebsite/exec/view.cgi?archive=10&num=26433. Accessed 13 Jun 2017

Awoko (2014) Sierra Leone news: Gambia Bird resumes twice-weekly flights to Freetown. Awoko. http://awoko.org/2014/10/07/sierra-leone-news-gambia-bird-resumes-twice-weekly-flights-to-freetown/. Accessed 7 Oct 2014

Barbaro M, Santora M (2014) Nurse held in Ebola quarantine will be allowed to go home Christie says. New York Times. http://www.nytimes.com/2014/10/28/nyregion/nurse-in-newark-to-be-allowed-to-finish-ebola-quarantine-at-home-christie-says.html?_r=0. Accessed 27 Oct 2014

Barbash F (2014) NBC says cameraman tested positive for Ebola. Entire crew to be flown home. The Washington Post. http://www.washingtonpost.com/news/morning-mix/wp/2014/10/02/nbc-says-cameraman-tested-positive-for-ebola-entire-crew-to-be-flown-home/, Accessed 2 Oct 2014

BBC (2014a) Ebola outbreak: 'five infected every hour' in Sierra Leone. BBC. http://www.bbc.com/news/world-africa-29453755. Accessed 2 Oct 2014

BBC (2014b) Ebola screening for NHS 111 calls announced. BBC. http://www.bbc.com/news/uk-29591561. Accessed 12 Oct 2014

BBC (2014c) Ebola Royal Navy prepare RFA Argus to sail to W Africa. BBC. http://www.bbc.com/news/uk-29617647. Accessed 14 Oct 2014

BBC (2014d) Ebola crisis Spanish nurse tests negative for virus. BBC. http://www.bbc.com/news/world-europe-29683616. Accessed 19 Oct 2014

Beaubien J (2014a) In Liberia, how to gear for Ebola still an issue. NPR. http://www.npr.org/2014/10/25/358898029/in-liberia-how-to-gear-for-ebola-still-an-issue. Accessed 25 Oct 2014

Beaubien J (2014b) Ebola researchers banned from medical meeting in New Orleans. NPR, WXPR. http://wxpr.org/post/ebola-researchers-banned-medical-meeting-new-orleans. Accessed 30 Oct 2014

Begley S, Abutaleb Y (2014) Cities, states scramble after Dallas's Ebola missteps expose planning gaps. Reuters. http://in.reuters.com/article/2014/10/12/health-ebola-planning-idIN-L2N0S70R220141012. Accessed 12 Oct 2014

Bendavid N (2014) EU appoints Ebola response coordinator. The Wall Street Journal. http://online.wsj.com/articles/eu-appoints-ebola-response-coordinator-1414100467. Accessed 23 Oct 2014

Bennett M (2014) Spain isolates 3 more, puts 52 under observation, as Spaniards report botched Ebola crisis response. The Spain Report. https://www.thespainreport.com/11672/spain-isolates-three-puts-52-ebola-observation-spaniards-report-botched-crisis-response/. Accessed 7 Oct 2014

Benowitz I, Ackelsberg J, Balter SE et al (2014) Surveillance and preparedness for Ebola virus disease – New York City, 2014. Morb Mortal Wkly Rep 63:934–936

Berlinger J, Smith-Spark L, Hoije K (2014) Reports: first confirmed Ebola patient in Mali dies. CNN. http://www.cnn.com/2014/10/24/world/africa/mali-ebola/. Accessed 24 Oct 2014

Berman M (2014) Ebola stricken health care worker flew on a passenger plane a day before being diagnosed. The Washington Post. http://www.washingtonpost.com/news/post-nation/wp/2014/10/15/ebola-stricken-nurse-flew-on-a-passenger-plane-a-day-before-being-diagnosed/. Accessed 15 Oct 2014

Bogoch II, Creatore MI, Cetron MS et al (2015) Assessment of the potential for international dissemination of Ebola virus via commercial air travel during the 2014 west African outbreak. Lancet 385:29–35

Boseley S (2014a) Ebola vaccine trialled in Mali. The Guardian. http://www.theguardian.com/world/2014/oct/10/ebola-vaccine-mali-trialled-health-workers. Accessed 10 Oct 2014

Boseley S (2014b) WHO warns 10,000 new cases of Ebola a week are possible. The Guardian. https://www.theguardian.com/world/2014/oct/14/who-new-ebola-cases-world-health-organisation. Accessed 28 May 2017

Botelho G, Smith-Spark L, Maestro LP (2014) Hospital worker: Spaniard exposed in ER for 8 hours after positive Ebola test. CNN. http://www.cnn.com/2014/10/08/world/europe/ebola-spain/. Accessed 14 May 2017

Brinded L (2014) Ebola outbreak: hundreds of dead farmers leads to 24% jump in food prices. International Business Times. http://www.ibtimes.co.uk/ebola-outbreak-hundreds-dead-farmers-leads-24-jump-food-prices-1470570. Accessed 31 May 2014

Brumfield B, Levs J (2014) Spain has outbreak's 1st known case of contracting Ebola outside of Africa. CNN. http://www.cnn.com/2014/10/06/health/ebola-us/index.html?hpt=hp_t2. Accessed 6 Oct 2014

Burns R (2014) Pentagon orders 21-day Ebola quarantine for troops. Associated Press, ABC News. http://abcnews.go.com/Politics/wireStory/hagel-approves-21-day-ebola-quarantine-troops-26541976?page=2. Accessed 29 Oct 2014

Business Journals (2014) Dallas residents flock to Twitter to discuss Ebola. The Business Journals. http://www.bizjournals.com/dallas/news/2014/10/01/twitterverse-a-sample-of-the-reaction-to-the-ebola.html. Accessed 1 Oct 2014

Casert R (2014) EU wants massive increase in staff to fight Ebola. Associated Press, NBC 29. http://www.nbc29.com/story/27025247/eu-wants-massive-increase-in-staff-to-fight-ebola. Accessed 27 Oct 2014

Casule K (2014) Macedonia checking for Ebola after Briton dies, hotel sealed off. Reuters. http://in.reuters.com/article/2014/10/09/health-ebola-macedonia-idINKCN0HY24220141009. Accessed 9 Oct 2014

CBS DC and Associated Press (2014a) Report: 75 hospital workers who came in contact with Ebola patient placed on no-fly list. CBS DC. http://washington.cbslocal.com/2014/10/17/report-75-hospital-workers-who-came-in-contact-with-ebola-patient-placed-on-no-fly-list/. Accessed 17 Oct 2014

CBS DC and Associated Press (2014b) Ebola scare at Pentagon after woman who was recently in Africa vomits on tour bus. CBS DC. http://washington.cbslocal.com/2014/10/17/ebola-scare-at-pentagon-after-woman-who-was-recently-in-africa-vomits-on-tour-bus/. Accessed 17 Oct 2014

CBS DWF (2014a) Uncertainty continues at apartments where Ebola patient stayed. CBS DFW. http://dfw.cbslocal.com/2014/10/01/uncertainty-continues-at-apartments-where-ebola-patient-stayed/. Accessed 1 Oct 2014

CBS DFW (2014b) Family of U.S. Ebola carrier moves into donated home. CBS DFW. http://dfw.cbslocal.com/2014/10/03/family-of-u-s-ebola-carrier-moves-into-donated-home/. Accessed 3 Oct 2014

CBS DWF (2014c) Dallas County deputy recounts Ebola scare. CBS DFW. http://dfw.cbslocal.com/2014/10/10/dallas-county-deputy-recounts-ebola-scare/. Accessed 10 Oct 2014

CBS DWF (2014d) CDC plane safely transports Ebola patient Nina Pham to Maryland. CBS DFW. http://dfw.cbslocal.com/2014/10/16/presbyterian-hospital-prepares-to-move-ebola-patient-nina-pham/. Accessed 28 May 2017

CBS New York and Associated Press (2014) New York, New Jersey set up mandatory quarantine requirement amid Ebola threat. CBS New York, Associated Press. http://newyork.cbslocal.com/2014/10/24/new-york-new-jersey-set-up-mandatory-quarantine-requirement-amid-ebola-threat/. Accessed 24 Oct 2014

CBS News (2014a) Ebola could cost global economy $32.6B, World Bank says. CBS News, CBC News. http://www.cbc.ca/news/business/ebola-could-cost-global-economy-32-6b-world-bank-says-1.2792485. Accessed 8 Oct 2014

CBS News (2014b) Dallas officials vow to care for Ebola patient Nina Pham's dog. CBS News. http://www.cbsnews.com/news/dallas-officials-vow-to-care-for-ebola-patient-nina-phams-dog/. Accessed 25 May 2017

CBS News (2014c) U.S. soldiers returning from Liberia monitored for Ebola in Italy. CBS News. http://www.cbsnews.com/news/ebola-outbreak-u-s-soldiers-returning-from-liberia-placed-in-isolation-in-italy/. Accessed 27 Oct 2014

Centers for Disease Control and Prevention (2014a) Enhanced Ebola screening to start at five U.S. airports and new tracking program for all people entering U.S. from Ebola-affected countries. 8 Oct 2014

Centers for Disease Control and Prevention (2014b) CDC Expands Passenger Notification. 16 Oct 2014

Centers for Disease Control and Prevention (2014c) Tightened guidance for U.S. healthcare workers on personal protective equipment for Ebola. 20 Oct 2014

Centers for Disease Control and Prevention (2014d) Interim U.S. guidance for monitoring and movement of persons with potential Ebola virus exposure. 27 Oct 2014

Charlton C (2014) Liberian officials accused of muzzling reporters trying to draw worldwide attention to Ebola crisis after banning journalists from health clinics. The Daily Mail. http://www.dailymail.co.uk/news/article-2789350/liberian-officials-accused-muzzling-reporters-trying-draw-worldwide-attention-ebola-crisis-banning-journalists-health-clinics.html. Accessed 12 Oct 2014

Chazan D (2014) France introduces Ebola screening at airport. The Telegraph. http://www.telegraph.co.uk/news/worldnews/ebola/11171620/France-introduces-Ebola-screening-at-airport.html. Accessed 31 May 2017

Chicago Tribune (2014) Illinois orders mandatory Ebola quarantine for high-risk travelers. Chicago Tribune. http://www.chicagotribune.com/news/local/breaking/chi-illinois-ebola-quarantine-20141025-story.html. Accessed 25 Oct 2014

Chuck E (2014) National survey of nurses shows heightened Ebola concerns. NBC News. http://www.nbcnews.com/storyline/ebola-virus-outbreak/national-survey-nurses-shows-heightened-ebola-concerns-n224491. Accessed 13 Oct 2014

Cooper C, Morris N, Walker T (2014) Ebola outbreak: Britain sending 750 soldiers and medics to Western Africa. The Independent. http://www.independent.co.uk/life-style/health-and-families/health-news/ebola-outbreak-britain-sends-750-soldiers-and-medics-to-western-africa-9783010.html. Accessed 16 May 2017

Cowell A (2014) Health worker who may have had contact with Ebola is on a cruise ship. New York Times. http://www.nytimes.com/2014/10/18/us/ebola-cruise-ship-dallas.html?_r=0. Accessed 17 Oct 2014

Cutlack G (2014) UK government orders 500,000 Ebola protection suits. Gizmodo. http://www.gizmodo.co.uk/2014/10/uk-government-orders-500000-ebola-protection-suits/. Accessed 13 Oct 2014

Dallas News (2014) UPDATE: Ebola patients family being moved as officials lower number of potential contacts from 100 to 50. Dallas News. http://thescoopblog.dallasnews.com/2014/10/hazmat-cleanup-crew-welcomes-chance-to-clean-up-ebola-with-open-arms.html/. Accessed 3 Oct 2014

Dastin J (2014) U.S. airline group to meet with health officials on Ebola. The Star, Reuters. http://www.thestar.com.my/News/World/2014/10/07/US-airline-group-to-meet-with-health-officials-on-Ebola/. Accessed 6 Oct 2014

Day PK (2014) Media react to NBC News' Dr. Nancy Snyderman violating Ebola quarantine. LA Times. http://www.latimes.com/entertainment/tv/showtracker/la-et-st-media-reacts-nbc-news-nancy-snyderman-ebola-violation-20141014-story.html. Accessed 14 Oct 2014

Diarra A, Diagana K (2014) Mauritania closes border with Mali over Ebola fears. Reuters. http://www.reuters.com/article/2014/10/25/us-health-ebola-mali-idUSKCN0IE0GM20141025. Accessed 25 Oct 2014

DiLorenzo S (2014) WHO: number of Ebola-linked cases passes 10,000. Associated Press, Wane. http://wane.com/2014/10/25/who-number-of-ebola-linked-cases-passes-10000/. Accessed 3 Jun 2017

Dinan S (2014) State Department plans to bring foreign Ebola patients to U.S. The Washington Times. http://www.washingtontimes.com/news/2014/oct/28/state-department-plans-to-bring-foreign-ebola-pati/?page=3. Accessed 29 Oct 2014

Djuric B (2014) Many NY hospital staff call in sick after Ebola patient arrives. Newswire http://newswire.net/newsroom/news/00085750-a-number-of-ny-hospital-staff-call-in-sick-after-ebola-patient-arrives.html. Accessed 26 Oct 2014

Donahue C, Tensa K (2014) Connecticut prepares after Yale student shows Ebola-like symptoms. Ridgefield Daily Voice. http://ridgefield.dailyvoice.com/news/connecticut-prepares-after-yale-student-shows-ebola-symptoms. Accessed 16 Oct 2014

Donnelly L, Knapton S (2014) Ebola: NHS hospitals put on standby. The Telegraph. http://www.telegraph.co.uk/news/worldnews/ebola/11146375/David-Cameron-to-hold-emergency-meeting-over-Ebola.html. Accessed 7 Oct 2014

Douglas S (2014) Ebola Sierra Leone is fighting a war against an unseen proliferating virus. The Guardian. http://www.theguardian.com/commentisfree/2014/oct/12/ebola-sierra-leone-fighting-war-against-unseen-virus. Accessed 12 Oct 2014

Douglas J, Owens M (2014) Dog under surveillance while nurse quarantined for Ebola. WMAZ, WFAA. http://www.13wmaz.com/story/news/health/2014/10/14/dog-under-surveillance-while-nurse-quarantined-for-ebola/17246863/. Accessed 14 Oct 2014

Dowsett S (2014) Spain seeks answers as seven more enter Ebola hospital. Reuters. http://www.reuters.com/article/2014/10/10/us-health-ebola-spain-idUSKCN0HZ0U920141010. Accessed 10 Oct 2014

Dribben M (2014) Visitors tell of Ebola struggles in Sierra Leone. Philadelphia Inquirer. http://www.philly.com/philly/health/20141005_Visitors_tell_of_Ebola_struggles_in_Sierra_Leone.html. Accessed 5 Oct 2014

Du Lac FJ, Phillip A, Dennis B (2014) Dallas health worker who tested positive for Ebola wore 'full' protective gear. The Washington Post. http://www.washingtonpost.com/news/post-nation/wp/2014/10/12/dallas-health-care-worker-who-treated-thomas-eric-duncan-has-tested-positive-for-ebola/. Accessed 12 Oct 2014

Dwyer D (2014) President Obama convenes emergency Ebola meeting at White House. ABC News. http://abcnews.go.com/Politics/president-obama-convene-emergency-ebola-meeting-white-house/story?id=26214911. Accessed 15 Oct 2014

Eiserer T (2014) Sheriff's officers entered quarantined Ebola patient's apartment. ABC 10. http://www.news10.net/story/news/nation/2014/10/03/sheriffs-officers-entered-quarantined-ebola-patients-apartment/16634315/. Accessed 3 Oct 2014

Evans H, Karni A (2014) Bellevue Hospital ICU patients head to NYU Langone to free up staff for Ebola cases: sources. New York Daily News. http://www.nydailynews.com/new-york/bellevue-patients-head-nyu-center-free-space-ebola-cases-article-1.1989007. Accessed 27 Oct 2014

Evans H, Parascandola R, Smith GB et al (2014) Boy, 5, who traveled to West Africa tests negative for Ebola at Bellevue Hospital. New York Daily News. http://www.nydailynews.com/new-york/boy-5-returned-west-africa-tested-ebola-bellevue-hospital-article-1.1988468. Accessed 7 Jun 2017

Fernandez M, Sack K, Santora M (2014) In Dallas schools, fear of possible Ebola exposure. New York Times. https://www.nytimes.com/2014/10/03/us/dallas-schools-worry-about-ebola.html?_r=0. Accessed 7 May 2017

Fink S (2014) In Liberia, a good or very bad sign: empty hospital beds. New York Times. http://www.nytimes.com/2014/10/29/world/africa/in-liberia-a-good-or-very-bad-sign-empty-beds-.html. Accessed 28 Oct 2014

Flegenheimer M, Shear MD, Barbaro M (2014) Under pressure, Cuomo says Ebola quarantines can be spent at home. New York Times. https://www.nytimes.com/2014/10/27/nyregion/ebola-quarantine.html?_r=0. Accessed 4 Jun 2017

Fox M (2014) CDC promises special Ebola response reams. NBC News. http://www.nbcnews.com/storyline/ebola-virus-outbreak/cdc-promises-special-ebola-response-teams-n225636. Accessed 14 Oct 2014

Fox News (2014a) Health care worker at Dallas hospital tests positive for Ebola. Fox News. http://www.foxnews.com/health/2014/10/12/health-care-worker-at-dallas-hospital-tests-positive-for-ebola/. Accessed 12 Oct 2014

Fox News (2014b) Family identifies Amber Vinson as 2nd health care worker infected with Ebola. Fox News. http://www.foxnews.com/health/2014/10/15/family-identifies-2nd-health-care-worker-infected-with-ebola/. Accessed 15 Oct 2014

Fox News (2014c) New York Gov. Cuomo loosens Ebola quarantine restrictions after criticism. http://www.foxnews.com/politics/2014/10/27/new-york-gov-cuomo-loosens-ebola-quarantine-restrictions-after-criticism/. Accessed 27 Oct 2014

Freyer FJ (2014) R.I. journalist headed to Nebraska for Ebola treatment. The Boston Globe. http://www.bostonglobe.com/metro/2014/10/03/ebola-stricken-journalist-from-rhode-island-headed-nebraska-for-treatment/9ZJ4SdIKR3allmUjAuPqHO/story.html. Accessed 4 Oct 2014

Gallagher J (2014) Ebola nurse, William Pooley returns to Sierra Leone. BBC. http://www.bbc.com/news/health-29680400. Accessed 19 Oct 2014

Garza LM, Valdmanis R (2014) Dallas Ebola patient on ventilator and receiving kidney dialysis. Reuters, Yahoo News. http://news.yahoo.com/jesse-jackson-meet-family-ebola-patient-dallas-153326316.html. Accessed 7 Oct 2014

Gbandia S, Gale J (2014) Ebola now reported across Sierra Leone after cases in Koinadugu. Bloomberg. http://www.bloomberg.com/news/2014-10-16/ebola-now-reported-across-sierra-leone-after-cases-in-koinadugu.html. Accessed 15 Oct 2014

Ghebremedhin S, Battiste N, Keneally M (2014) Texas Ebola watch eyes 50 people, 10 at 'high risk'. ABC News. http://abcnews.go.com/Health/texas-ebola-watch-eyes-50-people-10-high/story?id=25938924. Accessed 3 Oct 2014

Giles C (2014) Husband of Spanish Ebola survivor 9 others leave hospital as 21-day observation period ends. Associated Press, 680 News. http://www.680news.com/2014/10/27/husband-of-spanish-ebola-survivor-9-others-leave-hospital-as-21-day-observation-period-ends/. Accessed 27 Oct 214

Goodwyn W (2014) First U.S. Ebola case confirmed In Dallas. NPR. http://www.npr.org/2014/10/01/352925378/first-u-s-ebola-case-confirmed-in-dallas. Accessed 30 Apr 2017

Govan F (2014) Ebola medics 'better trained in Sierra Leone than Spain'. The Telegraph. http://www.telegraph.co.uk/news/worldnews/ebola/11155840/Ebola-medics-better-trained-in-Sierra-Leone-than-Spain.html. Accessed 11 Oct 2014

Grogan K (2014) GSK chief Ebola vaccine will come too late for outbreak. PharmaTimes. http://www.pharmatimes.com/Article/14-10-17/GSK_chief_Ebola_vaccine_will_come_too_late_for_outbreak.aspx. Accessed 17 Oct 2014

Guardian (2014a) Gatwick begins Ebola screening. The Guardian. http://www.theguardian.com/world/2014/oct/21/gatwick-begins-ebola-screening. Accessed 21 Oct 2014

Guardian (2014b) Ebola case reported in Mali. The Guardian. http://www.theguardian.com/world/2014/oct/23/mali-first-case-ebola. Accessed 24 Oct 2014

Guynn J (2014) Mark Zuckerberg gives $25M to fight Ebola. USA Today. http://www.usatoday.com/story/tech/2014/10/14/mark-zuckerberg-facebook-ebola/17244621/. Accessed 14 Oct 2014

Harper J (2014) Tallmadge home where Ebola patient Amber Vinson stayed cordoned off by police. Cleveland.com. http://www.cleveland.com/akron/index.ssf/2014/10/tallmadge_home_where_ebola_pat.html. Accessed 15 Oct 2014

Hartmann M (2014) Everything we know about New York City's Ebola patient. New York Magazine. http://nymag.com/daily/intelligencer/2014/10/what-we-know-about-new-york-citys-ebola-patient.html. Accessed 24 Oct 2014

Hartocollus A (2014) 9 in Connecticut being watched for symptoms of Ebola. New York Times. http://www.nytimes.com/2014/10/23/nyregion/9-in-connecticut-being-watched-for-symptoms-of-ebola.html?action=click&contentCollection=Health&module=RelatedCoverage&region=Marginalia&pgtype=article. Accessed 22 Oct 2014

Hatton B, Giles C (2014) Ebola escapes Europe's defenses; pet dog must die. Associated Press, Lubbock Avalanche-Journal. http://lubbockonline.com/filed-online/2014-10-07/ebola-escapes-europes-defenses-pet-dog-must-die#.VDQuWrd0zix. Accessed 7 Oct 2014

Health Site (2014) Latest Ebola news: Germany treats the third Ebola patient. The Health Site. http://www.thehealthsite.com/news/latest-ebola-news-germany-treats-the-third-ebola-patient/. Accessed 10 Oct 2014

Hellenic Shipping News (2014) Ports tighten ship entry procedures as Ebola fears spread. 9 Oct 2014

Herriman R (2014) Ashoka Mukpo receives Brincidofovir at Nebraska, NIH releases exposed patient. Outbreak News Today. http://outbreaknewstoday.com/ashoka-mukpo-receives-brincidofovir-at-nebraska-nih-releases-exposed-patient-39826/. Accessed 15 May 2017

Hickox K (2014) UTA grad isolated at New Jersey hospital as part of Ebola quarantine. The Dallas Morning News. http://www.dallasnews.com/ebola/headlines/20141025-uta-grad-isolated-at-new-jersey-hospital-as-part-of-ebola-quarantine.ece. Accessed 26 Oct 2014

Hirschler B (2014) Drugmakers to join forces to make millions of Ebola vaccine doses. Reuters. http://www.reuters.com/article/2014/10/22/us-health-ebola-johnson-johnson-idUSKCN0IB0N420141022. Accessed 22 Oct 2014

Höije K (2014) Mali rushes to contain Ebola after its first case. The Guardian. http://www.theguardian.com/global-development/2014/oct/28/mali-rushes-contain-ebola-first-case. Accessed 28 Oct 2014

Houston Chronicle (2014) State: Ebola test negative for North Texas deputy. The Houston Chronicle. http://www.houstonchronicle.com/news/texas/article/Hospital-No-signs-of-Ebola-in-Dallas-area-officer-5811988.php#/0. Accessed 9 Oct 2014

Hsu SS, Henderson N-M (2014) No mandatory Ebola quarantine for health workers coming to Washington area. The Washington Post. http://www.washingtonpost.com/national/health-science/no-mandatory-ebola-quarantine-for-health-workers-coming-to-washington-area/2014/10/25/71a9a8c8-5c68-11e4-bd61-346aee66ba29_story.html. Accessed 25 Oct 2014

Hume J (2014) Canada to screen body temperatures of incoming West African passengers. Well and Tribune. http://www.wellandtribune.ca/2014/10/08/canada-to-screen-body-temperatures-of-incoming-west-african-passengers. Accessed 8 Oct 2014

Hussain M, Arsenault C (2014) Food crisis looms as Ebola rampages through West Africa. Reuters. http://af.reuters.com/article/topNews/idAFKCN0HR1P420141002?sp=true. Accessed 2 Oct 2014

Hylton H (2014) Dallas keeps calm and carries on after Ebola arrives. Time. http://time.com/3452341/dallas-ebola-texas-ground-zero/. Accessed 1 Oct 2014

Independent.ie (2014) Ebola woman touched face with glove. Independent.ie. http://www.independent.ie/world-news/ebola-woman-touched-face-with-glove-30649259.html. Accessed 14 May 2017

Infection Control Today (2014) Free Ebola online courses available from UNMC Nebraska Medicine. Infection Control Today. http://www.infectioncontroltoday.com/news/2014/10/free-ebola-online-courses-available-from-unmc-nebraska-medicine.aspx. Accessed 27 Oct 2014

James D (2014) CDC Ebola response team converges on New York City. Pharmacy Times. http://www.pharmacytimes.com/news/CDC-Ebola-Response-Team-Converges-on-New-York-City?utm_source=GoogleNews&utm_medium=GoogleNews&utm_campaign=PharmacyTimesNews. Accessed 24 Oct 2014

Jansing C (2014) Samantha Power travels to Guinea amid Ebola outbreak. NBC News. http://www.nbcnews.com/storyline/ebola-virus-outbreak/samantha-power-travels-guinea-amid-ebola-outbreak-n234081. Accessed 26 Oct 2014

JTA (2014) Israeli agency sends mobile clinics to Africa to fight Ebola. JTA. http://www.jta.org/2014/10/05/news-opinion/israel-middle-east/israeli-agency-sends-mobile-clinics-to-africa-to-fight-ebola. Accessed 5 Oct 2014

Kalter L (2014) Doctor details life in Ebola-torn Liberia. The Boston Herald. http://www.bostonherald.com/news_opinion/local_coverage/2014/10/doctor_details_life_in_ebola_torn_liberia. Accessed 19 Oct 2017

Kamara A (2014) Ebola burial teams in Sierra Leone go back to work. USA Today. https://www.usatoday.com/story/news/world/2014/10/08/ebola-sierra-leone-spain/16898253/. Accessed 15 May 2017

Karimi F (2014) From Guinea to the U.S.: timeline of first Ebola patient in New York City. CNN. http://www.cnn.com/2014/10/24/health/new-york-ebola-timeline/. Accessed 24 Oct 2014

Karimi F, Sutton J (2014) Dallas Ebola patient is in critical condition, hospital says. CNN. http://www.cnn.com/2014/10/04/health/ebola-us/. Accessed 10 May 2017

Kassam A (2014a) Spanish nurse's Ebola infection blamed on substandard equipment. The Guardian. http://www.theguardian.com/world/2014/oct/07/ebola-crisis-substandard-equipment-nurse-positive-spain. Accessed 7 Oct 2014

Kassam A (2014b) Nurse reported Ebola symptoms many times before being quarantined. The Guardian. http://www.theguardian.com/world/2014/oct/08/spanish-ebola-nurse-symptoms-quarantine. Accessed 8 Oct 2014

Kassam A (2014c) Spanish Ebola patient's condition worsens as seven people are quarantined. The Guardian. https://www.theguardian.com/world/2014/oct/09/ebola-outbreak-six-quarantined-in-spain-madrid-hospital-ramos. Accessed 16 May 2017

Kassam A (2014d) Madrid hospital staff quit over Ebola fears. The Guardian. http://www.theguardian.com/world/2014/oct/10/madrid-hospital-staff-quit-ebola. Accessed 10 Oct 2014

Kelto A (2014) CDC issues new Ebola screening protocols for U.S. airports. NPR. http://www.npr.org/2014/10/08/354639728/cdc-issues-new-ebola-screening-protocols-for-u-s-airports. Accessed 8 Oct 2014

Keneally M (2014a) US journalist believes he got Ebola while cleaning infected car. ABC News. http://abcnews.go.com/Health/us-journalist-ebola-nebraska-treatment/story?id=25987193. Accessed 6 Oct 2014

Keneally M (2014b) Ebola scare sends Caribbean cruise ship back home. ABC News. http://abcnews.go.com/Health/ebola-scare-sends-caribbean-cruise-ship-back-home/story?id=26276019. Accessed 31 May 2017

Keneally M, Battiste N (2014) Texas Ebola patient Thomas Eric Duncan now getting experimental drug. ABC News. http://abcnews.go.com/Health/texas-ebola-patient-thomas-eric-duncan-now-experimental/story?id=25998659. Accessed 14 May 2017

Kent J (2014) TSA agent at Cleveland Hopkins Airport patted down Ebola patient; now on paid leave. http://www.clevelandleader.com/node/23242. Accessed 18 Oct 2014

Kesling B (2014) Ohio bans international travel for residents being monitored for Ebola. The Wall Street Journal. http://online.wsj.com/articles/ohio-bans-international-travel-for-residents-being-monitored-for-ebola-1413687948. Accessed 19 Oct 2014

Killough A (2014) New York governor on Ebola fears: I'll ride the subway today. CNN. http://www.cnn.com/2014/10/24/politics/andrew-cuomo-ebola/. Accessed 4 Jun 2017

Kocherga A (2014) Fort Bliss families worry as troops prepare to head to West Africa. KHOU. http://www.khou.com/story/news/health/2014/10/01/families-of-us-soldiers-worry-as-troops-prepare-for-deployment-in-west-africa-to-fight-ebola-epidemic/16567449/. Accessed 2 Oct 2014

Korte G, Vanden Brook T (2014) Obama may call on reserves to deal with Ebola in Africa. USA Today. http://www.usatoday.com/story/news/politics/2014/10/16/obama-ebola-reserves/17363251/. Accessed 16 Oct 2014

Larson K (2014) Liberia short on ambulances for Ebola patients. US World & News Report. https://www.usnews.com/news/world/articles/2014/10/01/liberia-short-on-ambulances-for-ebola-patients. Accessed 30 Apr 2017

Leitsinger M (2014) The E-Team: pentagon announces special Ebola support squad. NBC News. http://www.nbcnews.com/news/us-news/e-team-pentagon-announces-special-ebola-support-squad-n229266. Accessed 19 Oct 2014

Leitsinger M, Jamieson A (2014) Texas Ebola watch ends for 48 contacts of Thomas Eric Duncan. NBC News. http://www.nbcnews.com/storyline/ebola-virus-outbreak/texas-ebola-watch-ends-48-contacts-thomas-eric-duncan-n229491. Accessed 20 Oct 2014

Levy A (2014) 101st Airborne to take over in Africa deployment. http://www.14news.com/story/26883766/101st-airborne-to-take-over-in-africa-deployment. Associated Press, 14 News. Accessed 24 Oct 2014

Liping G (2014) China pledges 500m yuan Ebola aid to Africa. China Daily, ECNS. http://www.ecns.cn/2014/10-25/139949.shtml. Accessed 24 Oct 2014

Livingston D, Powell C (2014) Ebola patient who visited Summit County might have been contagious longer than first believed; 7 in county quarantined. Akron Beacon J. http://www.ohio.com/news/break-news/ebola-patient-who-visited-summit-county-might-have-been-contagious-longer-than-first-believed-7-in-county-quarantined-1.532246#. Accessed 30 May 2017

Loftus M (2015) The long, extraordinary recovery of Ian Crozier. Emory Med Spring 2015:9

Lomax S (2014) Liberia health workers abandon Ebola ETU in Bong County over pay. AllAfrica. http://allafrica.com/stories/201410061344.html. Accessed 4 Oct 2014

Lopez R (2014) Confusion concern where Ebola patient stayed. WFAA. http://www.wfaa.com/story/news/health/2014/10/01/ivy-apartments-ebola-reaction/16569917/. Accessed 1 Oct 2014

Lupkin S (2014) Texas health workers use Tabasco to help train for Ebola. ABC News. http://abcnews.go.com/Health/texas-health-workers-tabasco-train-ebola/story?id=26385702. Accessed 23 Oct 2014

Malo S (2014) Ebola screening starts at New York's JFK airport. Reuters. http://www.reuters.com/article/us-health-ebola-jfk-idUSKCN0I004U20141011. Accessed 17 May 2017

Mangan D (2014) Texas college rejects Nigerian applicants, cites Ebola cases. NBC News. http://
    www.nbcnews.com/storyline/ebola-virus-outbreak/texas-college-rejects-nigerian-applicants-
    cites-ebola-cases-n226291. Accessed 15 Oct 2014
Marcos C (2014) Lawmakers call for official Ebola response coordinator. The Hill. http://thehill.
    com/blogs/floor-action/house/219936-lawmakers-call-for-official-ebola-response-coordinator.
    Accessed 7 Oct 2014
Margason G (2014) Texas juvenile arrested after posting false Ebola report on Twitter. NewsOK.
    http://newsok.com/frisco-student-arrested-for-creating-false-ebolascare/article/5348040.
    Accessed 2 Oct 2014
Marowits R (2014) Air Canada allows flight attendants to wear gloves to protect against Ebola.
    Canadian Occupation Safety. http://www.cos-mag.com/emergency-management/emergency-
    management-stories/4162-air-canada-allows-flight-attendants-to-wear-gloves-to-protect-
    against-ebola.html. Accessed 20 Oct 2014
Martin B (2014) Travel shares drop on Ebola fears. The Telegraph. http://www.telegraph.co.uk/
    finance/markets/11145573/Travel-shares-drop-on-Ebola-fears.html. Accessed 15 May 2014
Martinez M (2014) U.S. Ebola patients partner quarantined in apartment with family members.
    CNN.   http://www.cnn.com/2014/10/02/us/texas-woman-quarantine-ebola-thomas-duncan/
    index.html?hpt=hp_t1. Accessed 2 Oct 2014
Mathis-Lilley B (2014) Kaci Hickox still doesn't have Ebola, might move out of Maine. The
    Slatest. http://www.slate.com/blogs/the_slatest/2014/11/10/kaci_hickox_ebola_nurse_likely_
    not_infected_may_leave_state.html. Accessed 10 Nov 2014
Mazumdar T (2014) Devastating news from the Ebola clinic. BBC. http://www.bbc.com/news/
    health-29507673. Accessed 7 Oct 2014
McGuirk R (2014) Australia lifts Ebola donation to $16 million but won't send personnel for
    fear of infection. Daily Journal. http://www.dailyjournal.net/view/story/ba2f515e3c6045de-
    b3761047e5e8728c/AS--Australia-Ebola/. Accessed 2 Oct 2014
McNeil DG Jr (2014) Second Ebola outbreak in Mali eclipses early success. New York Times.
    https://www.nytimes.com/2014/11/13/health/mali-reports-a-second-larger-ebola-outbreak.
    html?_r=0. Accessed 4 Jun 2017
McNeil DG Jr, Shear MD (2014) U.S. plans 21-day watch of travelers from Ebola-hit nations.
    New York Times. http://www.nytimes.com/2014/10/23/health/us-to-monitor-travelers-from-
    ebola-hit-nations-for-21-days.html?_r=0. Accessed 22 Oct 2014
Médecins Sans Frontières (2014) Ebola: Norwegian MSF staff member infected in Sierra Leone.
    6 Oct 2014
Miles T (2014) Update 1 – Mali Ebola victim had contact with 141 people, 57 still sought.
    Reuters.   http://af.reuters.com/article/commoditiesNews/idAFL5N0SQ3VO20141031?sp=t
    rue. Accessed 31 Oct 2014
MINA (2014) Foreigner dies at Clinic of Infectious Disease, doctors think he had Ebola. MINA,
    Macedonia Online. http://macedoniaonline.eu/content/view/26226/2/. Accessed 9 Oct 2014
Minder R, Belluck P (2014) Spain, amid protests, kills dog of Ebola-infected nurse. New York
    Times. http://www.nytimes.com/2014/10/09/science/ebola-dog-excalibur-nurse-spain.html?_
    r=0. Accessed 8 Oct 2014
Minder R, Grady D (2014) Ebola Infects Spanish Nurse, a First in West. New York Times. https://
    www.nytimes.com/2014/10/07/world/europe/spain-reports-first-case-of-ebola-contracted-out-
    side-west-africa.html. Accessed 24 Sept 2017
Monnier O, Rihouay F (2014) WHO said to track 111 people in Mali after Ebola death. Bloomberg.
    http://www.bloomberg.com/news/2014-10-28/who-said-to-track-111-people-in-mali-after-
    ebola-death.html. Accessed 27 Oct 2014
Morozova D (2014) Woman who fell ill in Pentagon parking lot doesn't have Ebola. http://news-
    maine.net/21056-woman-who-fell-ill-pentagon-parking-lot-doesnt-have-ebola. Accessed 18
    Oct 2014

Morris S (2014) Husband of Spanish nurse quarantined. IOL, Reuters. http://www.iol.co.za/news/world/husband-of-spanish-nurse-quarantined-1.1761458#.VDPqqLd0ziw. Accessed 7 Oct 2014

Murray L (2014) Revenue plummets 25 percent at Texas Health Presbyterian after Ebola cases. Dallas Business Journal. http://www.bizjournals.com/dallas/blog/morning_call/2014/10/revenue-plummets-25-percent-at-texas-health.html?utm_source=feedburner&utm_medium=feed&utm_campaign=Feed%3A+industry_6+(Industry+Health+Care). Accessed 23 Oct 2014

Nadeau BL (2014) Ebola contracted in Madrid hospital could spread in Europe. The Daily Beast. http://www.thedailybeast.com/articles/2014/10/07/ebola-contracted-in-madrid-hospital-could-spread-in-europe. Accessed 7 Oct 2014

NBC DFW (2014) Ebola patient contacted CDC before flight, agency says. NBC DFW. http://www.nbcdfw.com/news/local/Ebola-Patient-Contacted-CDC-Before-Flight-Agency-Says-279365622.html. Accessed 15 Oct 2014

NBC News (2014a) Texas Ebola patient had contact with school age kids Perry Says. NBC News. http://www.nbcnews.com/storyline/ebola-virus-outbreak/texas-ebola-patient-had-contact-school-age-kids-perry-says-n215976. Accessed 1 Oct 2014

NBC News (2014b) NBC News freelancer in Africa diagnosed with Ebola. NBC News. http://www.nbcnews.com/storyline/ebola-virus-outbreak/nbc-news-freelancer-africa-diagnosed-ebola-n217271. Accessed 7 May 2017

NBC News (2014c) U.S. close to solution for how hospitals must dispose of Ebola waste. NBC News. http://www.nbcnews.com/storyline/ebola-virus-outbreak/u-s-close-solution-how-hospitals-must-dispose-ebola-waste-n216596. Accessed 2 Oct 2014

NBC News (2014d) Ebola survivor Dr. Kent Brantly donates blood to Ashoka Mukpo. NBC News. http://www.nbcnews.com/storyline/ebola-virus-outbreak/ebola-survivor-dr-kent-brantly-donates-blood-ashoka-mukpo-n220811. Accessed 8 Oct 2014

NBC News (2014e) Ebola-infected nurse Amber Vinson arrives at Emory for treatment. NBC News. http://www.nbcnews.com/storyline/ebola-virus-outbreak/ebola-infected-nurse-amber-vinson-arrives-emory-treatment-n226976. Accessed 28 May 2017

NBC News (2014f) Airline: CDC warned 'possibility' Ebola nurse had symptoms on plane. NBC News. http://www.nbcnews.com/storyline/ebola-virus-outbreak/airline-cdc-warned-possibility-ebola-nurse-had-symptoms-plane-n227046. Accessed 16 Oct 2014

NBC News (2014g) Dallas considers disaster declaration due to Ebola. NBC News. http://www.nbcnews.com/storyline/ebola-virus-outbreak/dallas-considers-disaster-declaration-due-ebola-n227571. Accessed 16 Oct 2014

Nelson S (2014) Ebola hotline launched in Illinois. WQAD. http://wqad.com/2014/10/17/ebola-hotline-launched-in-illinois/. Accessed 17 Oct 2014

Neuman S (2014) Mali's first Ebola case in current outbreak is 2-year-old girl. NPR, Wyoming Public Media. http://wyomingpublicmedia.org/post/malis-first-ebola-case-current-outbreak-2-year-old-girl. Accessed 24 Oct 2014

New Haven Register (2014) Yale grad student who traveled to Liberia hospitalized with Ebola-like symptoms in New Haven. http://www.ctnewsjunkie.com/archives/entry/yale_grad_student_who_traveled_to_liberia_hospitalized_with_ebola-like_symp. Accessed 16 Oct 2014

Newcastle Herald (2014) Ebola epidemic: Australian aid worker Brett Adamson's despair. Newcastle Herald. http://www.theherald.com.au/story/2603201/ebola-epidemic-horrific-says-aussie-aid-worker-poll/?cs=305. Accessed 3 Oct 2014

Nossiter A (2014a) A hospital from hell in a city swamped by Ebola. New York Times. http://www.nytimes.com/2014/10/02/world/africa/ebola-spreading-in-west-africa.html?_r=0. Accessed 1 Oct 2014

Nossiter A (2014b) Ebola help for Sierra Leone is nearby, but delayed on the docks. New York Times. http://www.nytimes.com/2014/10/06/world/africa/sierra-leone-ebola-medical-supplies-delayed-docks.html?_r=0. Accessed 6 Oct 2014

Nossiter A (2014c) Officials admit a defeat by Ebola in Sierra Leone. New York Times. http://www.nytimes.com/2014/10/11/world/africa/officials-admit-a-defeat-by-ebola-in-sierra-leone.html?_r=0. Accessed 11 Oct 2014

NPR (2014) An Ebola success story in northern Liberia. NPR. http://www.npr.org/2014/10/26/359065316/an-ebola-success-story-in-northern-liberia. Accessed 7 Jun 2017

NYC Health + Hospitals (2014) Statement on patient at Bellevue Hospital. 23 Oct 2014

O'Carroll L (2014a) Ebola: Sierra Leone hospitals running out of basic supplies, say doctors. The Guardian. http://www.theguardian.com/world/2014/oct/03/ebola-sierra-leone-epidemic. Accessed 3 Oct 2014

O'Carroll L (2014b) British nurse who survived Ebola on his way back to Sierra Leone. The Guardian. http://www.theguardian.com/world/2014/oct/15/british-nurse-ebola-survivor-sierra-leone-return. Accessed 15 Oct 2014

O'Carroll L (2014c) Sierra Leone's fight against Ebola infection: 'the world is not safe.' The Guardian. http://www.theguardian.com/world/2014/oct/30/ebola-sierra-leone-fight-who-disease-fight. Accessed 30 Oct 2014

Ohio Department of Health (2014) Ohio Department of Health: 16 October 2014. 16 Oct 2014

Ohlheiser A (2014) Cut off from school, children in Ebola-stricken Sierra Leone get lessons by radio. The Washington Post. http://www.washingtonpost.com/news/to-your-health/wp/2014/10/09/cut-off-from-school-children-in-ebola-stricken-sierra-leone-get-lessons-by-radio/. Accessed 9 Oct 2014

Ohlheiser A, Phillip A (2014) As Spanish Ebola patient's health deteriorates, two doctors who treated her are under observation. The Washington Post. http://www.washingtonpost.com/news/to-your-health/wp/2014/10/09/as-spanish-ebola-patients-health-deteriorates-two-doctors-who-treated-her-are-under-observation/. Accessed 9 Oct 2014

Olu-Mammah J, Giahyue JH (2014) Sierra Leone residents clash with police over Ebola response. Reuters. http://www.globalpost.com/dispatch/news/thomson-reuters/141014/sierra-leone-residents-clash-police-over-ebola-response. Accessed 14 Oct 2014

Onishi N (2014) U.S. patient aided pregnant Liberian, then took ill. New York Times. http://www.nytimes.com/2014/10/02/world/africa/ebola-victim-texas-thomas-eric-duncan.html. Accessed 2 Oct 2014

Page J (2014) Judge rejects strict limits on U.S. nurse who treated Ebola patients. Reuters. http://www.reuters.com/article/2014/10/31/us-health-ebola-usa-idUSKBN0II1SP20141031. Accessed 31 Oct 2014

Paye-Layleh J (2014a) Liberia leader seeks more power to fight Ebola, but critics decry measures as heavy handed. Associated Press, 660 News. http://www.660news.com/2014/10/10/liberia-leader-seeks-more-power-to-fight-ebola-but-critics-decry-measures-as-heavy-handed/. Accessed 10 Oct 2014

Paye-Layleh J (2014b) Beds at Ebola treatment units empty in Liberia. Associated Press, SF Gate. http://www.sfgate.com/news/medical/article/Cremation-fears-leave-empty-Ebola-beds-in-Liberia-5843034.php. Accessed 24 Oct 2014

Paye-Layleh J (2014c) Liberia opens 1 of largest Ebola treatment centers. Associated Press, ABC News. http://abcnews.go.com/International/wireStory/liberia-opens-largest-ebola-treatment-centers-26597737. Accessed 31 Oct 2014

Paye-Layleh J, Giles C (2014) U.S. military planes deliver more marines into Ebola hot zone; African leaders plead for help. Associated Press, Democratic Underground. https://www.democraticunderground.com/1014914460. Accessed 16 May 2017

Paye-Layleh J, Roy-Macaulay C (2014) Dozens quarantined for Ebola in Liberia threaten to break out of isolation for lack of food. US News & World Report. https://www.usnews.com/news/world/articles/2014/10/23/threat-to-break-isolation-in-liberia-over-food. Accessed 23 Oct 2014

Penty C, Munoz M (2014) Spanish Ebola patients doctor lays out procedure shortfalls. Associated Press, The Daily Herald. http://www.dailyherald.com/article/20141009/news/141008329/. Accessed 9 Oct 2014

Perez C (2014) 5 kids linked to Ebola case held in isolation. The New York Post. http://nypost. com/2014/10/01/texas-ebola-victim-may-have-infected-another-person. Accessed 1 Oct 2014

Phillip A, Ferdman RA (2014) After nurse contracts Ebola Spanish health workers raise concerns about protective equipment. The Washington Post. http://www.washingtonpost.com/news/ to-your-health/wp/2014/10/07/after-nurse-contracts-ebola-spanish-health-workers-raise-concerns-about-protective-equipment/. Accessed 7 Oct 2014

Pinckard C (2014) Horseshoe Casino Cleveland customer arrested after comment about Ebola. Cleveland.com. http://www.cleveland.com/metro/index.ssf/2014/10/horseshoe_casino_cleveland_cus.html. Accessed 28 May 2014

Power S (2014) Twitter, 28 Oct 2014. https://twitter.com/AmbPower44/ status/527070625882726400?ref_src=twsrc%5Etfw&ref_url=http%3A%2F%2Fwww. masslive.com%2Fnews%2Findex.ssf%2F2014%2F10%2Fgood_ebola_news_out_of_west_ af.html. Accessed 8 Jun 2017

Pudelek J (2014) DEC launches Ebola appeal. Civil Society News. http://www.civilsociety.co.uk/ fundraising/news/content/18468/dec_launches_ebola_appeal. Accessed 29 Oct 2014

Rahmanzadeh S, Mohney G (2014) Deputy who delivered Ebola quarantine order in hospital ER. ABC News. http://abcnews.go.com/Health/deputy-delivered-ebola-quarantine-order-hospital-er/story?id=26055781. Accessed 8 Oct 2014

Rainone C (2014) Ebola in Dallas: what we know about 2nd case diagnosed in U.S. NBC, NBC Bay Area. http://www.nbcbayarea.com/news/national-international/Ebola-Dallas-Health-Worker-278937901.html. Accessed 12 Oct 2014

Rajagopalan M (2014) China is sending an elite army unit to Ebola-hit Liberia. Business Insider. http://www.businessinsider.com.au/r-china-to-send-elite-army-unit-to-help-fight-ebola-in-liberia-2014-10. Accessed 30 Oct 2014

Reuters (2014a) US stocks – Wall St. falls on Ebola concerns; airlines tumble. Reuters, The Daily Mail. http://www.dailymail.co.uk/wires/reuters/article-2776495/US-STOCKS-Wall-St-falls-Ebola-concerns-airlines-tumble.html. Accessed 1 Oct 2014

Reuters (2014b) Dallas Ebola patient throwing up all over the place on way to hospital. Retuers, The Baltimore Sun. http://www.baltimoresun.com/health/chi-ebola-patient-america-20141002,0,4611727.story. Accessed 2 Oct 2014

Reuters (2014c) First French Ebola patient leaves hospital. Reuters. http://in.reuters.com/article/2014/10/04/health-ebola-france-idINL6N0RZ0DC20141004. Accessed 4 Oct 2014

Reuters (2014d) Canada sending second mobile Ebola lab scientists to Sierra Leone. Reuters, Canoe.com. http://cnews.canoe.ca/CNEWS/Canada/2014/10/04/21985931.html. Accessed 4 Oct 2014

Reuters (2014e) Sierra Leone records 121 Ebola deaths in a single day. Reuters. http://www. reuters.com/article/2014/10/06/us-health-ebola-leone-idUSKCN0HU0ZT20141006. Accessed 6 Oct 2014

Reuters (2014f) High risk Ebola could reach France and UK by end-October, scientists calculate. Reuters, NDTV. http://www.ndtv.com/article/world/high-risk-ebola-could-reach-france-and-uk-by-end-october-scientists-calculate-602254. Accessed 5 Oct 2014

Reuters (2014g) Norway will fly its first Ebola patient back from Sierra Leone. Reuters. http:// www.reuters.com/article/us-heatlh-ebola-norway-idUSKCN0HV1IT20141006. Accessed 14 May 2017

Reuters (2014h) Liberian healthcare workers want hazard pay. Reuters, Eyewitness News. http:// ewn.co.za/2014/10/07/Ebola-health-care-workers-want-hazard-pay. Accessed 7 Oct 2014

Reuters (2014i) Ebola burial teams in Sierra Leone on strike over hazard pay. Reuters, The Huffington Post. http://www.huffingtonpost.com/2014/10/07/sierra-leone-ebola-strike_n_5948192.html. Accessed 7 Oct 2014

Reuters (2014j) U.N. medic in Liberia tests positive for Ebola. Retuers. http://www.trust.org/ item/20141008110012-vjk35/?source=fiOtherNews2. Accessed 8 Oct 2014

Reuters (2014k) Britain says to start screening passengers for Ebola. Reuters. http://af.reuters. com/article/sierraLeoneNews/idAFL6N0S44D720141009. Accessed 9 Oct 2014

Reuters (2014l) Spanish Ebola victim conscious and sitting unaided. Reuters. http://www.reuters. com/article/2014/10/11/us-health-ebola-spain-idUSKCN0HZ0U920141011. Accessed 11 Oct 2014

Reuters (2014m) Healthcare crippled as Ebola overwhelms hospitals in Liberia. Reuters, Fox News. http://www.foxnews.com/health/2014/10/10/healthcare-crippled-as-ebola-overwhelms-hospitals-in-liberia/. Accessed 10 Oct 2014

Reuters (2014n) Third Ebola patient released from Atlanta's Emory University Hospital. Reuters. http://www.reuters.com/article/us-health-ebola-usa-emory-idUSKCN0I927720141020. Accessed 2 Jun 2017

Reuters (2014o) US restricts entrants from Ebola hit nations to five airports. Reuters, KFGO. http://kfgo.com/news/articles/2014/oct/21/us-restricts-entrants-from-ebola-hit-nations-to-five-airports/. Accessed 21 Oct 2014

Reuters (2014p) As virus spreads insurers exclude Ebola from new policies. Reuters, Jamestown Sun. http://www.jamestownsun.com/content/virus-spreads-insurers-exclude-ebola-new-policies. Accessed 22 Oct 2014

Reuters (2014q) Liberians fast, pray for three days to break Ebola 'curse.' Reuters, Fox News. http://www.foxnews.com/health/2014/10/30/liberians-fast-pray-for-three-days-to-break-ebola-curse/. Accessed 30 Oct 2014

Ritchie A (2014) Ebola is 'disaster of our generation' says aid agency. AFP, Yahoo News. http://news.yahoo.com/obama-calls-end-ebola-hysteria-110006011.html. Accessed 18 Oct 2014

Robinson M (2014) British Army medics from 22 Field Hospital in Aldershot arrive in Sierra Leone as part of UK's response in fight against Ebola crisis. The Daily Mail. http://www.dailymail.co.uk/news/article-2795151/british-army-medics-22-field-hospital-aldershot-arrive-sierra-leone-uk-s-response-fight-against-ebola-crisis.html. Accessed 16 Oct 2014

Román D (2014) Spain struggles to address concern over Ebola case. The Wall Street J. http://online.wsj.com/articles/spain-struggles-to-address-concern-over-ebola-case-1412678870. Accessed 7 Oct 2014

Rudra G (2014) Ebola-infected doctor's fiancee back in their home. ABC News. http://abcnews.go.com/Health/ebola-infected-doctors-fiancee-back-home/story?id=26450510. Accessed 25 Oct 2014

Saavedra M (2014) Photos offer insight after Ebola decontamination. KHOU. http://www.khou.com/story/news/local/texas/2014/10/21/photos-offer-insight-after-ebola-decontamination/17655803/. Accessed 21 Oct 2014

Sannoh B (2014) Ebola – as seen through the eyes of a 13-year-old from Sierra Leone. The Guardian. http://www.theguardian.com/world/2014/oct/11/bintu-sannoh-ebola-sierra-leone-eyewitness. Accessed 12 Oct 2014

Santora M (2014a) Doctor in New York City is sick with Ebola. New York Times. http://www.nytimes.com/2014/10/24/nyregion/craig-spencer-is-tested-for-ebola-virus-at-bellevue-hospital-in-new-york-city.html?_r=0. Accessed 24 Oct 2014

Santora M (2014b) New York State offers protections for medical workers joining Ebola fight. New York Times. http://www.nytimes.com/2014/10/31/nyregion/new-york-state-offers-protections-for-medical-workers-joining-ebola-fight.html?_r=0. Accessed 30 Oct 2014

Schechter D (2014) Dallas diocese provided secret Ebola isolation home. WFAA. http://www.wfaa.com/story/news/health/2014/10/20/ebola-isolation-duncan-family-catholic-church/17637929/. Accessed 21 Oct 2014

Schieffelin JS, Shaffer JG, Goba A et al (2014) Clinical illness and outcomes in patients with Ebola in Sierra Leone. N Engl J Med 371:2092–2100

Schluz S (2014) New Ebola containment facility comes to north Texas. NBC DFW. http://www.nbcdfw.com/news/health/Perry-to-Announce-Change-to-Texas-Ebola-Preparedness-Response-279914872.html. Accessed 21 Oct 2014

Schnirring L (2014) Feds unveil Ebola screening steps; Texas patient dies. CIDRAP. http://www.cidrap.umn.edu/news-perspective/2014/10/feds-unveil-ebola-screening-steps-texas-patient-dies. Accessed 15 May 2017

Schwartz C (2014) Nurse under Ebola quarantine hires civil rights lawyer. The Huffington Post. http://www.huffingtonpost.com/2014/10/26/kaci-hickox-lawyer_n_6050450.html. Accessed 4 Jun 2017

Serna J (2014) California issues quarantine policy for Ebola Exposure. LA Times. http://www.latimes.com/local/lanow/la-me-ln-california-orders-ebola-quarantine-protocols-20141029-story.html. Accessed 8 Jun 2017

Shankar S (2014) Sierra Leone peacekeepers quarantined after one soldier tests positive for Ebola. International Business Times. http://www.ibtimes.com/sierra-leone-peacekeepers-quarantined-after-one-soldier-tests-positive-ebola-1704488. Accessed 14 Oct 2014

Sharkov D (2014) Spanish nurse infected with Ebola receives blood transfusion from recovered patient. Newsweek. http://www.newsweek.com/spanish-nurse-infected-ebola-receives-blood-transfusion-recovered-patient-275813. Accessed 15 May 2017

Sheets CA (2014) US government Has Ebola 'do not fly list' of exposed people: report. International Business Times. http://www.ibtimes.com/us-government-has-ebola-do-not-fly-list-exposed-people-report-1705808. Accessed 28 May 2017

Shoichet CE (2014) Nurses' union slams Texas hospital for lack of Ebola protocol. CNN. http://www.cnn.com/2014/10/15/health/texas-ebola-nurses-union-claims/index.html?hpt=hp_t1. Accessed 15 Oct 2014

Shoichet CE, Levs J, Yan H (2014) CDC: U.S. health worker with Ebola should not have flown on commercial jet. CNN. http://www.cnn.com/2014/10/15/health/texas-ebola-outbreak/index.html?hpt=hp_t1. Accessed 15 Oct 2014

Sia SJ (2014) What movie night means to patients in an Ebola ward. http://qz.com/287442/what-movie-night-means-to-patients-in-an-ebola-ward/?utm_medium=App.net&utm_source=PourOver. Quartz, International Medical Corps. Accessed 27 Oct 2014

Sickles J (2014) Ebola quarantine ends for Thomas Eric Duncan's fiancee, but not her heartache. Yahoo News. https://news.yahoo.com/ebola-quarantine-ends-for-thomas-eric-duncans-financee-but-not-grief-163314541.html. Accessed 20 Oct 2014

Sieff K (2014) As Ebola patients vanish in Liberia's health system, survivors go on a desperate search. The Washington Post. http://www.washingtonpost.com/world/africa/as-ebola-patients-vanish-in-liberias-health-system-survivors-go-on-a-desperate-search/2014/10/20/274acf48-08dd-4a76-9f58-8c35dfb22312_story.html. Accessed 20 Oct 2014

Sifferlin A (2014) Emory's 'sickest' Ebola patient, now in recovery, reveals identity. Time. http://time.com/3622735/ebola-emory-university-hospital-ian-crozier/. Accessed 7 Dec 2014

Silver M (2014) Ebola diary: the grave diggers, the mistress, the man on the porch. NPR. http://www.npr.org/blogs/goatsandsoda/2014/10/12/354626252/ebola-diary-the-grave-diggers-the-mistress-the-man-on-the-porch. Accessed 12 Oct 2014

Sputnik International (2014) Liberia suspends senate elections amid Ebola outbreak: reports. Sputnik International. http://en.ria.ru/society/20141009/193869208/Liberia-Suspends-Senate-Elections-Amid-Ebola-Outbreak-Reports.html. Accessed 9 Oct 2014

Stanglin D (2014a) Liberia says Dallas Ebola patient lied on exit documents. USA Today. http://www.usatoday.com/story/news/nation/2014/10/02/liberia-ebola-patient-thomas-duncan-airport-screening/16591753/. Initially accessed 2 Oct 2014

Stanglin D (2014b) Rwanda to screen US visitors for Ebola. USA Today. http://www.usatoday.com/story/news/world/2014/10/21/rwanda-united-statees-ebola-screening/17653947/. Accessed 21 Oct 2014

Styles R (2014) Shunned by their families evicted from their homes and paid next to nothing: plight of African nurses risking their lives to treat Ebola patients revealed. The Daily Mail. http://www.dailymail.co.uk/femail/article-2810935/Shunned-families-evicted-homes-paid-Plight-African-nurses-risking-lives-treat-ebola-patients-revealed.html. Accessed 28 Oct 2014

Sullivan P (2014) House Dems call for US troops to give direct Ebola care. The Hill. http://thehill.com/blogs/blog-briefing-room/220832-house-dems-call-for-us-troops-to-give-direct-ebola-care. Accessed 15 Oct 2014

Sun L, Dennis B, Achenbach J (2014) Rate of new Ebola infections in Liberia is slowing, WHO says. The Washington Post. https://www.washingtonpost.com/national/health-science/rate-of-new-ebola-infections-in-west-africa-is-slowing-who-says/2014/10/29/74e70a86-5fa0-11e4-9f3a-7e28799e0549_story.html?utm_term=.d23874794eac. Accessed 28 May 2017

Svan JH, DeMotts J (2014) Germany-based aircraft take supplies to Liberia for Ebola fight. Stars and Stripes. http://www.stripes.com/news/germany-based-aircraft-take-supplies-to-liberia-for-ebola-fight-1.307072. Accessed 7 Oct 2014

Szabo L (2014a) Family of Dallas Ebola patient quarantined. USA Today. https://www.usatoday.com/story/news/nation/2014/10/02/ebola-family-quarantined/16579953/. Accessed 30 Apr 2017

Szabo L (2014b) Doctors: school closings in Texas, Ohio, unnecessary. USA Today. https://www.usatoday.com/story/news/nation/2014/10/16/solon-ohio-ebola-school-closings/17343431/. Accessed 28 May 2017

Szabo L (2014c) Cameraman declared Ebola free after treatment. USA Today. http://www.usatoday.com/story/news/nation/2014/10/21/ebola-cameraman-tweeting/17678173/. Accessed 22 Oct 2014

Tapper J (2014) Obama will name Ron Klain as Ebola Czar. CNN. http://www.cnn.com/2014/10/17/politics/ebola-czar-ron-klain/index.html. Accessed 17 Oct 2014

Tharoor I (2014) The awful lack of Ebola supplies in Liberia. The Washington Post. http://www.washingtonpost.com/news/morning-mix/wp/2014/10/15/liberia-needs-79940-more-body-bags/. Accessed 17 Oct 2014

The Health Site (2014) Ebola in Sierra Leone Norwegian doctor with Ebola cured and discharged. http://www.thehealthsite.com/news/ebola-in-sierra-leone-norwegian-doctor-with-ebola-cured-and-discharged/. Accessed 21 Oct 2014

The Local (2014) Germany has 50 beds ready for Ebola cases. The Local. http://www.thelocal.de/20141013/germany-has-50-beds-ready-for-ebola-cases-liberia. Accessed 13 Oct 2014

Tommy E (2014) Sierra Leone news: cumulative number of 8,478 households under isolation since May. Awareness Times. http://news.sl/drwebsite/publish/article_200526320.shtml. Accessed 3 Oct 2014

Townsend M (2014) Ebola deaths in Liberia are far higher than reported' as officials downplay epidemic. The Guardian. http://www.theguardian.com/world/2014/oct/19/ebola-liberia-death-toll-data-sorious-samura. Accessed 18 Oct 2014

Tsiaperas T (2014) First person to come out of quarantine after direct contact with Ebola patient Thomas Eric Duncan. The Scoop Blog, Dallas News. http://thescoopblog.dallasnews.com/2014/10/hospital-workers-who-cared-for-countrys-first-ebola-patient-asked-to-limit-movement.html/. Accessed 18 Oct 2014

Udland M (2014) Hazmat suit company goes wild. The Business Inside. http://www.businessinsider.in/Hazmat-Suit-Company-Goes-Wild/articleshow/44634220.cms. Accessed 7 Oct 2014

United Nations (2014) Ebola: back from outbreak epicentre, UN official says survivors now helping with care. 17 Oct 2014

UNMEER (2014a) UN Mission for Ebola Emergency Response statement for clarification: no threat that Ebola is airborne. 3 Oct 2014

UNMEER (2014b) UN mission for Ebola response: external situation report. 8 Oct 2014

Vanden Brook T, Jackson D (2014) More U.S. troops being sent to battle Ebola. USA Today. http://www.usatoday.com/story/news/world/2014/10/03/ebola-pentagon/16650617/. Accessed 3 Oct 2014

Villacorta N (2014) Hundreds of calls, but no new US Ebola cases – Did a computer raise risks of Ebola's spread? Politico. http://www.politico.com/politicopulse/1014/politicopulse15564.html. Accessed 6 Oct 2014

Wagner M (2014) Dr. Nancy Snyderman, Ebola-exposed NBC News crew violates self-quarantine, placed in mandatory isolation. Daily News. http://www.nydailynews.com/life-style/health/ebola-exposed-nbc-news-crew-violates-self-quarantine-isolation-article-1.1970958. Accessed 11 Oct 2014

Warner G (2014) Africa's Switzerland bans Ebola – but at what cost? NPR, WKNO. http://wknofm. org/post/africas-switzerland-bans-ebola-what-cost. Accessed 1 Oct 2014

Washington Examiner (2014) CDC now watching 125 people for Ebola signs. Washington Examiner, NewsOK. http://newsok.com/cdc-now-watching-125-people-for-ebola-signs/article/5353833. Accessed 15 Oct 2014

Wayne A (2014) Bill for Ebola adds up as care costs $1,000 an hour. Bloomberg. http://www. bloomberg.com/news/2014-10-07/bill-for-ebola-adds-up-as-care-costs-1-000-an-hour.html. Accessed 8 Oct 2014

Wheaton O (2014) Spain threatens to kill dog of nurse infected with Ebola sparking campaign to save it. Metro. http://metro.co.uk/2014/10/08/outcry-as-spanish-government-threatens-to-kill-dog-of-nurse-infected-with-ebola-4897216/. Accessed 8 Oct 2014

Whitely J (2014) Paramedics, ER staff under Ebola observation in Dallas. First Coast News. http:// www.firstcoastnews.com/story/news/health/2014/10/01/paramedics-er-staff-ebola-observation-dallas/16520713/. Accessed 1 Oct 2014

Wiley J (2014) Dallas Ebola patient mourned as others are monitored for signs of disease. Sacramento Bee, Fort Worth Star-Telegram. http://www.sacbee.com/2014/10/09/6771916/dallas-ebola-patient-mourned-as.html. Accessed 9 Oct 2014

Wines M (2014) Waste from Ebola poses challenge to hospitals. New York Times. http://www. nytimes.com/2014/10/18/us/waste-from-ebola-poses-challenge-to-hospitals.html?_r=0. Accessed 17 Oct 2014

Winter M (2014) Family: Amber Vinson free of Ebola virus. USA Today. https://www.usatoday. com/story/news/nation/2014/10/22/ebola-amber-vinson-recovery/17742417/. Accessed 3 Jun 2017

WKYC (2014) Ebola patient had CDC OK to fly to Cleveland. http://www.wkyc.com/story/news/local/akron/2014/10/15/ebola-patient-who-was-in-akron-identified/17304331/. Accessed 15 Oct 2014

Wolter O (2014) Lying about Ebola could bring $300k fine says Masse. Windsorite. http://windsorite.ca/2014/10/lying-about-ebola-could-bring-300k-fine-says-masse/. Accessed 20 Oct 2014

Wonacott P (2014) In Sierra Leone, ambulances carry Ebola patients, big questions. Wall Str J. http://online.wsj.com/articles/in-sierra-leone-ambulances-carry-ebola-patients-big-questions-1414686785. Accessed 30 Oct 2014

Worland J (2014) Obama hugs nurse who survived Ebola. Time. http://time.com/3537430/obama-hugs-nurse-ebola-survivor/. Accessed 4 Jun 2017

World Health Organization (2014a) Ebola response roadmap situation report. 1 Oct 2014

World Health Organization (2014b) Ebola response roadmap situation report. 3 Oct 2014

World Health Organization (2014c) Ebola response roadmap situation report. 8 Oct 2014

World Health Organization (2014d) Ebola response roadmap update. 10 Oct 2014

World Health Organization (2014e) WHO Director-General's speech to the Regional Committee for the Western Pacific. 13 Oct 2014

World Health Organization (2014f) Are the Ebola outbreaks in Nigeria and Senegal over? Ebola situation assessment. 14 Oct 2014

World Health Organization (2014g) Ebola response roadmap situation report. 15 Oct 2014

World Health Organization (2014h) Ebola response roadmap update. 17 Oct 2014

World Health Organization (2014i) The outbreak of Ebola virus disease in Senegal is over. 17 Oct 2014

World Health Organization (2014j) WHO congratulates Senegal on ending Ebola transmission. 17 Oct 2014

World Health Organization (2014k) Nigeria is now free of Ebola virus transmission. 20 Oct 2014

World Health Organization (2014l) Ebola response roadmap situation report. 22 Oct 2014

World Health Organization (2014m) Mali confirms its first case of Ebola. 24 Oct 2014

World Health Organization (2014n) Mali case, Ebola imported from Guinea. 10 Nov 2014

World Health Organization (2014o) Ebola response roadmap situation report. 29 Oct 2014

World Health Organization (2014p) Ebola response roadmap situation report. 31 Oct 2014

World Health Organization (2014q) Personal protective equipment in the context of filovirus disease outbreak response, rapid advice guideline. October 2014

WSOCTV (2014) Charlotte Ebola survivor donates plasma to NYC doc with virus. WSOCTV. http://www.wsoctv.com/news/update-charlotte-ebola-survivor-donates-plasma-nyc/113029728. Accessed 4 Jun 2017

Wulfhorst E, Malo S (2014) Doctor with Ebola in New York hospital after return from Guinea. Yahoo News. http://news.yahoo.com/york-doctor-tests-positive-ebola-ny-times-004857476.html. Accessed 24 Oct 2014

Yan H (2014a) 1st Ebola diagnosis in the United States: should we worry? CNN. http://www.cnn.com/2014/10/01/health/ebola-us-no-reason-to-panic/. Accessed 7 Apr 2017

Yan H (2014b) 2nd health care worker tests positive for Ebola at Dallas hospital. CNN. http://www.cnn.com/2014/10/15/health/texas-ebola-outbreak/index.html?hpt=hp_t1. Accessed 15 Oct 2014

Yan H, Shoichet CE (2014) Texas hospital official: we are 'deeply sorry' about Ebola mistakes. CNN. http://www.cnn.com/2014/10/16/health/us-ebola/index.html?hpt=hp_t1. Accessed 16 Oct 2014

Zeeble (2014) Following 2nd Ebola nurse diagnosis, Dallas' village reacts with caution, Concern. KERA News. http://keranews.org/post/following-2nd-ebola-nurse-diagnosis-dallas-village-reacts-caution-concern. Accessed 28 May 2017

Zoroya G (2014) Pentagon builds units to transport Ebola patients. USA Today. https://www.usa-today.com/story/news/world/2014/10/26/ebola-transport-military-patients-aircraft-phoenix-air/17669025/. Accessed 7 Jun 2017

Zwirko W (2014) CDC: 114 people tested for Ebola in Texas. KHOU. http://www.khou.com/story/news/local/texas/2014/10/04/cdc-114-people-tested-for-ebola-in-texas/16718861/. Accessed 4 Oct 2014

Chapter 6
Beginning of the Decline (November–December 2014)

Abstract In November and December 2014, the Ebola outbreak began to follow different paths in different countries. Liberia experienced a significant drop in cases. The apparent declines seen in Liberia in October 2014 were real. Hospitals that were once filled beyond capacity now had only a few cases. By November 13, 2014, conditions had improved so much that Liberia let its state of emergency expire. In Guinea, caseloads remained relatively stable. Sierra Leone became the epicenter of the outbreak. During November 2014, case numbers in Sierra Leone rapidly increased and the disease reached parts of the country that had not yet been affected. Sierra Leone's healthcare system was hard-hit. By December 14, 2014, 12 Sierra Leone doctors had been infected. In other parts of the world, the outbreak also presented a mixed picture. The outbreaks in the United States and Spain were over. In Mali, a second Ebola cluster flared up in mid-November. Ebola reached Scotland on December 29, 2014. Despite the increasing number of cases in Sierra Leone and the intermittent sparks around the world, healthcare officials began to think the worst of the outbreak might be over. Trend lines started to point downward.

6.1 Day-by-Day Outbreak Entries (November–December 2014)

November 1, 2014 (Saturday)
Experts at the WHO think the number of Ebola cases in West Africa may be leveling off. Instead of the exponential growth that has been occurring up until now, they think there may begin to be a steady addition of about 1000 new cases a week (Gallagher 2014a).

María Teresa Romero Ramos has been released from isolation at Carlos III Hospital in Spain (Heckle 2014). She is no longer isolated, but she is still in the hospital.

A UN employee has contracted Ebola in Sierra Leone and been evacuated to France for treatment (Landauro 2014).

© Springer International Publishing AG, part of Springer Nature 2018   173
S. G. Bullard, *A Day-by-Day Chronicle of the 2013-2016 Ebola Outbreak*,
https://doi.org/10.1007/978-3-319-76565-5_6

November 2, 2014 (Sunday)

The number of Ebola cases in Sierra Leone appears to be increasing. There are now six to nine times more cases each week in Sierra Leone than there were 2 months ago (Al Jazeera 2014a).

Another Sierra Leone doctor, Dr. Godfrey George, has contracted Ebola. Dr. George is the medical superintendent of the Kambia Government Hospital (Associated Press 2014a). He is the fifth Sierra Leone doctor to become infected. The other four have died from the disease.

Health officials stress that it is important for people to remain vigilant and not become overconfident in dealing with Ebola. Missing even a single case can trigger a widespread outbreak. For example, an Ebola victim recently traveled from Monrovia to Nimba County, Liberia. He rode on the back of a motorcycle and arrived at a refugee camp for citizens of the Ivory Coast. Within hours he had physical contact with over 28 people (Sieff 2014a).

The United Kingdom is setting up three new laboratories in Sierra Leone to help with the Ebola outbreak (Press Association 2014a).

Coming Attractions Bridal & Formal will reopen on Tuesday, November 4, 2014. This is the bridal store Amber Vinson visited in Akron, Ohio (Associated Press 2014b).

November 3, 2014 (Monday)

About 30 residents of the village of Kigbal, Sierra Leone, have recently died from Ebola. This is roughly 10% of the population. The village chief says there are bodies everywhere (Harding 2014a).

Infected Sierra Leone doctor, Dr. Godfrey George, has died (ABC News 2014).

Sierra Leone radio talk show host David Tam Baryoh was arrested in Freetown after a guest on his show criticized President Koroma's handling of the Ebola outbreak. It is unclear what Baryoh will be charged with, but his arrest warrant was signed by the President himself (Committee to Protect Journalists 2014).

Many West African Ebola survivors are suffering long-term debilitating effects from the disease. Doctors are calling it post-Ebola syndrome. Symptoms include body aches, chest pain, headache, fatigue, and vision problems. Visual impairment is often the most significant problem. Some victims report cloudy vision; others experience progressive vision loss. At least two people in Kenema, Sierra Leone, have gone blind (Neporent 2014).

MSF says few healthcare workers are willing to work in newly opened Ebola clinics in West Africa (Vogel 2014).

UNICEF will double its staff in Guinea, Sierra Leone, and Liberia to 600 (Roy-Macaulay 2014a)

Forty-two people in Ohio have ended their observation periods after being exposed to Ebola victim Amber Vinson (Associated Press 2014c).

November 4, 2014 (Tuesday)

Ebola has recently infected numerous people in Koinadugu District, Sierra Leone. The district had been free of the disease until mid-October 2014. The Red Cross collected 30 bodies from Koinadugu District today (O'Carroll 2014a).

   Throughout Sierra Leone, many people are forced to break quarantine to search for food. Food deliveries to quarantined households have been intermittent and unreliable (Al Jazeera 2014b).

   It is estimated that 1126 Ebola treatment beds are currently available in West Africa. However, 4388 are needed (Gale and Kitamura 2014).

   Shipping companies are adding Ebola clauses to their contracts. The clauses state where goods should be delivered to if the intended port is closed due to Ebola (Reuters 2014a).

   Australia appears ready to send healthcare workers to West Africa. A deal has reportedly been reached where infected Australians will be sent to Britain or Germany for treatment (Australian Associated Press 2014).

   The Philippines plans to quarantine 110 Filipino peacekeepers returning from Liberia. The troops will be isolated on an island in Luzon (Romero 2014).

November 5, 2014 (Wednesday)

Total cases: 13,042 (−525 new)   Fatalities: 4818 (−133 new)
                            (World Health Organization 2014a)

   The WHO continues to adjust its Ebola figures. This has led to another decrease in the official numbers.

   The number of Ebola cases in Sierra Leone continues to increase. 24.6% of all Sierra Leone Ebola cases have occurred within the last 21 days. In contrast, no new Ebola cases were reported in Guéckédou, Guinea, during the past week (World Health Organization 2014a).

   María Teresa Romero Ramos has been released from Carlos III Hospital in Spain (Press Association 2014b).

   US personnel in Liberia are not allowed to have direct contact with Ebola patients. However, 70 healthcare workers with the US Public Health Service Commissioned Corps will treat patients (Zoroya 2014a). All of the workers have volunteered for the assignment and they will only treat infected local medical workers (Zoroya 2014a). About 1300 US troops are currently in Liberia (Beaubien 2014a). Separately, President Obama has asked Congress for $6.2 B to fight Ebola (Zoroya 2014a).

   The United Kingdom has opened the Kerry Town treatment center in Sierra Leone (Myall 2014). The 80-bed facility is the first of six planned British treatment centers.

   German doctors have treated two Ebola patients with the experimental heart medicine FX06. The drug is designed for heart attack patients, but doctors think it could help Ebola patients too. FX06 reduces the loss of plasma through blood vessels. To date, the drug's effectiveness on Ebola patients is unclear. One of the patients treated with the drug has recovered. The other died from massive bleeding (Taylor 2014).

   It has now been 21 days since Amber Vinson visited Northeast Ohio. Because no new Ebola cases have been detected in the region, local health officials now consider the area to be Ebola-free (WTAM 2014). With the US Ebola outbreak seemingly contained, Americans do not seem as interested in the overall Ebola outbreak. Today on Twitter, there were about 200 Ebola mentions per minute. This is down from a recent average of 1000 per minute (Haglage 2014a).

Due to transportation and customs difficulties, many US research groups are having a hard time obtaining live samples of Ebola virus. Ebola mutates rapidly, so it is critical for researchers to experiment with up-to-date samples. Universities and research groups are working closely with the CDC and foreign governments to obtain the virus. For example, this week Tulane University received 900 blood samples from Sierra Leone Ebola patients. To get the samples, several Sierra Leone officials, including the country's President, had to sign off on the shipment. The CDC also had to provide a permit to allow the samples to be received in the United States (Steenhuysen 2014).

China will send another 1000 healthcare workers to West Africa to fight Ebola (Daily Times 2014).

November 6, 2014 (Thursday)
There are currently 357 people being monitored for Ebola in New York City. Some had contact with Dr. Spencer, but most are recent arrivals from West Africa (Stuart 2014).

Port officials in Freetown, Sierra Leone, say the port is conducting normal vessel operations. However, the temperature is taken from everyone who boards a ship and hand-washing and PPE are required (presumably not full-body PPE) (Finnan 2014).

The WHO believes the Ebola vaccines undergoing trials will probably cost about $100 a dose when they become available (Boakye-Yiadom 2014).

Children's Healthcare of Atlanta at Egleston is building a special care unit to treat Ebola-infected children (Schneider 2014).

November 7, 2014 (Friday)

Total cases: 13,268 (226 new)   Fatalities: 4960 (142 new)
                                 (World Health Organization 2014b)

MSF confirms that the number of Ebola cases in Liberia is declining. One MSF treatment center in Liberia currently has no patients (BBC 2014a). Effective burial practices are thought to have helped reduce Ebola transmission in Liberia (Miles 2014a). In August 2014, Liberian burials typically occurred 3 days after death. Now they usually take place within 24 h (Miles 2014a). Because the bodies of Ebola victims are highly infectious, rapid burial greatly limits the risk for postmortem exposure from corpses.

Guinea continues to experience high levels of Ebola transmission. Marc Poncin, the Response Coordinator for MSF, thinks most of the Ebola cases in Guinea are being imported from Sierra Leone and Liberia. He says people fleeing disease flare-ups in those countries are returning to their families in Guinea. Some of the returnees are infected and pass Ebola onto their relatives (Beaubien 2014b).

It is unclear how many children have been orphaned by Ebola. Officials in Sierra Leone think there are about 2600 Ebola orphans in the country. NGOs like UNICEF believe the number is closer to 7000 (O'Carroll 2014b).

Texas is on its way to becoming Ebola-free. It has been 21 days since the last Texan was placed under surveillance. None of the 177 people being monitored have developed Ebola (Lupkin 2014a).

The WHO has issued a booklet describing how to conduct safe and dignified burials for West African Ebola victims (World Health Organization 2014c). The guidelines include cultural instructions for burying Christian and Muslim victims (World Health Organization 2014c). The procedures for burying a Muslim Ebola victim are:

The team leader will explain the safe and dignified process of burial.

Ask the family if there are any specific requests in regard to the process of a dignified burial, for example, do they want to perform a dry ablution on the body prior to burial?

Deceased Muslims should not be cremated or placed in the body bag naked.

A dry ablution can be performed by a Muslim member of the burial team on the deceased patient before being placed in the body bag. Otherwise a Muslim person/family member can perform this simple procedure once they have been placed in the body bag (see next page information for dry ablution).

The deceased patient is shrouded by wrapping in a plain white cotton sheet before being placed in the body bag. The shroud should be knotted at both ends. The BMT [body management team] should provide a shroud for the family or they provide one themselves.

If there are female members of the Burial team, they should shroud deceased female patients prior to placing in a body bag (see next page information for shrouding).

Permission can be sought in advance from the Imam that the body bag can be used to represent a shroud. White body bags should be used for Muslim patients.

Dry ablution

(To be only carried out by a Muslim person or Muslim faith representative).

A short Arabic prayer of intention is said over the deceased.

The hand of the Muslim Burial team member carrying out the dry ablution (in PPE), softly strikes their hands on clean sand or stone and then gently passes over the hands and then the face of the deceased. This symbolically represents the ablution that would normally have been done with water.

A short Arabic prayer is said over the deceased.

The body bag is closed if no request for shrouding has been made.

Dry ablution can also be carried out over the deceased in the body bag if a Muslim Burial team member is not available and it was not possible to perform directly on the body.

This process takes about 1–2 minutes only.

Shrouding

A plain unstitched white cotton sheet (scented with musk, camphor or perfumed) is placed on top of the opened body bag.

The deceased is lifted by the Burial team and placed on top of the shroud.

The extended side edges of the shroud are pulled over the top of the deceased to cover the head, body, legs and feet.

Three strips cut from the same fabric are used to tie and close up the shroud. One for above the head, one for below the feet and one for around the middle of the body. It is knotted at both ends.

If there are female members of the Burial team, they should shroud the deceased female patients.

The body bag is closed. (World Health Organization 2014c)

US troops are currently being quarantined in Italy after serving in West Africa. In the future, many troops will undergo their quarantine periods at US bases. The bases involved will include Fort Hood (Texas), Fort Bliss (Texas), Fort Bragg (North Carolina), Joint Base Lewis-McChord (Washington state), and Joint Base Langley-Eustis (Virginia). Depending on the location of their next deployment, some troops may still be quarantined in Italy or in Germany (Associated Press 2014d).

The CDC is preparing 50 Ebola PPE kits that can be sent to US hospitals that have newly identified Ebola patients. Each kit contains enough material to take care of one Ebola patient for 5 days. The kits include gowns, coveralls, aprons, boot covers, gloves, face shields, hoods, N95 respirators, powered air-purifying respirators, and disinfectant wipes (Centers for Disease Control and Prevention 2014a).

Former President George W. Bush met with Ebola survivor Amber Vinson today (NBC News 2014a).

November 8, 2014 (Saturday)

There have been no new Ebola cases in Mali since the arrival of Fanta Condé (Monnier 2014). Not even Condé's grand aunt, who brought Condé to Mali and cared for her while she was sick, has developed the disease (Monnier 2014; World Health Organization 2014d).

Photojournalist John Moore of Getty Images recently returned to the United States from Liberia. He is currently undergoing quarantine at his home in Connecticut. He was asked to describe the circumstances surrounding one of his photographs that has become an iconic image from the Ebola outbreak. In the picture, the sister of a deceased Ebola victim is reaching toward her sister's body bag as it is being carried away by members of a burial unit. Moore said the sister was trying to throw soil onto the body bag (Haglage 2014b). Ebola victims in Liberia are cremated, not buried. Burial is the cultural norm in Liberia, so the soil might have been meant as a symbolic burial.

Morocco has refused to host the 2015 Africa Cup of Nations soccer tournament due to concerns about Ebola (RT 2014).

November 9, 2014 (Sunday)

Rural communities in Sierra Leone often receive little assistance from the central government and have to handle the Ebola outbreak themselves. In the Lokamasama region, 3 h northeast of Freetown, local chief Maro Lamina Angbathor has taken measures into his own hands. He has ordered the construction of a 90-bed isolation ward in the village school and has quarantined the hard-hit village of Kigbal; 31 of village's 200 residents have recently died from Ebola. It is hoped that more help, especially an ambulance, will be sent from nearby Port Loko. If not, the community will do its best to control the outbreak and isolate the sick (Chaon 2014).

When survivors are released from one Ebola center in Liberia, they dip their hands into paint and press their hands against a wall. The center has been open for a long time, but the survivor wall is very small (Eiklor 2014).

Eighteen thousand California nurses are planning to stage a walkout from Kaiser Permanente healthcare facilities on November 11, 2014. A variety of factors are contributing to strike. One concern is that the company has not implemented robust

Ebola preparedness measures. The strike will affect 21 hospitals and 65 clinics (Holloway 2014).

November 10, 2014 (Monday)

The number of Ebola cases in Liberia continues to decline. A 250-bed MSF treatment center in Monrovia has only 50 patients (Gallagher 2014b). The MSF center in Foya has not had any patients since October 30, 2014. Because of the drop in cases, MSF will adopt a new strategy in the country. It will create quick-response teams that will be sent to contain flare-ups of the disease as they arise (Gallagher 2014b). Although cases are falling, the United States has just opened the first of 17 planned 100-bed treatment centers in Liberia (Paye-Layleh 2014a). The treatment center is located in Tubmanburg, about 40 miles north of Monrovia (Paye-Layleh 2014a).

The Liberian village of Jene-Wonde, near the Sierra Leone border, has been heavily impacted by Ebola. About 10% of the population has died since late September 2014, and the disease continues to rage in the community. Village resident Momo Sheriff says about two people are being buried each day. Sheriff's own son has died from the disease (Williams 2014).

In Koinadugu District, Sierra Leone, 50 people have died from Ebola since mid-October 2014 (AFP 2014a).

Mali believes it has contained the Ebola outbreak which started with 2-year-old Fanta Condé. No one under surveillance has developed symptoms, and 108 people will complete their 21-day quarantine by November 14, 2014 (McNeil and Höijenov 2014; Miles 2014b). At one point, Condé's 5-year-old sister developed a fever. But she had malaria, not Ebola (McNeil and Höijenov 2014).

An Indian national has been quarantined at the New Delhi airport. The man is an Ebola survivor who contracted the disease in Liberia. The treatment center that released him gave him documents saying he was no longer infected. However, when he arrived in India, active virus particles were found in his semen. He will be isolated until he tests negative (Reuters 2014b).

Dr. Craig Spencer is now Ebola-free (Szabo 2014a). Kaci Hickox has completed her 21-day observation period in Fort Kent, Maine (Mathis-Lilley 2014).

Canada will quarantine high-risk people for 21 days. It is unclear whether health-care workers returning from West Africa will be considered high risk (Branswell 2014).

SES, a satellite service company, has started broadcasting an educational channel about Ebola. The free channel provides people with information about the disease and tips about how to prevent it (Clarke 2014).

November 11, 2014 (Tuesday)

Several Ebola threats have been made in New Zealand. A Jihadist group sent a package to the New Zealand Herald newspaper today containing a small vial of liquid labeled "Ebola" (Chang 2014; New Zealand Herald 2014). It is assumed to be a hoax, but even so, the package was carefully handled and samples have been sent for testing. The paper's newsroom was evacuated and cleaned (Chang 2014). A similar package arrived at the New Zealand Parliament building causing a brief lockdown (New Zealand Herald 2014).

Ebola cases continue to increase in Sierra Leone. On Saturday, November 8, 2014, 45 new cases were reported in the country (Spickernell 2014). On Sunday, 111 new cases were reported. Most of the new cases are in Freetown and Port Loko (Spickernell 2014). The government of Sierra Leone will provide $5000 to the families of healthcare workers who die fighting Ebola (Reuters 2014c).

A sixth Sierra Leone doctor, Dr. Martin Salia, has contracted Ebola (Roy-Macaulay 2014b). Dr. Salia was infected in Freetown (Roy-Macaulay 2014b).

Thirty members of Fanta Condé's family have been released from quarantine in Mali (Ahmed 2014). None developed Ebola.

Dr. Craig Spencer has been released from Bellevue Hospital in New York City (Lupkin 2014b). He has been cautioned to avoid having sex for at least 3 months (Long and Peltz 2014). With his release, there are no active Ebola cases in the United States.

In California, nurses at Kaiser Permanente have begun a 2-day strike. The strike is partly due to concerns about the company's lack of Ebola preparedness (Smith 2014b).

Ireland will send a limited number of troops to Sierra Leone to fight Ebola (O'Connor 2014).

Morocco will not be allowed to participate in the Africa Cup of Nations soccer tournament. Morocco had refused to host the event out of fear of Ebola (Bisson 2014).

November 12, 2014 (Wednesday)

Total cases: 14,098 (830 new)   Fatalities: 5160 (200 new)
                              (World Health Organization 2014e)

A new Ebola death has occurred in Mali's capital, Bamako (World Health Organization 2014f). The case is not believed to be connected to Fanta Condé. Officials say a 25-year-old nurse named Saliou Diarra has died from Ebola (AFP 2014b). Diarra became infected at the Pasteur Clinic after treating a 70-year-old Muslim Grand Imam (AFP 2014b; World Health Organization 2014f). A doctor at the clinic may also be infected (AFP 2014b). The Pasteur Clinic is now quarantined along with at least 30 people who had contact with the victims (AFP 2014b). Overall, three people are thought to have died in this flare-up: the Grand Imam, nurse Diarra, and a friend of the Grand Imam who recently died (AFP 2014b; World Health Organization 2014f). There is some confusion about the Grand Imam's name. An early report by AFP (2014b) identified him as Goita Sekou, but this report also stated that he was 66 years old. Later reports (i.e., Reuters 2014i) identified him as Oussa Koita, and this is likely his correct name. To avoid confusion, he will simply be referred to as the Grand Imam (e.g., World Health Organization 2014f). The Grand Imam recently came to Mali from Guinea. He was suffering from kidney failure and had Ebola-like symptoms. He died on October 27, 2014, but was not tested for Ebola (World Health Organization 2014f). Because he was a Grand Imam, he was buried according to traditional Muslim customs. His body was washed and touched by numerous people (World Health Organization 2014f).

Healthcare workers at a MSF Ebola clinic in Bandajuma, Sierra Leone, have gone on strike because they have not received their $100 a week hazard pay. About 60 patients are currently at the clinic. MSF says they may have to close the center if the strike continues (BBC 2014b).

The Anti-Corruption Commission and the Sierra Leone Police have arrested three men who tried to sell fake chlorine powder. Chlorine is commonly used to clean Ebola-contaminated surfaces. The men were arrested after trying to sell an inspector a large amount of fake powder for $23,600 (Anti-Corruption Commission 2014).

In Liberia, the rate of new Ebola cases has fallen from about 500 a week to about 50 a week (Daniel 2014). Due to the drop in cases, the United States says it will probably not need to deploy all 4000 troops to the country (Cooper and Tavernise 2014). At present there are about 2100 US troops in Liberia (Cooper and Tavernise 2014).

The US embassy in Wellington, New Zealand, has received a suspicious package similar to the ones sent to the New Zealand Parliament and the New Zealand Herald newspaper yesterday. It is believed the packaged arrived on Tuesday like the others. However, the US embassy was closed in honor of Veterans Day, so the package was not found until today (Finley 2014).

The US nonprofit agency American Refugee Committee is setting up an Ebola treatment center in Fish Town, Liberia, near the border of the Ivory Coast (Associated Press 2014e).

In North Carolina, the Carolinas Poison Control Center has launched a new Ebola hotline number (844) 836–8714. Numerous callers have been contacting the agency about Ebola. To date, 279 calls have been received about the disease (News & Observer 2014).

November 13, 2014 (Thursday)
Liberia has ended its state of emergency. The existing state of emergency was set to expire and needed to be renewed if it was to continue. President Ellen Johnson Sirleaf has decided not to extend it, so this effectively ends Liberia's state of emergency. President Sirleaf says the Ebola outbreak is not over, but there have been recent successes in fighting the disease (Reuters 2014d).

A doctor at the Pasteur Clinic in Mali has tested positive for Ebola. The body of a young girl is also being tested for Ebola. She died at an isolation center in Bamako today (Schnirring 2014a).

Corpses continue to be a source of infection in Sierra Leone. The burials provided by Ebola burial teams do not always fit with local customs. As a result, relatives sometimes go to the graves at night and exhume the corpses. They wash and prepare the bodies according to traditional methods and rebury them (Awoko 2014a). If the deceased person died from Ebola, this can lead to infection.

Clinical trials of three potential Ebola treatments will begin at MSF clinics in Guinea and Liberia next month. Brincidofovir will be tested in Monrovia, Liberia.

Favipiravir will be tested in Guéckédou, Guinea. Transfusions with convalescent blood will be tested in Conakry, Guinea. All of these treatments have shown promise in small-scale trials and with US and Spanish Ebola victims (Karimi 2014).

November 14, 2014 (Friday)

Total cases: 14,413 (315 new)   Fatalities: 5177 (17 new)
(World Health Organization 2014g)

Five people have been diagnosed with Ebola in Mali (Rihouay and Bennett 2014). One is a woman who washed the body of the deceased Grand Imam (Gayle 2014). A sixth person, the girl who died on Thursday, is also thought to have had Ebola (Rihouay and Bennett 2014). Officials are working to trace the contacts of all known and suspected cases. At least 200 people have been identified as potential contacts (Rihouay and Bennett 2014).

Infected Sierra Leone doctor, Dr. Martin Salia, will be flown to the United States for treatment. Dr. Salia is a permanent US resident and normally lives with his wife in Maryland. He will be treated in Nebraska (Stobbe and Roy-Macaulay 2014).

Healthcare workers have gained the trust of residents in Liberia. Locals were initially afraid of healthcare workers because they wore frightening-looking PPE and took sick people away to walled treatment centers from which they did not return. Medical personnel have worked hard to demystify their work. For example, in Foya, the walls of the treatment center have been replaced with transparent fences so residents can look into the facility and see what the workers are doing (Sun 2014a).

The California Department of Public Health and the California Division of the Occupational Safety and Health Administration have issued new guidelines for California healthcare workers. The new requirements say that all people working with Ebola patients must have PPE that covers the entire body and prevents the passage of fluids. Additionally, all the pieces of PPE must be compatible with each other (California Department of Industrial Relations 2014). It is unclear what role the recent nurse's strike played in the development of the new requirements. It is likely that the strike added pressure to the agencies to change the current guidelines.

The lack of tourism and suspension of commercial flights has reduced the government Sierra Leone's access to foreign currency (AFP 2014c).

France has advised against nonessential travel to Bamako and Kayes, Mali (Reuters 2014e).

Senegal has reopened its transportation links with Ebola-affected countries. Senegal will now allow planes and ships to arrive from West Africa. However, the country's land border with Guinea remains closed (Reuters 2014f).

November 15, 2014 (Saturday)
Dr. Martin Salia has arrived in Nebraska (Schubert 2014). He is critically ill and was not able to walk off the plane by himself (NBC News 2014b). Dr. Salia's wife, Isatu

Salia, will pay the estimated $100,000 for his evacuation from West Africa (Martinez and Mohney 2014).

Two more people are believed to have died from Ebola in Mali. Both died in a house that held the body of the Grand Imam (News Ghana 2014).

The British intelligence agency MI5 says the Islamic State may try to send Ebola-infected terrorists to England (Ward 2014). No specific threat appears to have been detected, but the agency considers this hazard as a possibility.

France will begin screening air passengers arriving from Mali for Ebola (France 24 2014).

A team of 160 Chinese healthcare workers arrived in Liberia today. They will staff a new treatment center (Reuters 2014g).

November 16, 2014 (Sunday)
Liberia has set an ambitious goal. It hopes to end Ebola transmission and have no Ebola new cases by Christmas 2014 (VOA News 2014a).

Dr. Martin Salia's medical condition continues to worsen. He is now in extremely critical condition. Dr. Salia's Ebola infection incubated longer than other infected US healthcare workers. He was given an Ebola test when he first developed symptoms. The results were negative, but his condition continued to decline. After about a week, a second test was conducted. It was positive. The first test was wrong – he had had Ebola all along. The treatment center where Dr. Salia worked has been closed and three of his close colleagues are under quarantine (Sieff 2014b).

Dr. Javid Abdelmoneim has been treating Ebola patients in Kailahun, Sierra Leone, for about a month. He says most of the people who die from the disease arrive at the clinic in very bad shape and die very quickly. Those who survive have more energy, even when they first arrive. Over the next few days, they become lethargic and have no appetite. They are so weak they cannot stand or feed themselves. After 4 or 5 days, they start to get better. Their appetite returns and they become ravenously hungry. The average time from admittance to release is 15 days for a survivor (Abdelmoneim 2014).

The United States will begin screening passengers arriving from Mali for Ebola. Screening will start on Monday, November 17, 2014. There are no direct flights to the United States from Mali, but 15–20 people arrive in the United States each day from Mali after making connecting flights in other countries (Centers for Disease Control and Prevention 2014b).

About 170 Kansas National Guard Soldiers from the 891st Engineer Battalion Headquarters will be deployed to West Africa (KSN 2014).

Concerns about Ebola are prompting many countries to begin preparedness measures, even countries that are far away from the ongoing West African outbreak. For example, Jamaica is constructing a four-bed Ebola treatment center at the Cornwall Regional Hospital in St. James (Jamaica Observer 2014).

November 17, 2014 (Monday)
Dr. Martin Salia died at the Nebraska treatment facility at approximately 0400 h this morning (Aizenman 2014a; Fox News 2014). He had been treated with ZMapp and received plasma transfusions from an Ebola survivor, but these could not reverse the

course of the disease. Dr. Salia had lost kidney function, was having difficulty breathing, and was unresponsive (Aizenman 2014a).

There are currently 442 people under surveillance in Mali (AFP 2014d).

EU Ebola coordinator Christos Stylianides and Commissioner of Health Vytenis Andriukaitis have completed a 4-day mission to West Africa. Their trip has prompted the EU to contribute an additional $36 M to Ebola-fighting efforts (PR Newswire 2014).

The head of UNMEER in Guinea, Marcel Rudasingwa, unexpectedly died of natural causes. He is not thought to have had Ebola (Reuters 2014h).

It is difficult to recruit healthcare workers to work in West Africa. The French Red Cross says 60% of their volunteers back out due to pressure from family and friends (Associated Press 2014f).

November 18, 2014 (Tuesday)
A seventh Sierra Leone doctor has died from Ebola. Dr. Moses Kargbo died at the Hastings Treatment Center today. He was retired but had volunteered to help with the outbreak (News OK 2014).

There are normally 377 native medical doctors in Sierra Leone. Given Sierra Leone's population of 6 M, this means there is only one doctor for every 15,544 people (Awoko 2014b). It also illustrates the impact Ebola is having on Sierra Leone's medical infrastructure. So far, seven Sierra Leone doctors have died from Ebola. This is 1.8% of the country's total doctoral pool.

Sierra Leone still has too few beds for Ebola patients. Forty people called the country's Ebola hotline today requesting transport to a treatment center. Due to the lack of space, 11 of these people could not be accommodated and had to remain at home (Sieff 2014c).

UNICEF has opened two new Ebola isolation centers in Sierra Leone. They are both in Bombali District, in the towns of Pate-Bana and Mapakie (Awoko 2014c).

Due to the declining number of Ebola cases in Liberia, the United States will build fewer treatment centers than originally planned. Instead of 17 100-bed treatment centers, the United States will build 10 centers, most with 50 beds (Zoroya 2014b).

The border between Liberia and the Ivory Coast is ill-defined and porous. Even so, Ebola has not reached the Ivory Coast. Before the outbreak, people easily moved back and forth between the two countries. Now, Ivory Coast villagers mount community-based patrols to prevent Liberians from crossing. The unarmed militia take their jobs very seriously. Members of one militia say a provincial deputy told them that if a single Ivory Coast villager developed Ebola, the entire affected village would be burned to the ground (Warner 2014).

The World Bank estimates that 25% of farmers in Sierra Leone, Liberia, and Guinea have not planted crops because of the Ebola outbreak. The Bank is concerned that this could lead to famine in the region (The News 2014).

The cost for treating the three Ebola patients at the Nebraska Medical Center has totaled at least $1.16 M (Sun 2014b).

The University of Mississippi Medical Center is renovating a vacant building to serve as a treatment site for any future Mississippi Ebola cases (Associated Press 2014g).

November 19, 2014 (Wednesday)

Total cases: 15,145 (732 new)   Fatalities: 5420 (243 new)
(World Health Organization 2014h)

A Cuban doctor, Dr. Felix Baez, has tested positive for Ebola in Sierra Leone (Trotta 2014). He will be sent to Geneva, Switzerland, for treatment. There are currently 256 Cuban medical workers in West Africa (Trotta 2014). So far during the outbreak, a total of 568 healthcare workers have contracted Ebola, and 329 of them have died (World Health Organization 2014h).

A 34-year-old Liberian nurse died at the US clinic in Monrovia, Liberia, today. She is the first person to die at the facility. Dr. Russ Bowman, one of the clinic's physicians, says the nurse was unresponsive when she arrived, so there was little the staff could do for her (Zoroya 2014c).

Thieves in Guinea held up a minibus carrying blood samples being taken for Ebola testing. A cooler full of blood samples was stolen. It is unclear why the thieves wanted the blood. It may have been taken by mistake. Radio announcements are asking the robbers to return the samples (Associated Press 2014h).

Given the current downward trends in West African Ebola case numbers, CDC Director Thomas Frieden says it is unlikely the worst-case scenario projections made during the summer will come true. Some of the early models had predicted that 1.4 M people could be infected by mid-January 2015 (Stobbe 2014).

University Hospital in Frankfurt, Germany, has released Ugandan doctor Dr. Michael Mawanda. He was admitted with Ebola on October 3, 2014 (Frankfurter Allgemeine 2014).

November 20, 2014 (Thursday)
In Bamako, Mali, the doctor who treated the infected Grand Imam has died from Ebola (Reuters 2014i).

A 38-year-old nurse in Bamako, Mali, was attacked by her neighbors after they learned that patients at her clinic had died from Ebola. A crowd gathered at her door chanting "Rita has Ebola." Stones were thrown at her, but she was not injured. The children of some of the clinic's workers have been harassed at school or sent home (MENAFN 2014).

The Macaulay Street Holding Unit in Freetown, Sierra Leone, isolates patients before they are sent to clinics for treatment. About 25% of arriving patients die before they can be sent for care. New facilities are opening in Sierra Leone, but it takes time for them to be fully staffed. For example, the United Kingdom recently opened a 92-bed center in Kerry Town, but many of the beds remain empty while the British train local healthcare workers to run the facility (Sieff 2014c).

A memorial service for Dr. Martin Salia will be held at St. Mary's Church in Landover Hills, Maryland, on November 28, 2014, from 1800 to 2000 h. His funeral will be on November 29 at 1300 h (CBS Baltimore 2014).

Infected Cuban doctor, Dr. Felix Baez, has been transported to Switzerland for treatment (Reuters 2014j).

Because of the Ebola outbreak, the United States will grant temporary protected status to people from Guinea, Liberia, and Sierra Leone who are currently in the US. Residents of the three countries can apply for protection from deportation and for work permits. The documents will be valid for 18 months. It is thought the move will affect about 8000 people (Reuters 2014k).

India will deploy 24 additional thermal scanners at its international airports. The scanners assess arriving passengers for fevers. Eighteen scanners are currently in use (IANS 2014a).

November 21, 2014 (Friday)

Total cases: 15,315 (206 new)   Fatalities: 5459 (39 new)
                                (World Health Organization 2014i)

The Hastings Treatment Center in Sierra Leone has been vigorously rehydrating Ebola patients. The extreme vomiting and diarrhea caused by Ebola rapidly dehydrates victims. Standard rehydration techniques include providing patients with IV drips. However, because of the risk of accidental needlesticks, IVs are not generally used with Ebola patients. Despite the danger, the staff at Hastings started using IVs in mid-September. The results have been very encouraging. The fatality rate for patients in standard treatment centers is about 64%. At the Hastings Treatment Center, the fatality rate is 40%. Equally encouraging is the fact that none of the center's healthcare workers using the IVs have contracted Ebola (Aizenman 2014b).

The Magbente Ebola Treatment Unit near Makeni, Sierra Leone, has started operations (Kamara 2014).

The Liberian finance minister predicts Liberia's economy will shrink by 0.4% in 2014. This is in contrast to the 5.9% increase Liberia experienced in 2013. The reduction is almost entirely due to the Ebola outbreak (Leadership 2014a).

A female Spanish healthcare worker is being flown to Carlos III Hospital in Madrid, Spain, for observation. She was treating a confirmed Ebola patient in Mali when she suffered a needlestick injury (Payne 2014).

The US Food and Drug Administration says it will start stockpiling blood plasma from Ebola survivors for use in future patients (Palmer 2014).

Nepal is asking all Nepalese peacekeepers returning from Liberia to abstain from sex for 3 months to prevent the spread of Ebola (Poudel 2014).

November 22, 2014 (Saturday)
A new Ebola case has been confirmed in Mali. The new patient is a friend of the nurse who died from Ebola (Reuters 2014l).

Infected Cuban doctor, Dr. Felix Baez, has begun treatment with ZMapp. He is currently in stable condition (Associated Press 2014i).

Phoenix Air Group, Incorporated, is playing a pivotal role in US Ebola efforts. The company specializes in providing unique air transport capabilities. It has worked with the CDC for about 9 years. In 2005, the CDC asked Phoenix Air Group if the company could develop a way to transport critically ill, highly infectious patients. This led to the successful development of an air-transportable isolation chamber. It also preadapted the company to be ready to help with the Ebola outbreak. So far, Phoenix Air Group has transported all of the infected Ebola patients to the United States (Haglage 2014c).

A group of 30 UK volunteer healthcare workers from the NHS is on their way to Sierra Leone to fight Ebola (Associated Press 2014j).

November 23, 2014 (Sunday)
BBC reporter Tulip Mazumdar and her news team recently made an overland journey from Freetown, Sierra Leone, to Conakry, Guinea. While traveling to Sierra Leone's border, the group passed through numerous Ebola checkpoints. At each site, the team had their temperatures taken. One checkpoint had prepared a novel hand-washing device. It was composed of suspended chlorine wash bottles connected to a stick. When a user stepped on the stick, the bottles tipped over and disinfectant poured onto their hands. As the team crossed the border and entered Guinea, they found that conditions in Guinea were dramatically different from Sierra Leone. In addition to having lower-quality infrastructure, such as having unpaved rather than paved roads, many Guineans were in denial about Ebola. At the town of Maferiah, several hours from Conakry, villagers said they had heard of Ebola, but many did not believe the disease actually existed (Mazumdar 2014).

UNMEER is opening an office in Mali to help with the country's Ebola outbreak (Clottey 2014).

US troops have finished building a third Ebola treatment center in Liberia. The new unit is in the town of Buchanan in Grand Bassa County (Worzi 2014a).

The Smith Barracks in Germany will be used as an isolation center for US troops returning from West Africa. Efforts have been made to make the barracks comfortable. It has been well stocked with sofas and televisions. A pool table and foosball games are also available. The facility can accommodate up to 180 troops (NBC News 2014c).

A UN worker has recovered from Ebola and has been discharged from the Begin Military Hospital in Paris (Reuters 2014m).

November 24, 2014 (Monday)
Liberia continues to see declines in the number of Ebola cases. Currently, about 20 new cases are being identified in the country each day, compared to 80 a day in September 2014 (Farge 2014a). Given these drops, Brigadier General Frank Tate has confirmed that the United States will not build two of its proposed treatment centers (Farge 2014a). Liberian President Ellen Johnson Sirleaf praised her country's Ebola-fighting efforts (AFP 2014e). She said:

A few months ago Ebola was chasing us, today we are chasing Ebola. Right now our people are out there doing contact tracing. Communities are taking responsibility and they are taking ownership.

They are going in every home to see who is sick so they can take the sick to the treatment centre. They are going to see those who have been abandoned so they can see what they can do for them.

And those who have been freed from the disease... those people are now being integrated into their communities so we are calling on all the communities to walk with them. (AFP 2014e)

Although Liberian Ebola cases are in decline, pockets of the disease continue to flare up in the country. In Rivercess County in the southeastern part of Liberia, 24 Ebola deaths have occurred. Local healthcare worker Lorenzo Dorr says the disease reached the region when a sick woman came from Monrovia on October 21, 2014. She treated her illness using traditional methods but died. Officials told people they should not touch her corpse, but she was given a traditional burial and her body was bathed. A few days later, people who helped with her funeral started becoming sick (Bloch 2014).

An eighth Sierra Leone doctor, Dr. Aiah Solomon Konoyeima, has tested positive for Ebola. Dr. Konoyeima has been working at the Children's Hospital in Freetown (Paye-Layleh and Roy-Macaulay 2014).

Irish burial experts from the Glasnevin Trust, in partnership with Concern Worldwide, are helping manage the burial records of Ebola victims in Freetown, Sierra Leone. The group is supervising ten burial teams at two cemeteries. Graves are marked with small white crosses and families are provided with maps so they can find their loved ones (Cullen 2014).

An Italian doctor [Fabrizio Pulvirenti] working for Emergency in Sierra Leone has contracted Ebola (Reuters 2014n; Sylvers 2014). He will be transported to Rome for treatment (Sylvers 2014).

High demand has companies struggling to produce enough PPE to deal with the Ebola outbreak. Increased demand from US consumers (such as hospitals and the CDC) has reduced the number of PPE suits available for shipment to Africa. For example, DuPont has tripled its production of hazmat suits, but it still is not producing enough to meet the demand. As a result, the company has prioritized buyers. It has placed customers who have direct contact with Ebola victims at the top of the list (Hinshaw 2014).

To date, 99 people in Britain have been tested for Ebola. Only William Pooley has tested positive (Perring 2014).

November 25, 2014 (Tuesday)
Burial workers left 15 bodies at the main hospital in Kenema, Sierra Leone, today. The workers say they have not received their hazard pay for October or November. The bodies have been removed, but the workers are now on strike (BBC 2014c).

Dan Baschiera, an Australian volunteer healthcare worker, has been helping Ebola patients in Sierra Leone. He has seen many patients die. He says rigor mortis sets in very quickly with Ebola victims, frequently within minutes. The faces of the dead often become frozen in painful grimaces. He also says Red Cross burial teams are finding entire villages empty (Baschiera 2014).

The UN says it will not meet its initial Ebola roadmap target by December 1, 2014. The goal was to have 70% of Ebola patients under treatment and 70% of Ebola victims safely buried by this date. The recent increase in Ebola cases in Sierra Leone has contributed to the missed deadline (Al Jazeera 2014c).

In Mali, the WHO says that 99% of the people who had contact with the recent Ebola patients have been identified and traced. The agency is hopeful the outbreak in Mali can be contained. Even so, two new Ebola cases have been identified in the Country. These include the 23-year-old fiancée of deceased nurse Saliou Diarra (Schnirring 2014b).

Police in Thailand are looking for a 31-year-old Sierra Leone man named Samuel Sesay. Sesay arrived in Thailand 2 weeks ago but has stopped reporting for his mandatory 21-day observation checks. Officials do not think Sesay has Ebola, but failing to check in with health officials is a crime (Straits Times 2014).

In the city of Guangzhou, China, travelers coming from Ebola-affected countries are being quarantined. About 150 people arrive in the city each day from countries with Ebola. All foreign visitors from these countries are required to stay at a single hotel, the Hotel Canton. They stay free of charge for their 21-day quarantine period. Visitors under quarantine can travel around the city, but only if they agree to carry a GPS-equipped cell phone and report for twice daily medical checkups. The hotel discards the mattresses of guests after they check out. In an odd twist, travelers are apparently not told they have to stay in the Hotel Canton when they arrive in Guangzhou. Instead, they often have travel from hotel to hotel until they learn they can only stay at the Hotel Canton (Ide 2014).

China has opened a 100-bed, Ebola treatment center in Monrovia, Liberia (Paye-Layleh and Roy-Macaulay 2014).

Illinois has ended its Ebola hotline. Interest in the disease has faded in Illinois and the number of calls to the hotline has fallen (WAND 2014).

November 26, 2014 (Wednesday)

Total cases: 15,935 (584 new)   Fatalities: 5689 (230 new)
                           (World Health Organization 2014j)

Over the last 3 weeks, Sierra Leone's Ebola fatality rate has more than doubled from 52 people per week to 131 per week (Awoko 2014d). Last week, there were 385 new Ebola cases in the country (World Health Organization 2014j). Of these, 118 were in Freetown, 72 in Port Loko, 55 in the Western Area Rural, 54 in Bombali, 31 in Tonkolili, 16 in Kono, 14 in Bo, 10 in Moyamba, 2 in Kailahun, and 1 in Kenema (World Health Organization 2014j). Despite the new cases, Sierra Leone's Information Minister believes the disease may have peaked and could be on the verge of slowing down (Roy-Macaulay and Schemm 2014).

Ledgerwood et al. (2017) describe the initial results of the GlaxoSmithKline Ebola vaccine trials (the preliminary report was published online today; the full article was published March 3, 2017). Assays to assess the safety and efficacy of the vaccine began at Bethesda, Maryland, in September 2014. No significant adverse effects were detected in 20 vaccinated volunteers, although two people developed transient fevers after being vaccinated. All of the volunteers developed Ebola antibodies within 4 weeks of vaccination. Those given higher vaccine doses (2×10^{11} particle units versus 2×10^{10}) produced more antibodies. Volunteers receiving higher vaccine doses also produced disease-fighting T cells, whereas those receiving lower doses generally did not (Ledgerwood et al. 2017).

Tests indicate that the nurse who died at the US clinic in Liberia on November 19, 2014, did not have Ebola (Zoroya 2014d). She remains the first person to die at the site, but she did not die from Ebola.

South Korea plans to send a team of ten healthcare workers to Goderich, Sierra Leone, to fight Ebola. Britain has agreed to treat any infected Koreans and will evacuate them to a European hospital for treatment (Reuters 2014o).

The six US Ebola survivors, Dr. Kent Brantly, Dr. Rick Sacra, Ashoka Mukpo, Nina Pham, Amber Vinson, and Nancy Writebol, met together today for an interview on the *Today* show. It is the first time all six survivors have come together (Kim 2014).

November 27, 2014 (Thursday)
Another Sierra Leone doctor, Dr. Komba Songu-M'Briwa, has contracted Ebola. Dr. Songu-M'Briwa treated Dr. Martin Salia at the Hastings Treatment Center before Salia was transported to the United States for treatment. It is unclear how Dr. Songu-M'Briwa became infected. He is now being treated at the Hastings Ebola Treatment Center himself. Dr. Songu-M'Briwa is the ninth Sierra Leone doctor to become infected (Sieff 2014d).

In Liberia, an inaccurate death certificate has led to a new cluster of Ebola cases. A man named Solomon King Pour of the Rock Hill community recently died. His relatives thought he might have died from Ebola, but his official death certificate said he had died from other causes. Consequently, community members washed and prepared his body according to local customs. Since his burial, at least eight people associated with the funeral have developed Ebola; one has died. As word of the exposure has spread, community members have voluntarily isolated themselves to prevent further infections (Karmo 2014).

The British Ebola treatment center in Kerry Town, Sierra Leone, remains underutilized. The 92-bed center opened 3 weeks ago, but currently only 11 patients are being treated at the site. Overall, the center has treated 28 patients (Watt 2014).

Germany has developed a dedicated medevac plane for Ebola patients. Lufthansa and the Robert Koch Institute retrofitted an Airbus A340-300 with an isolation unit, two airlocks, an air filtration system, and a cabin for medical workers to decontaminate their PPE. The plane will allow healthcare workers to provide in-flight intensive care to Ebola patients (Paye-Layleh 2014b). Previous medevac aircraft were too small to allow for complex patient care.

A group of 17 Australian healthcare workers has been deployed to Sierra Leone to help with the Ebola outbreak (Medhora 2014).

November 28, 2014 (Friday)
French President Francois Hollande traveled to Guinea today. He is in the country for a 1-day visit designed to show support for Guinea's Ebola-fighting efforts. Hollande is the first western head of state to visit an Ebola-affected country during the outbreak (BBC 2014d).

US nonprofit group EduNation, in conjunction with other agencies, is delivering food to quarantined houses in Sierra Leone. Households with more than ten quarantined individuals receive a food package containing two 50 kg bags of rice, five gallons of palm oil, 25 kg of onions, fish, hot peppers, Maggie seasoning, a bag of salt, a box of soap, sanitary items, and bundles of water (Gbenda 2014).

The WHO is advising male Ebola survivors to abstain from sex for 3 months after they recover from the disease. It also encourages survivors to maintain good personal hygiene after masturbation. Data indicate that Ebola can remain in semen for 82 days after a person develops Ebola symptoms (CBC News 2014).

Researchers have developed a portable, solar-powered Ebola detection lab that can diagnose Ebola in as little as 15 min. Healthcare workers have long wanted a quick and accurate Ebola test. Trials of the experimental lab will begin at a clinic in Conakry, Guinea (VOA News 2014b).

India will require all Ebola survivors to produce a certificate saying no virus is present in any of their body fluids before they can enter the country. Survivors without a certificate will have to wait 90 days after treatment before they can enter India (PTI 2014a).

Infected Cuban doctor, Dr. Felix Baez, is reported to be improving (Reuters 2014p).

November 29, 2014 (Saturday)
Schools in Sierra Leone remain closed, so the country continues to broadcast educational programs over the radio. The programs are considered a simple, relatively effective way to educate children during the crisis. Though helpful, the approach is not perfect. Some students complain that they cannot ask questions. Students are encouraged to call teachers by phone, but not all of them can afford to do so (Kamara and Collins 2014).

There are no active Ebola cases in Mali. There are 285 people under surveillance, but none of them have symptoms of the disease (Reuters 2014q).

A funeral mass was held today for Dr. Martin Salia. Dr. Salia's body was cremated, so his wife carried a small black box containing his ashes into the church (Nuckols 2014).

The condition of the Italian doctor who contracted Ebola in Sierra Leone is deteriorating. He is being treated at the Lazzaro Spallanzani Institute in Rome. The institute issued a statement today saying the doctor has nausea, vomiting, diarrhea, and a fever over 102.2 °F (AFP 2014f).

November 30, 2014 (Sunday)
Criticism continues to mount about the UK's Ebola clinic in Kerry Town, Sierra Leone. Locals and foreign aid workers say the clinic lacks a sense of urgency. Staff at the facility say these concerns are unfounded and are upset by the allegations. On

a positive note, a 21-year-old student named Kadiatu Sesay was recently discharged from the clinic. She is the third survivor to be released from the facility (Harding 2014b).

NPR reporter Kelly McEvers is in Monrovia, Liberia (Weekend Edition 2014). She describes the current conditions on the ground:

> *KELLY MCEVERS: Well, because I wasn't here during the worst time, and that was August and September, it's hard to say how things have changed. But what I do know are the stories that people have been telling us about what it was like during that time. And it sounds really, really grim. You know, the Ebola treatment units were full. There weren't enough beds. People were being turned away, literally, you know, dying in the streets. You had slums, like West Point, which I'm looking over right now. I'm sort of up on a hill looking down over that West Point slum in Monrovia, the capital, where things were very dire.*
>
> *Things are different now. There's an election going on. People are kind of letting their guard down. You get a sense that because the numbers are going down, people are relaxing. But what you are hearing from health officials is that people need to remain vigilant. What's happening now is you see Ebola cases popping up in the rural areas again. So that means that the sickness has spread from the city here and people are going back out into their villages and getting sick there.* (Weekend Edition 2014)

She also describes reports from teams sent to investigate infected rural communities:

> *MCEVERS: I mean, but we heard crazy stories. You know, one team went into a really remote village and all they found when they got there were 22 fresh graves. I mean, that's still happening. So I think everyone's saying, look, you know, we're working on it, but we've got more to do.* (Weekend Edition 2014)

December 1, 2014 (Monday)

Sierra Leone continues to have very high levels of Ebola transmission (Heilprin 2014). The large number of deaths in and around Freetown has officials scrambling to handle numerous Ebola-infected bodies. The size of the crisis is almost of industrial scale. At one of Freetown's cemeteries (almost certainly King Tom Cemetery), workers dig graves, while bulldozers clear space for additional burials. In one afternoon, about 20 bodies arrived for burial (BBC 2014e).

Sierra Leone's military has opened a new 40-bed treatment center at the 34 Military Hospital in Freetown. Separately, since it opened on September 19, 2014, the Hastings Treatment Center has admitted 585 patients, discharged 363, and had 155 deaths (Awareness Times 2014).

The WHO says Guinea and Liberia have both reached the roadmap goal of isolating 70% of infected victims and safely burying 70% of Ebola fatalities. Sierra Leone has not reached these goals, but the WHO thinks the prognosis for Sierra Leone is very good. This is because new treatment facilities are opening and the number of available beds in the country will soon increase (Miles 2014c).

MSF says the international response to Ebola has been slow and uneven. There continues to be too few trained staff from first world countries in West Africa (Médecins Sans Frontières 2014a).

Two elite UK schools, Cheadle Hulme School and Withington Girls' School, will send their students on an annual 1-week trip to The Gambia despite the ongoing

Ebola outbreak in neighboring countries. Not all parents are happy with this decision. One father (a doctor) says he will not only prevent his daughter from going on the December 13–21, 2014, trip, but he will also keep her home from school for the 21-day incubation period after the other students return (Fitzgerald 2014).

Ebola has not reached Connecticut, but state hospitals have already spent $5 M in planning and preparing for possible Connecticut Ebola cases (Hladky 2014).

Nigeria is training 250 healthcare volunteers to assist with the West African outbreak (Leadership 2014b).

December 2, 2014 (Tuesday)

Today marks the 1 year anniversary of the start of the Ebola outbreak.

The WHO has congratulated Spain for containing its Ebola outbreak. It has been 42 days since the last, and only, infected Spanish national tested negative for the disease. Because no one else has developed the disease, the Spanish Ebola outbreak is now considered over (World Health Organization 2014k).

Infected Sierra Leone doctor, Dr. Komba Songu-M'Briwa, continues to undergo treatment at the Hastings Treatment Center. He has been given a private room, but his treatment is the same as the other patients at the facility. He receives antibiotics, an IV drip, and a nutritious diet (Associated Press 2014k).

A story has emerged from the Caldwell community in Liberia about a teacher named Nancy Freeman and her family. It is being used to illustrate the potential dangers of hiding Ebola patients. In November 2014, several people in Freeman's family died from Ebola. The neighbors were not told. Freeman's stepmother then became sick and Freeman took care of her privately. Eventually the stepmother became so sick she had to go to the hospital. When Freeman returned from the facility, she told the neighbors her stepmother had jaundice. She then cleaned the house with bleach. A few days later, Freeman became sick. She remained at home. When she vomited, she cleaned the area with bleach. Eventually she was taken to the hospital where she died from Ebola (Smith 2014a).

The World Bank says the economies of Guinea, Sierra Leone, and Liberia have been crippled by the Ebola outbreak. The agency predicts that Guinea's economy will grow by 0.5% this year, Sierra Leone's by 4.0%, and Liberia's by 2.2%. All of these values are less than half of last year's growth rate. In the case of Guinea, it is only about 10% of last year's growth (Paye-Layleh and Dilorenzo 2014).

Massachusetts General Hospital in Boston admitted a suspected Ebola patient (Scalese and Tedesco 2014). The person had been in Liberia and arrived at the hospital with Ebola-like symptoms (Scalese 2014). It was later determined that the person had malaria, not Ebola (Scalese 2014).

The United States has identified 35 hospitals that will act as Ebola treatment centers for future US Ebola cases. Together, these facilities have a 53-bed capacity (Sun 2014c).

December 3, 2014 (Wednesday)

Total cases: 17,145 (1210 new)   Fatalities: 6070 (381 new)
(World Health Organization 2014l)

The 21-day surveillance period has ended for 114 New York City healthcare workers who helped take care of Dr. Craig Spencer. None of them developed Ebola. There are currently 222 people still under surveillance in New York. Most of these are people who recently arrived from Ebola-affected countries (Ferris 2014).

Anthony Banbury, the head of UNMEER, says there continues to be high levels of Ebola transmission in and around Freetown, Sierra Leone. However, conditions in most of West Africa are significantly better than they were 2 months ago. The current rate of infection is also much lower than what had been predicted. Banbury describes one image that stays with him from the outbreak. He visited a graveyard next to a treatment center. Many of the graves are filled with children and young adults. Even more disturbing, there were numerous unfilled graves waiting to receive victims (Morning Edition 2014a).

An 11th Sierra Leonean doctor, Dr. Dauda Koroma, has tested positive for Ebola. He is being treated at a military hospital in Freetown (Roy-Macaulay 2014c).

There are currently only eight patients at the ELWA-3 Ebola treatment center in Monrovia, Liberia. ELWA-3 is one of the largest Ebola hospitals, with a 250-bed capacity (Beaubien 2014c). The fact that so few patients are being treated at the facility is a dramatic illustration of the drop in Liberian Ebola cases.

Doctors at the Nebraska Biocontainment Unit have prepared a paper describing the way they dealt with the waste generated by Ebola patients (Park 2014). Each patient produced about 1010 lb of solid waste at the rate of about four to eight bags a day (Lowe et al. 2014). Most of the solid waste was composed of towels, linens, bedding, and caregiver PPE. Liquid waste from the patient's toilets was sterilized with hospital-grade disinfectant before it was flushed (Lowe et al. 2014).

Nigeria is providing special insurance for the 250 Nigerian healthcare workers going to West Africa to fight Ebola. The insurance will provide $96,000 for personal accident and disability and $190,000 for medical expenses. It will pay $100,000 to the beneficiary of any worker who dies (Osayande 2014).

US Africa Command's General David Rodriguez says that given the drop in Liberian Ebola cases, many US troops deployed in West Africa may soon be able to return home. The troops are not expected to be needed in Sierra Leone or Guinea (Carroll 2014).

The United Nations Development Programme is working with West African governments and UNMEER to develop a system to coordinate payments to healthcare workers and burial teams in Guinea, Sierra Leone, and Liberia (AllAfrica 2014a).

A US healthcare worker in West Africa may have been exposed to Ebola. They are being transferred to Emory University Hospital for observation (Reuters 2014r).

December 4, 2014 (Thursday)
Sierra Leone's Ebola Czar, Palo Conteh, held a press conference today to describe the country's Ebola-fighting efforts (Conteh 2014). He says that although the number of cases continues to rise, additional treatment beds are coming online which should help the situation. Ninety burial teams are now working in Sierra Leone. He also shared the results of a mid-October Ebola survey. On the positive side, 90% of respondents said that they would go to a hospital if they suspected they had Ebola.

Most also said that they would welcome an Ebola survivor back into their community. On the negative side, about one-third of respondents said they would not accept alternatives to traditional burial for a family member, 10% said they would touch the body of a loved one, and 13% said they would not wait for a burial team to bury the corpse of a loved one (Conteh 2014). Separately, it is reported that Conteh plans to jail anyone who is caught washing a body in Sierra Leone (APA 2014a).

Sierra Leone's National Ebola Response Centre has asked the Mayor of Freetown to prepare a new cemetery. The city's King Tom Cemetery is currently the only facility authorized to accept the bodies of Ebola victims. At the rate fatalities are occurring, the cemetery will soon be filled to capacity (APA 2014b).

The Mayor of Kenema, Sierra Leone, says his city is Ebola-free. The central government says this declaration is premature and such statements should be avoided (APA 2014c).

The US healthcare worker who may have been exposed to Ebola in West Africa has arrived in Atlanta. They arrived at 0545 h on a Phoenix Air Group jet (Martin 2014).

The cost needed to control the Ebola outbreak in Dallas, Texas, has been totaled. The Texas Department of State Health Services spent about $1.28 M on control efforts (NBC DFW 2014). Dallas County spent $384,000 (NBC DFW 2014). The City of Dallas spent $155,000 for the general outbreak and $27,000 to care for Nina Pham's dog "Bentley" (NBC News 2014d).

Mali has received its first mobile Ebola-testing laboratory (Associated Press 2014l).

December 5, 2014 (Friday)
Officials in Sierra Leone say 80–100 new Ebola cases are occurring in the country each day. The largest number of cases are in northern and western parts of Sierra Leone. At present, there are four functioning treatment centers in the country (Lederer 2014).

Two more Sierra Leone doctors, Dr. Dauda Koroma and Dr. Thomas Rogers, have died from Ebola. Dr. Rogers worked at Connaught hospital in Freetown and was being treated at the British clinic in Kerry Town (Roy-Macaulay 2014d).

Infected Cuban doctor, Dr. Felix Baez, has recovered from Ebola and no longer tests positive for the virus. He will be released from Geneva University Hospital in Switzerland (AFP 2014g).

A Nigerian UN peacekeeper has contracted Ebola in Liberia. He will be transported to the University Medical Center Utrecht in the Netherlands for treatment (Paye-Layleh and Corder 2014).

About 100 US marines have completed their deployment in Liberia. They are preparing to go to Germany for their 21-day observation period (Seck 2014).

The CDC says that when Ebola was active in the United States, the US healthcare system was somewhat hypervigilant and tended to over-identify possible Ebola cases. Of 650 people identified as being possibly infected, only four tested positive (0.6%) (Associated Press 2014m).

December 6, 2014 (Saturday)

With the US Ebola outbreak apparently over, US Ebola Czar, Ron Klain, will leave his post and return to his jobs as president of Case Holdings and general counsel for Revolution LLC. He expects to be back at his regular jobs by March 1, 2015 (Newmyer 2014).

Another Sierra Leone doctor, Dr. Aiah Solomon Konoyeima, has died from Ebola. Dr. Konoyeima worked at a children's hospital in Freetown and was being treated at the Hastings Treatment Center (Roy-Macaulay 2014e).

US troops have built seven Ebola treatment centers in Liberia. Ten more centers are expected to be finished by the end of December 2014 (Beardsley 2014).

Numerous false Ebola alarms continue to occur around the world. Some cases appear to be deliberate hoaxes. For example, a 19-year-old man in Taiwan claimed that he had been vomiting and had diarrhea since he returned from Nigeria where he had eaten bat meat. He tested negative for Ebola. However, Taiwanese records show that the man had never actually left Taiwan (IANS 2014b).

December 7, 2014 (Sunday)

New Zealand is sending 82 healthcare volunteers to Sierra Leone to fight Ebola (IANS 2014c).

December 8, 2014 (Monday)

Liberia is optimistic about its downward trend in Ebola cases. Currently about 10–12 new Ebola cases are occurring in Liberia each day. While still rather high, these numbers are well below the massive numbers that were occurring several months ago. To try to end the outbreak, the government is launching a "no new cases" campaign. Its goal is to eradicate Ebola from Liberia by the end of 2014. Officials worry that as the number of Ebola cases falls, citizens may become complacent and stop practicing rigorous protection measures. Residents are warned to stay vigilant until the caseload drops to zero (Morning Edition 2014b).

To help Liberian Ebola survivors relax and come to terms with their recent experiences, US Christian group Young Life has opened a weekend camp. Recently, more than 100 survivors took part in camp activities (Worzi 2014b).

Throughout West Africa, signs warn of the dangers of Ebola. A banner in Monrovia, Liberia, reads (transcribed from a photograph taken by James Giahyue Reuters 2014s, punctuation and spacing as on the original banner):

Stop
The stigma against
Ebola survivors!!!
Ebola is still real
Protect yourself and
your family.

Members of Sierra Leone's Junior Doctors Association have gone on strike. They are demanding better treatment for Ebola-infected healthcare workers. In particular, they want to make sure that critical equipment, like dialysis machines, are available to treat infected workers. The doctors note that 10 of 11 infected Sierra Leone doctors have died from Ebola, while only one US-treated healthcare worker has died.

They believe access to high-quality medical support and equipment is the key to surviving Ebola (Roy-Macaulay 2014f).

December 9, 2014 (Tuesday)
Liberian President Ellen Johnson Sirleaf says there have been no Ebola deaths in 9 of Liberia's 15 counties in recent days (AllAfrica 2014b).

Kilmarx et al. (2014) find that healthcare workers in Sierra Leone are 103 times more likely to contract Ebola than ordinary Sierra Leone citizens. Between May 23, 2014, and October 31, 2014, there were 3854 laboratory-confirmed Ebola cases in Sierra Leone. Of these, 199 were in healthcare workers. As of 2009, there were 2402 total healthcare workers in Sierra Leone. Assuming similar numbers of healthcare workers in 2014, this means that over 8%, or 1 in 12, Sierra Leone healthcare workers have contacted Ebola (e.g., Kilmarx et al. 2014).

Much of the money pledged to fight Ebola has not yet been delivered. Of eight leading countries, the United States has delivered the highest percentage of pledged dollars. The United States has delivered $420 M of a promised $572 M. In contrast, China has only delivered about $10 M of a promised $123 M (Caulderwood 2014).

The United States continues to screen passengers arriving from West African for Ebola. So far, no cases have been identified using these techniques. The CDC says 1933 passengers were screened between October 11, 2014, and November 10, 2014. Seven of these were referred for additional screening, but none of them had Ebola. Given the epidemiology of the disease and its incubation period, many disease experts think airport screening is ineffective (Szabo 2014b).

The US HHS says it will provide drug companies with immunity from legal claims related to the manufacturing, testing, development, distribution, and administration of the three Ebola vaccines currently under development. It is hoped that this will speed up the development of the vaccines. These protections do not apply outside the United States. (Reuters 2014t).

December 10, 2014 (Wednesday)

Total cases: 17,942 (797 new)   Fatalities: 6388 (318 new)
(World Health Organization 2014m)

Time magazine has named the "Ebola fighters" its person of the year (McLaughlin 2014; Von Drehle and Baker 2014). The magazine has been printed with five different covers, each featuring a different Ebola healthcare worker (Laurent 2014). The covers include Dr. Kent Brantly, Dr. Jerry Brown (a medical director in Monrovia, Liberia), Salome Karwah (an Ebola survivor and caregiver in a MSF clinic in Monrovia, Liberia), Ella Watson-Stryker (a MSF volunteer health promoter), and Foday Gallah (a 37-year-old ambulance supervisor and Ebola survivor in Monrovia, Liberia) (McLaughlin 2014; Von Drehle and Baker 2014).

Sierra Leone has begun a 2-week lockdown of Kono District in the eastern part of the country. The lockdown started today and will last until December 23, 2014. No one will be allowed in or out of the area, but residents can move around freely within the district. Witnesses say shops are open, but most people are staying indoors. The WHO says 87 bodies have been buried in Kono District in the last 11 days (AFP 2014h).

Liberian President Ellen Johnson Sirleaf made a video-linked address to US Senators today. She thanked America for helping with the outbreak and encouraged US lawmakers to continue their support. In particular she urged the leaders, as well as her own people, to not let their guard down as the number of Ebola cases in Liberia falls (Neergaard 2014).

December 11, 2014 (Thursday)
The last Ebola victim in Mali has recovered and left the hospital. There are now no known cases in the country (Reuters 2014u).

A WHO response team in Kono, Sierra Leone, has discovered the bodies of 25 Ebola victims in a closed off section of a local hospital. The team says healthcare workers at the site are doing all they can to fight the disease and help patients. They are simply overwhelmed by the scale of the crisis (BBC 2014f).

Officials in Sierra Leone say a new Ebola case has occurred in Kailahun District. It has been 11 days since the last known case in the district. The new patient works for MSF and provides psychological counseling for Ebola patients. He has been transferred to Freetown for treatment (Samba 2014).

Clinical trials of an Ebola vaccine have been ended because some participants reported joint pains. Trials of the Merck and NewLink vaccine started in Switzerland on November 10, 2014. The trials were stopped when 4 of the 59 participants complained of pain in their hands and feet. Researchers are investigating the cause. If the symptoms are harmless and temporary, a new trial with 15 people will begin on January 5, 2015 (Reuters 2014v).

The Global Alliance for Vaccines and Immunization says it will buy up to $300 M worth of Ebola vaccine as soon as one is recommended by the WHO (AFP 2014i).

UN Secretary-General Ban Ki-moon has appointed Ismail Ould Cheikh Ahmed as the next leader of UNMEER (AFP 2014j). Though it is somewhat unclear, it appears that UNMEER will have rotating leadership with each head serving for about 2 months. Ahmed will succeed Anthony Banbury.

An American nurse was exposed to Ebola in Sierra Leone. They have been placed under observation at the NIH in Bethesda, Maryland (Bethesda Magazine 2014).

December 12, 2014 (Friday)
Photojournalist Michel du Cille of the *Washington Post* has died from a heart attack in Liberia. Du Cille captured many images of the Ebola outbreak. He collapsed while hiking out of a remote village in Bong County (Eversley 2014).

Families are sending about 3000 lb of mail each week to US soldiers deployed in West Africa. Mail provides a significant morale boost to recipients, especially during the holiday season (Byrne 2014).

Preliminary results of the US Agency for International Development's Ebola Grand Challenge were announced today. The contest started in October 2014. Its goal was to aid the development of novel Ebola-fighting equipment. About 1500 contestants participated. Many entrants produced new or better PPE. One submis-

sion was of an antibacterial gel called Zylast that kills bacteria for up to 6 h after it
has been applied (McNeil 2014).

December 13, 2014 (Saturday)
Sierra Leone has banned public Christmas and New Year's celebrations and will
impose curfews during the holiday season. Most of Sierra Leone's residents are
Muslim, but about 25% are Christian (Sabin 2014).

The Guinean government is setting up village watch committees in the mining
region of Guinea. Their mission is to provide communities with information about
Ebola and identify and contain new outbreaks. Each committee is composed of a
young person, a woman, a traditional healer, a religious leader, and a public health
representative (Guensburg 2014).

Ebola survivors continue to face significant stigma when they return to their
communities. Landlords do not want to rent to them, employers may not hire them,
and taxi drivers often avoid them. In Monrovia, Liberia, Vivian Rogers, a 40-year-
old Ebola survivor and government filing clerk, has been told to stay at home by her
boss. Rogers says she is glad she is still being paid, but feels useless and does not
understand why people are afraid of her when she is no longer contagious (Zoroya
2014e).

Réunion Island in the Indian Ocean hospitalized a suspected Ebola case today
(RFI 2014).

December 14, 2014 (Sunday)
Ebola cases continue to spike in Sierra Leone. In mid-October, there were approximately 35 burials a day in Freetown. There are now around 80. On the positive side,
current burials are taking place quickly. During November 2014, 95% of burials
took place within 24 h of a body being recovered (Boseley 2014a).

A 12th Sierra Leone doctor, Dr. Victor Willoughby, has contracted Ebola
(Associated Press 2014n).

December 15, 2014 (Monday)
CDC director, Dr. Thomas Frieden, is concerned that Ebola could become endemic
in West Africa (Doucleff 2014). If this happens, some level of the disease will
remain in the region for the foreseeable future. This would mean that there would be
a perpetual risk of Ebola cases being exported from the area to other countries.

In Sierra Leone, Dr. Fasineh Samura, the coordinator for the Koinadugu District
Ebola Response Center, has set the ambitious goal of eradicating Ebola from the
district within 45 days. Dr. Samura says officials have a list of all the inhabitants of
the Neine Chiefdom. They plan to check each household every day for sick individuals. The Paramount Chief of the region, Alimamy Lahai Mansaray V, also
requests that residents not host any visitors from outside the region because they
might be infected (Sierra Express Media 2014).

As part of a clinical trial, doctors at the ELWA Hospital in Monrovia, Liberia,
have begun treating patients with convalescent blood serum (BBC 2014g).

The coming 3-month West African dry season is seen as a double-edged sword
in the fight against Ebola. As conditions dry, roads will become more passable. This

will help healthcare workers and supplies get to remote locations more easily. On the other hand, it will increase the mobility of the population which could spread the virus (Tyson 2014).

Ebola has significantly reduced West Africa's air connectivity with the outside world. Compared to a year ago, there are 81% fewer airline seats available for passengers leaving Liberia, 75% less for Sierra Leone, and 39% less for Guinea (Jasper and Bennett 2014).

A large portion of Ebola survivors are experiencing post-Ebola syndrome. Symptoms include joint pain, sleep disorders, skin problems, reproductive problems, and vision problems. In terms of scale, 40% of survivors in Kenema, Sierra Leone, have developed eye problems. Over 33% have developed skin problems (Trenchard 2014a).

December 16, 2014 (Tuesday)
Sierra Leone will conduct house-to-house searches for Ebola victims in the western parts of the country, including Freetown (Roy-Macaulay 2014g). The campaign will be known as Operation *Western Area Surge*. It will start Wednesday, December 17, 2014 (Associated Press 2014o). During the campaign, healthcare workers will visit homes to find hidden Ebola cases (Roy-Macaulay 2014g). The government will also launch a large-scale information campaign at the same time (Boseley 2014b). The campaign will be similar to drunk-driving campaigns used in western countries. It will attempt to intentionally frighten people about Ebola. Officials hope the information campaign will scare people into taking more personal protective measures and make them more willing to report Ebola cases to the authorities (Boseley 2014b).

In Mali, the last 13 people under surveillance have been released from quarantine. None of them developed Ebola. There are no active cases in the country, and no one is under observation (Reuters 2014w).

Conakry, Guinea, has banned all public Christmas and New Year's celebrations due to the Ebola outbreak (AFP and JIJI 2014).

The position of "chlorine sprayer" is a critical part of an Ebola management team. When a team arrives at a site to pick up a patient or recover a body, the chlorine sprayer must first decontaminate the area. The chlorine sprayer approaches the site and methodically sprays the victim and the surrounding area with a 0.5% chlorine solution. Once done, the sprayer signals to the rest of the team that they can begin their work. If a body is being recovered, the outer layer of the body bag is sprayed after the corpse is placed inside (Médecins Sans Frontières 2014b).

Summers et al. (2014) examined the medical and logistical challenges posed by Ebola in four rural Liberian counties. The authors interviewed healthcare workers in Grand Cape Mount, Grand Bassa, Rivercess, and Sinoe counties in western Liberia from August to September 2014. The most significant problems facing workers were inadequate training, lack of supplies, low-quality transportation, and poor communication networks. For example, at the time of the assessment, there were no functioning ambulances in either Rivercess or Sinoe counties. Roads throughout the region were often impassable, especially during the rainy season. It took one team

8 h to walk to a community that had reported cases. Despite some improvements over the last months, it is still difficult to identify and transport Ebola cases in rural Liberia (Summers et al. 2014).

US Ebola survivor, Dr. Richard Sacra, plans to return to the ELWA Hospital in Monrovia, Liberia, in January 2015 (Marcelo 2014).

December 17, 2014 (Wednesday)

Total cases: 18,603 (661 new)   Fatalities: 6915 (527 new)
(World Health Organization 2014n)

Operation *Western Area Surge* has begun in Sierra Leone (Associated Press 2014o). During this 15-day campaign, healthcare workers and volunteers will go door to door to find hidden Ebola cases and distribute brochures about Ebola's signs and symptoms (AFP 2014k). Markets will be open from 0600 to 1800 h Monday through Friday and 0600–1200 h Saturdays. Markets will be closed on Sundays (AFP 2014k). By lunchtime today, 52 suspected Ebola cases had been found. Some were discovered by search teams; others were reported to the Ebola hotline number (Farge 2014b). Burial workers at King Tom Cemetery in Freetown buried 51 Ebola victims today (Robinson 2014). The government reminds people that public gatherings are banned during the holiday season. For New Year's celebration, officials say that church services should end by 1700 h December 31, 2014 (Farge 2014b). Violators will be punished (AFP 2014k).

In the past 21 days, there were 1261 new Ebola cases in Sierra Leone (World Health Organization 2014n). Despite the high levels of transmission, CDC director Tom Frieden says US troops are not needed in Sierra Leone because British troops are helping in the country (Associated Press 2014o).

Ebola is affecting the economies of many African countries, even those that have not had any Ebola cases. Tourism revenue in The Gambia is down to 65% compared to last year. This November 10,453 international visitors arrived in The Gambia, compared to 20,905 last November (Novelli 2014).

December 18, 2014 (Thursday)

The Magbente Ebola Treatment Unit near Makeni, Sierra Leone, has discharged 29 Ebola survivors. These are the first patients to be released from the center since it opened on November 21, 2014. So far, the unit has handled 92 Ebola cases and has had six deaths (Kamara 2014).

Sierra Leone doctor, Dr. Victor Willoughby, has died from Ebola. A dose of experimental ZMAb (related to ZMapp) had arrived for him, but he died before it could be administered. Dr. Willoughby was Sierra Leone's most senior doctor (Roy-Macaulay and Diallo 2014).

Even with the high level of Ebola transmission in Sierra Leone, many people still refuse to believe the disease is real. An operator at the country's 117 Ebola hotline number says many callers insist Ebola is a lie and are abusive to her (Bowden 2014).

In Guinea, a serious fire at the Conakry airport has destroyed a warehouse containing Ebola-fighting medicine and supplies (Roy-Macaulay and Diallo 2014). All of the material appears to have been lost.

December 19, 2014 (Friday)
The Red Cross has trained two new burial teams in Kono District, Sierra Leone. One team recently recovered the body of a possible Ebola case in the remote village of Kwandor. The victim was a 5-month-old baby. The case provides an excellent example of the social and medical procedures followed by Red Cross burial teams. When the team arrived at the village, one member asked about the victim and explained the burial procedures. The whole village watched as the body was collected and the victim's house was disinfected. The men of the village then came forward and said a prayer. When the villagers were ready, the body was taken to the cemetery and buried (Pattison 2014).

Despite the dangers posed by Ebola, residents of Kono District, Sierra Leone, seem fascinated by what they are calling "the Ebola saga." When a new body is discovered, people are attracted in great numbers. In one video posted by Reuters (2014x), a large crowd is seen clustering around the body of a man sprawled at the side of the road. Some people are within inches of the body. An eyewitness says the man had been riding a bicycle when he fell off, vomited, and died. Almost everyone in the crowd has their cellphone out recording the scene. When a recovery team arrives, one of the workers says that viewing Ebola bodies has become a hobby for residents (Reuters 2014x).

Ebola survivors are helping at many Sierra Leone Ebola treatment centers. They often take care of infected children. Survivors are immune to the disease, so they do not need to wear PPE. As a result, they do not look threatening to children. They can also stay in the infected area for a long time because they do not need to leave the area to cool down (Trenchard 2014b).

Officials are concerned that the holiday season could help spread Ebola in West Africa. In particular, they worry that city dwellers may carry the virus to their home villages when they return to see their relatives. It is thought that about half the residents of Freetown, Sierra Leone, will travel to remote villages during the holidays (Fox 2014).

UN Secretary-General Ban Ki-moon arrived in Liberia today for a 2-day tour of Ebola-affected countries. Ban wants to visit the countries himself so he can personally see the response to the disease (AFP and Reuters 2014).

The United Nations Development Programme plans to work with Guinea, Liberia, and Sierra Leone to provide cash payments to families affected by Ebola. Payments will go to families who have lost their main breadwinner, survivors who are out of a job, and those caring for Ebola orphans. It is unclear exactly how much each family will receive, but $50 would support a family of five for about a month (Sifferlin 2014).

The Nigerian peacekeeper who was being treated for Ebola at Utrecht University Teaching Hospital in the Netherlands has recovered (ANP 2014).

The nurse who arrived at the NIH on December 11, 2014, has been released. They have not developed symptoms and will complete the rest of their 21-day quarantine at their home in Virginia (CBS DC 2014).

December 20, 2014 (Saturday)
Liberia is holding senatorial elections today. Voting was originally supposed to take place in October 2014, but it was postponed due to the outbreak (BBC 2014h).

UN Secretary-General Ban Ki-moon has arrived in Guinea as part of his West African tour (Sky News 2014).

US Senator Chris Coons (Democrat, Delaware) is in Liberia to assess the US Ebola response (CBS Philly 2014).

December 21, 2014 (Sunday)
Resources are stretched thin in Kono District, Sierra Leone. There are only two ambulances in the district and two ambulance drivers have died from Ebola. Conditions at Ebola centers in the district are dire. Ten healthcare workers at one center have contracted Ebola, five of them have died. At another site, nurses are so worried about interacting with infected patients that they toss medicine to them rather than risk close-quarter contact (Farge 2014c).

Unsafe burials remain a source of infection in Sierra Leone. The government is threatening to jail people caught holding illicit funerals. Medical personnel are appealing to citizens to accept medical burials. Dr. Desmond Williams of the CDC is leading by example. He made a radio broadcast saying that if he died, he wanted his family to give him a safe medical burial (VOA News 2014c).

A woman named Memuna Janneh has launched an organization called LunchBoxGift. It delivers meals to Ebola victims and healthcare workers in Sierra Leone. Janneh lives in London but has ties to Sierra Leone. Each meal costs about $1–3 and comes packaged in a bamboo wrapper that can be burned with the trash at an Ebola treatment center. The group started operating in September 2014 (Nathanson 2014).

December 22, 2014 (Monday)
Street Child of Sierra Leone is providing supplies to Ebola orphans in nine Chiefdoms of Port Loko District. The group defines an Ebola orphan as a child under 18 who has lost the family breadwinner to Ebola. Orphans are provided with bags of rice, cooking condiments, cups, plates, spoons, toothbrushes and toothpaste, soap, and used clothing (AllAfrica 2014c).

Tekmira Pharmaceuticals will provide 100 courses of its experimental TKM-Ebola-Guinea treatment for clinical trials in West Africa (Reuters 2014y).

December 23, 2014 (Tuesday)
Working conditions in West African Ebola wards are very challenging. The extreme heat makes working in PPE very difficult. In Port Loko, Sierra Leone, medical workers work in pairs. If one team member becomes overheated, they flash a "T" signal to the other worker. Both team members then immediately leave the hot zone. If the team is in the middle of a procedure, it is left for an incoming team to complete. It is difficult to write notes inside an Ebola ward. The chlorine-rich

environment destroys notepaper, and paper becomes contaminated with infected body fluids. To record data, scribes are posted outside the safety fence and information is shouted to them by medical workers in the ward (Deahl 2014).

Surgeries are no longer performed at the Hastings Treatment Center in Sierra Leone. Many of the surgeons have died from Ebola, and the surviving staff is working too hard to perform operations (Farge 2014d).

The first person has been convicted for violating Sierra Leone's anti-Ebola regulations. Amadou Kargbo, the local chief of Bumpeh, was found guilty of burying an Ebola victim, hiding a sick person (his daughter), and harboring a stranger. He was fined $235 and will spend 6 months in jail after he completes his 21-day quarantine (APA 2014d).

The 50-bed German-Liberia Ebola Treatment Center has opened in Paynesville, Liberia. It is the first German-sponsored Ebola center in West Africa (Caldwell 2014).

December 24, 2014 (Wednesday)

Total cases: 19,497 (894 new)   Fatalities: 7588 (673 new)
                                 (World Health Organization 2014o)

An accident has occurred at a CDC laboratory in Atlanta, Georgia. A technician may have been exposed to Ebola on Monday, December 22, 2014 (Grady and McNeil 2014). Ebola-infected material from the BSL-4 Ebola research lab was accidentally transferred to a BSL-2 lab (Gorman 2014; Graef 2014). The BSL-4 lab had intended to send dead virus particles to the BSL-2 lab, but sent live virus instead (Gorman 2014). The technician in the BSL-2 lab used standard BSL-2 safety equipment (gloves and gown) to work with the samples instead of full PPE (Gorman 2014). The mistake was discovered Tuesday. The technician will be monitored for 21 days to see if they develop symptoms (Grady and McNeil 2014). Other workers who entered the BSL-2 lab are being assessed. The CDC stresses there is no risk to the general public (Sun and Achenbach 2014).

Nurses at the Magbente Hospital in Makeni, Sierra Leone, have gone on strike because they have not received their hazard pay (MENAFN and AFP 2014).

People in Mali remain worried about Ebola and continue to frequently wash their hands (Diarra 2014).

A UN peacekeeper, a Liberian national, has contracted Ebola in Liberia and been isolated (Associated Press 2014p).

Ansumana et al. (2014) note a decline in Ebola mortality in Sierra Leone. Of 581 patients admitted to the Hastings Treatment Center in Freetown since September 20, 2014, 183 have died (31.5%), including 38 who were dead on arrival. This fatality rate is sharply lower than the 74% mortality seen in May and June 2014 in Kenema, Sierra Leone. The patients in Freetown were treated with antibiotics, malaria medicines, ibuprofen, intravenous nutrients, and anti-nausea medicine and given supportive care (Ansumana et al. 2014).

December 25, 2014 (Thursday)

Sierra Leone has placed the country's northern region on lockdown. The lockdown is planned to last for 3 days but could be extended if needed. During the lockdown, markets will be closed and travel will be prohibited unless it is related to the Ebola outbreak (BBC 2014i).

Christmas activities have been subdued in Sierra Leone due to the ban on public gatherings. Some churchgoers have been seen in Freetown in formal attire, but unlike normal years, no boisterous parties are being held. Small-scale private cele-brations are taking place, but police are patrolling the streets with instructions to break up any gatherings and arrest the organizers. At the Ebola treatment center in Kenema, patients listened to Christmas carols on a cassette player (Reuters 2014z).

A special Christmas party was held at the Bong County Ebola Treatment Center in Liberia (Baldauf 2014). Four healthcare workers turned their PPE into festive costumes of Santa, two elves, and Frosty the Snow Man. The medics brought candy, sodas, toys, and patterned cloths called lappas to patients in the high-risk area. The patients were overjoyed and sang Christmas carols (Baldauf 2014). In contrast, resi-dents of Monrovia celebrated a quiet Christmas. Some residents said it was the worst Christmas they had ever seen because of the overshadowing epidemic (AFP 2014l).

China says its Academy of Military Medical Sciences has developed an Ebola vaccine that will soon begin clinical trials (PTI 2014b).

December 26, 2014 (Friday)

The CDC technician exposed to Ebola in Atlanta remains under observation, but has not developed symptoms. Eleven other workers who were in the laboratory have been interviewed about their risk of exposure. None are believed to require monitor-ing. CDC Director Dr. Tom Frieden has ordered a full investigation of the incident (NBC News 2014e).

December 27, 2014 (Saturday)

The Dutch relief ship *Karel Doorman* arrived in Guinea today. It will deliver Ebola supplies to Guinea and then make deliveries to Liberia and Sierra Leone (NU.nl 2014).

The AIDS Healthcare Foundation will sponsor a float in the Rose Bowl Parade to honor Ebola fighters. The float will feature floral portraits of African doctors Dr. Sheik Umar Khan and Dr. John Taban Dada who worked with the foundation and died from Ebola (Sklar 2014).

December 28, 2014 (Sunday)

Former US Ebola Czar Ron Klain defended the CDC following the Ebola accident in Atlanta. He says the agency has been studying Ebola for 20 years and its work has saved thousands of lives (Pengelly 2014).

December 29, 2014 (Monday)

Doctors at Gartnavel Hospital in Glasgow, Scotland, have confirmed Scotland's first Ebola case (BBC 2014j). A female nurse [Pauline Cafferkey] working for Save the Children in Kerry Town, Sierra Leone, contracted the virus while in Sierra Leone. Not knowing she was infected, she returned to Scotland yesterday and developed symptoms this morning (BBC 2014j; Johnson 2014). During her return trip, the nurse flew on Royal Air Maroc flight AT596 from Sierra Leone to Casablanca, Morocco. She then took Royal Air Maroc flight AT800 from Casablanca to Heathrow Airport, London (Johnson 2014; Thomas 2014). In the United Kingdom, she took British Airways flight BA 1478 from Heathrow to Glasgow. She arrived in Scotland about 2330 h Sunday (Johnson 2014). She began feeling unwell this morning and was isolated at 0750 h (BBC 2014j). British Airways officials are working with the NHS to identify potential contacts (Gill 2014). There were 71 other passengers on her British Airways flight. Officials think the risk of transmission to fellow passengers is low, but an emergency helpline has been established. Authorities are asking passengers to call 08000 858531 so their specific risk can be assessed (BBC 2014j; Gill 2014).

Liberia has purchased 50 acres of land in the Disco Hill community of Monrovia to be used as an Ebola cemetery. Up until now, Liberian victims have been cremated. Cremation is very unpopular in Liberia because it conflicts with local religious beliefs. The government will let families bury their dead in the new cemetery if they do so safely and do not touch the bodies (BBC 2014k).

December 30, 2014 (Tuesday)

The infected Scottish nurse has been identified as 39-year-old Pauline Cafferkey (Evening Edinburgh News 2014). She worked in Kerry Town, Sierra Leone, and may have become infected at a church service on Christmas Day (Evening Edinburgh News 2014). Cafferkey was transferred to the Royal Free Hospital in London this morning. She flew to London on a plane equipped with a quarantine tent (Telegraph 2014). As part of her treatment, Cafferkey will receive convalescent blood plasma (BBC 2014l). She currently is in stable condition (Telegraph 2014).

Two other people are being tested for Ebola in the United Kingdom. One is a female healthcare worker who recently returned from West Africa and has been staying at Torridon Youth Hostel in the Scottish Highlands (BBC 2014m). She will be transferred to the Aberdeen Royal Infirmary for testing (BBC 2014m). The other person is in quarantine at the Royal Cornwall Hospital in Truro (Cowell 2014). A total of 931 people have been screened for Ebola in the United Kingdom since airport checks began (Larner 2014).

Liberia reports a flare-up of Ebola cases near its border with Sierra Leone. Between December 1 and 25, 2014, 49 new cases were reported in western Grand Cape Mount County (Paye-Layleh 2014c).

December 31, 2014 (Wednesday)

Total cases: 20,206 (709 new)   Fatalities: 7905 (317 new)
(World Health Organization 2014p)

Infected British nurse Pauline Cafferkey is being treated with convalescent blood plasma and an unnamed, experimental antiviral drug (BBC 2014n; Borland et al. 2014). Cafferkey's family cannot physically touch her, but they can see and interact with her via an intercom system (Borland et al. 2014). In total, 203 people may have had contact with Cafferkey while she was traveling on December 28, 2014. Officials are getting in touch with these people. Cafferkey had a fever while she was at Heathrow Airport, and her temperature was checked seven times. However, her temperature remained within acceptable limits (below 99.5 °F) and did not trigger further Ebola assessments (Borland et al. 2014). In response to this apparent failure, the United Kingdom's Chief Medical Officer, Sally Davies, has requested that UK Ebola screening procedures be reviewed and improved (Associated Press 2014q).

Liberia will lift its 0000–0600 h curfew tonight to allow people to attend New Year's Eve church services. Participating churches are asked to avoid overcrowded conditions and have attendees practice safe personal protection practices such as hand-washing (Giahyue 2014).

As Ebola survivors leave the Maforki Ebola Treatment Centre in Port Loko, Sierra Leone, they tie a ribbon to a tree near the unit. Many colorful ribbons now adorn the tree (United Nations 2014).

Ebola is affecting many aspects of Sierra Leone's sociology, including the country's sex life. In terms of prostitution, customers fear prostitutes may be infected. They either avoid prostitutes or pay them very little. One sex worker says a customer recently offered $7 for her services when she would normally charge $40. Relationship-based sex also appears to be down. One condom provider says the hotels he serves normally require about 2000 condoms a month. Since spring 2014, however, none of the hotels have needed to replenish their stocks (Aizenman and Smith 2014).

UNICEF has donated ten ambulances to Guinea (United Nations 2014).

Some US troops are returning to their home bases after being deployed to West Africa. Returnees include 140 troops from Fort Campbell, Kentucky. They will undergo their 21-day quarantine at different sites before returning to their base. By mid-January, US Africa Command will decide whether the soldiers remaining in Liberia will move to other West African countries or return home (Associated Press 2014q).

References

ABC News (2014) Sierra Leone says another doctor dies of Ebola. ABC News. http://abcnews.go.com/Health/wireStory/sierra-leone-doctor-dies-ebola-26649996. Accessed 3 Nov 2014

Abdelmoneim J (2014) Dispatches from the Ebola zone: The traumas and successes of working in a Sierra Leone treatment centre. The Independent. http://www.independent.co.uk/news/world/africa/dispatches-from-the-ebola-zone-the-traumas-and-successes-of-working-in-a-sierra-leone-treatment-centre-9864120.html. Accessed 17 Nov 2014

AFP (2014a) Ebola virus death toll rises in remote Sierra Leone town. AFP, Manila Standard. http://manilastandardtoday.com/2014/11/10/ebola-virus-death-toll-rises-in-remote-sierra-leone-town/. Accessed 10 Nov 2014

AFP (2014b) Mali Ebola clinic in lockdown, doctor thought to have virus. AFP, Newsmax. http://www.newsmax.com/World/Africa/Health-Ebola-Mali-clinic/2014/11/12/id/606831/. Accessed 19 Jun 2017

AFP (2014c) Ebola wiping out Sierra Leone's post-war gains: study. AFP, The Daily Mail. http://www.dailymail.co.uk/wires/afp/article-2834844/Ebola-wiping-Sierra-Leones-post-war-gains-study.html. Accessed 19 Jun 2017

AFP (2014d) Fearing Ebola surge, Mali widens virus watch to 440 people. AFP, The Daily Mail. http://www.dailymail.co.uk/wires/afp/article-2837790/Mali-places-hundreds-watch-bid-stem-Ebola.html. Accessed 17 Nov 2014

AFP (2014e) Liberia 'chasing Ebola now', not other way around. AFP, Global Post. http://www.globalpost.com/dispatch/news/afp/141124/liberia-chasing-ebola-now-not-other-way-around. Accessed 24 Nov 2014

AFP (2014f) Ebola-infected Italian doctor's health worsens. AFP, The Straits Times. http://www.straitstimes.com/news/world/europe/story/ebola-infected-italian-doctors-health-worsens-20141129. Accessed 30 Nov 2014

AFP (2014g) Cuba says Ebola doctor to leave Swiss hospital. AFP, Medical Xpress. http://medicalxpress.com/news/2014-12-cuba-ebola-doctor-swiss-hospital.html. Accessed 5 Dec 2014

AFP (2014h) Ebola lockdown in eastern Sierra Leone mining district. AFP, The Daily Mail. http://www.dailymail.co.uk/wires/afp/article-2869123/Ebola-lockdown-eastern-Sierra-Leone-mining-district.html. Accessed 11 Dec 2014

AFP (2014i) Alliance set to buy millions of Ebola vaccine doses. AFP, Yahoo News. http://news.yahoo.com/alliance-set-buy-millions-ebola-vaccine-doses-142602341.html. Accessed 11 Dec 2014

AFP (2014j) New UN Ebola mission chief named. AFP. http://www.globalpost.com/dispatch/news/afp/141211/new-un-ebola-mission-chief-named. Accessed 11 Dec 2014

AFP (2014k) Sierra Leone launches stiff measures to fight Ebola surge. AFP, Yahoo News. https://uk.news.yahoo.com/sierra-leone-launches-stiff-measures-fight-ebola-surge-153229385.html#6I5s7AP. Accessed 17 Dec 2014

AFP (2014l) "Worst Christmas ever" in morose, Ebola-hit Liberia. AFP, The Straits Times. http://www.straitstimes.com/news/world/more-world-stories/story/worst-christmas-ever-morose-ebola-hit-liberia-20141226. Accessed 25 Dec 2014

AFP and JIJI (2014) Guinean capital follows Ebola-hit Freetown's lead, bans Christmas, New Year celebrations. AFP, The Japan Times. http://www.japantimes.co.jp/news/2014/12/17/world/science-health-world/guinean-capital-follows-ebola-hit-freetowns-lead-bans-christmas-new-year-celebrations/#.VJCNKbd0ziw. Accessed 16 Dec 2014

AFP and Reuters (2014) Ban Ki-moon travels to west Africa to assess Ebola crisis. AFP, Reuters, DW. http://www.dw.de/ban-ki-moon-travels-to-west-africa-to-assess-ebola-crisis/a-18141532. Accessed 19 Dec 2014

Ahmed B (2014) Mali no new Ebola cases, family ends quarantine. ABC News. http://abcnews.go.com/Health/wireStory/mali-ebola-cases-family-ends-quarantine-26829398. Accessed 11 Nov 2014

Aizenman N (2014a) In Sierra Leone, tears and wails mark the death of Dr. Martin Salia. NPR, WGBH. http://wgbhnews.org/post/sierra-leone-tears-and-wails-mark-death-dr-martin-salia. Accessed 17 Nov 2014

Aizenman N (2014b) An Ebola clinic figures out a way to start beating the odds. NPR. http://www.npr.org/blogs/goatsandsoda/2014/11/21/365715575/an-ebola-clinic-figures-out-a-way-to-start-beating-the-odds. Accessed 22 Nov 2014

Aizenman N, Smith G (2014) The prostitutes are not happy. Neither are brides. Sex, love and Ebola. NPR. http://www.npr.org/blogs/goatsandsoda/2014/12/31/374057299/the-prostitutes-are-not-happy-neither-are-brides-sex-love-and-ebola. Accessed 1 Jan 2015

Al Jazeera (2014a) Ebola cases 'surge' in rural Sierra Leone. Al Jazeera. Higher. http://www.aljazeera.com/news/africa/2014/11/ebola-cases-surge-rural-sierra-leone-2014112221854603455.html. Accessed 15 Jun 2017

Al Jazeera (2014b) Ebola quarantines violated in search of food. http://www.aljazeera.com/news/africa/2014/11/ebola-quarantines-violated-search-food-201411543857794804.html. Accessed 5 Nov 2014

Al Jazeera (2014c) UN: deadline to curb Ebola will not be met. Al Jazeera. http://www.aljazeera.com/news/africa/2014/11/deadline-curb-ebola-will-not-be-fully-met-2014112418512630314.html. Accessed 25 Nov 2014

AllAfrica (2014a) Liberia: pay Liberia Ebola workers – UNDP official says benefits essential. AllAfrica, Front Page Africa. http://allafrica.com/stories/201412031065.html. Accessed 3 Dec 2014

AllAfrica (2014b) Liberia: Ellen speaks on Ebola decline. AllAfrica, The News. http://allafrica.com/stories/201412091338.html. Accessed 9 Dec 2014

AllAfrica (2014c) Sierra Leone: street child boosts over 2,000 Ebola orphans in Port Loko. AllAfrica, Concord Times. http://allafrica.com/stories/201412231592.html. Accessed 23 Dec 2014

ANP (2014) Nigerian treated for Ebola in Utrecht makes full recovery. ANP, Dutch News. http://www.dutchnews.nl/news/archives/2014/12/nigerian-treated-for-ebola-in-utrecht-makes-full-recovery.php/. Accessed 19 Dec 2014

Ansumana R, Jacobsen KH, Sahr F et al (2014) Ebola in Freetown area, Sierra Leone – a case study of 581 patients. N Engl J Med 372:587–588

Anti-Corruption Commission (2014) ACC intelligence leads to police arrest of chlorine fraudsters. 21 Nov 2014

APA (2014a) Ebola: Sierra Leone to prepare new cemetery. APA, Star Africa. http://en.starafrica.com/news/ebola-sierra-leone-to-prepare-new-cemetery.html. Accessed 4 Dec 2014

APA (2014b) Sierra Leone: washing of dead bodies attracts jail term. APA, Star Africa. http://en.starafrica.com/news/sierra-leone-washing-of-dead-bodies-attracts-jail-term.html. Accessed 4 Dec 2014

APA (2014c) Row over 'Ebola-free' declaration in Sierra Leone. APA, Star Africa. http://en.starafrica.com/news/row-over-ebola-free-declaration-in-sierra-leone.html. Accessed 4 Dec 2014

APA (2014d) Local chief sentenced for flouting anti-Ebola measures. APA, Star Africa. http://en.starafrica.com/news/local-chief-sentenced-for-flouting-anti-ebola-measures.html. Accessed 23 Dec 2014

Associated Press (2014a) Sierra Leone doctor tests positive for Ebola. Associated Press, Item Live. http://www.itemlive.com/health/sierra-leone-doctor-tests-positive-for-ebola/article_a880560f-cf1b-5bba-89d0-011ef47df30c.html. Accessed 2 Nov 2014

Associated Press (2014b) Akron bridal shop visited by Dallas nurse who contracted Ebola set to reopen. Associated Press, Daily Journal. http://www.dailyjournal.net/view/story/40c7d4cc27e6491b948b23b5005258e5/OH--Ohio-Ebola-Dress-Shop/. Accessed 2 Nov 2014

Associated Press (2014c) 42 people removed from Ohio Ebola contact list. Associated Press, WCBE. http://wcbe.org/post/42-people-removed-ohio-ebola-contact-list. Accessed 3 Nov 2014

Associated Press (2014d) Military names 5 U.S. bases for troop Ebola quarantines. Associated Press, CBS News. http://www.cbsnews.com/news/military-names-5-u-s-bases-for-troop-ebola-quarantines/. Accessed 9 Nov 2014

Associated Press (2014e) Non-profit sets up Ebola treatment unit in Liberia. Associated Press, Independent. http://www.marshallindependent.com/page/content.detail/id/739382/Non-profit-sets-up-Ebola-treatment-unit-in-Liberia.html?isap=1&nav=5028. Accessed 12 Nov 2014

Associated Press (2014f) Red Cross officials: Ebola flaring anew in Africa. Associated Press, Town Hall. http://townhall.com/news/world/2014/11/17/red-cross-officials-ebola-flaring-anew-in-africa-n1919783. Accessed 17 Nov 2014

Associated Press (2014g) UMC renovating facility to serve as Ebola isolation unit. Associated Press, MS Business. http://msbusiness.com/blog/2014/11/18/umc-renovating-facility-serve-ebola-isolation-unit/. Accessed 18 Nov 2014

Associated Press (2014h) Bandits in Guinea steal suspected Ebola blood. Associated Press, Fox CT. http://foxct.com/2014/11/21/bandits-in-guinea-steal-suspected-ebola-blood/. Accessed 21 Nov 2014

Associated Press (2014i) Cuban doctor begins experimental Ebola treatment. Associated Press, 10 TV. http://www.10tv.com/content/stories/apexchange/2014/11/22/cb--cuba-ebola.html. Accessed 22 Nov 2014

Associated Press (2014j) UK volunteers fly to Sierra Leone to fight Ebola. Associated Press, KURV. http://www.kurv.com/world/10924. Accessed 22 Nov 2014

Associated Press (2014k) Sierra Leone doctor who beat Ebola will return to front lines. The Associated Press, Macleans. http://www.macleans.ca/politics/worldpolitics/sierra-leone-doctor-who-beat-ebola-will-return-to-front-lines/. Accessed 2 Dec 2014

Associated Press (2014l) Mali receives first mobile lab for testing Ebola. Associated Press, Yahoo News. https://news.yahoo.com/mali-receives-first-mobile-lab-testing-ebola-212902663.html. Accessed 4 Dec 2014

Associated Press (2014m) CDC report: Ebola reports rarely panned out. Associated Press, Chicago Defender. http://chicagodefender.com/2014/12/06/cdc-report-ebola-reports-rarely-panned-out/. Accessed 6 Dec 2014

Associated Press (2014n) Top Sierra Leonean physician contracts Ebola. Associated Press, News113. http://www.news1130.com/2014/12/14/top-sierra-leonean-physician-contracts-ebola/. Accessed 14 Dec 2014

Associated Press (2014o) House searches for Ebola in Sierra Leone capital. Associated Press, Town Hall. http://townhall.com/news/world/2014/12/17/search-for-ebola-in-sierra-leone-capital-begins-n1933005. Accessed 17 Dec 2014

Associated Press (2014p) Liberia's UN mission reports 4th Ebola case. Associated Press, Town Hall. http://townhall.com/news/world/2014/12/24/liberias-un-mission-reports-4th-ebola-case-n1935621. Accessed 24 Dec 2014

Associated Press (2014q) Top UK doctor Ebola screening should be improved. Associated Press, Lancaster Online. http://lancasteronline.com/news/world/top-uk-doctor-ebola-screening-should-be-improved/article_fe77e32c-0a07-5cc5-91a6-62f83ffaf014.html. Accessed 31 Dec 2014

Australian Associated Press (2014) The federal government has reportedly reached an agreement that would allow it to help Australian health workers fight the deadly Ebola virus. Australian Associated Press, The Daily Mail. http://www.dailymail.co.uk/news/article-2820484/The-federal-government-reportedly-reached-agreement-allow-help-Australian-health-workers-fight-deadly-Ebola-virus.html. Accessed 4 Nov 2014

Awareness Times (2014) Sierra Leone news: RSLAF opens new Ebola treatment centre. Awareness Times. http://news.sl/drwebsite/publish/article_200526786.shtml. Accessed 2 Dec 2014

Awoko (2014a) Sierra Leone news: bi-weekly allowances for health workers. Awoko. http://awoko.org/2014/11/13/sierra-leone-news-bi-weekly-allowances-for-health-workers/. Accessed 13 Nov 2014

Awoko (2014b) Sierra Leone news: budget exposes 1 doctor to15000 Sierra Leoneans. Awoko. http://awoko.org/2014/11/18/sierra-leone-news-budget-exposes1-doctor-to15000-sierra-leoneans/. Accessed 18 Nov 2014

Awoko (2014c) Sierra Leone news: UNICEF opens isolation care centers in Bombali. Awoko. http://awoko.org/2014/11/18/sierra-leone-news-unicef-opens-isolation-care-centers-in-bombali/. Accessed 18 Nov 2014

Awoko (2014d) Sierra Leone news: trends: Ebola deaths double in last 3 weeks. Awoko. http://awoko.org/2014/11/26/sierra-leone-news-trends-ebola-deaths-double-in-last-3-weeks/. Accessed 26 Nov 2014

Baldauf M (2014) Photos: Christmas in an Ebola ward. Quartz. http://qz.com/318038/photos-christmas-in-an-ebola-ward/. Accessed 25 Dec 2014

Baschiera D (2014) Ebola outbreak Darwin volunteer writes from Sierra Leone treatment centre, 'I just cry in my goggles.' ABC News Australia. http://www.abc.net.au/news/2014-11-26/darwin-ebola-volunteer-dan-baschiera-writes-from-sierra-leone/5919516. Accessed 25 Nov 2014

BBC (2014a) Ebola outbreak: MSF confirms case decline in Liberia. BBC. http://www.bbc.com/news/world-africa-29957338. Accessed 16 Jun 2017

BBC (2014b) Ebola crisis: Sierra Leone health workers strike. BBC. http://www.bbc.com/news/world-africa-30019895. Accessed 12 Nov 2014

BBC (2014c) Ebola outbreak: Sierra Leone workers dump bodies in Kenema. BBC. http://www.bbc.com/news/world-africa-30191938. Accessed 25 Nov 2014

BBC (2014d) Ebola crisis: French President Hollande visits Guinea. BBC. http://www.bbc.com/news/world-africa-30241374. Accessed 28 Nov 2014

BBC (2014e) Dangerous job of grave digging in Ebola hit Sierra Leone. BBC. http://www.bbc.com/news/health-30273824. Accessed 1 Dec 2014

BBC (2014f) Ebola crisis: Sierra Leone bodies found piled up in Kono. BBC. http://www.bbc.com/news/world-africa-30429360. Accessed 11 Dec 2014

BBC (2014g) Ebola serum supply reaches Liberia. BBC. http://www.bbc.com/news/health-30478512. Accessed 15 Dec 2014

BBC (2014h) Ebola crisis: Liberia holds senate postponed election. BBC. http://www.bbc.com/news/world-africa-30553837. Accessed 20 Dec 2014

BBC (2014i) Ebola crisis: Sierra Leone declares three-day lockdown in north. BBC. http://www.bbc.com/news/world-africa-30601523. Accessed 25 Dec 2014

BBC (2014j) Ebola case confirmed in Glasgow hospital. BBC. http://www.bbc.com/news/uk-scotland-30628349. Accessed 30 Dec 2014

BBC (2014k) Ebola outbreak: Liberia opens new cemetery. BBC. http://www.bbc.com/news/world-africa-30626732. Accessed 30 Dec 2014

BBC (2014l) Ebola nurse to be treated with recovered patients' plasma. BBC. http://www.bbc.com/news/uk-30637199. Accessed 30 Dec 2014

BBC (2014m) Second woman to be tested for Ebola in Scotland after Aberdeen transfer. BBC. http://www.bbc.com/news/uk-scotland-highlands-islands-30630768. Accessed 30 Dec 2014

BBC (2014n) Experimental drug for Ebola patient Pauline Cafferkey. BBC. http://www.bbc.com/news/uk-30644986. Accessed 31 Dec 2014

Beardsley S (2014) US troops in Ebola zones look ahead to next task as infection rates drop. Stars and Stripes. http://www.stripes.com/news/us-troops-in-ebola-zones-look-ahead-to-next-task-as-infection-rates-drop-1.317758. Accessed 7 Dec 2014

Beaubien J (2014a) U.S. military response to Ebola gains momentum In Liberia. NPR. http://www.npr.org/blogs/goatsandsoda/2014/11/05/361796044/u-s-military-response-to-ebola-gains-momentum-in-liberia. Accessed 5 Nov 2014

Beaubien J (2014b) Guinea is seeing more Ebola cases: can the trend be stopped? NPR. http://www.npr.org/blogs/goatsandsoda/2014/11/07/362062293/guinea-is-seeing-more-ebola-cases-can-the-trend-be-stopped?utm_medium=RSS&utm_campaign=news. Accessed 7 Nov 2014

Beaubien J (2014c) Startling statistic: only 8 patients in largest Ebola hospital. NPR. http://www.npr.org/sections/goatsandsoda/2014/12/03/368229279/startling-statistic-only-8-patients-in-largest-ebola-hospital. Accessed 3 Dec 2014

Bethesda Magazine (2014) NIH admitting patient today with 'exposure to Ebola virus.' Bethesda Magazine. http://www.bethesdamagazine.com/Bethesda-Beat/2014/NIH-Admitting-Patient-Today-with-Exposure-to-Ebola-Virus/. Accessed 11 Dec 2014

Bisson M (2014) Morocco thrown out of Africa Cup of Nations after withdrawing as host. World Football Insider. http://www.worldfootballinsider.com/Story.aspx?id=37385. Accessed 11 Nov 2014

Bloch H (2014) Ebola in remote Liberia, through the eyes of a local health worker. NPR. http://www.npr.org/blogs/goatsandsoda/2014/11/24/365689595/ebola-in-remote-liberia-through-the-eyes-of-a-local-health-worker. Accessed 24 Nov 2014

Boakye-Yiadom N (2014) Ebola vaccine to cost $100 per dose. Citifmonline. http://www.citifmonline.com/2014/11/06/ebola-vaccine-to-cost-100-per-dose/. Accessed 6 Nov 2014

Borland S, Taylor R, Harding E (2014) Nurse suffering from Ebola is sitting up and talking to her family after being treated with experimental drugs as doctor says the next few days will be crucial to her survival. The Daily Mail. http://www.dailymail.co.uk/news/article-2891870/

How-did-miss-ebola-nurse-sick-complained-fever-Heathrow-asked-tested-SEVEN-TIMES-revealed-caught-disease-hug-church.html. Accessed 31 Dec 2014

Boseley S (2014a) Ebola diary: burials go on as Christmas is 'cancelled' in Sierra Leone. The Guardian.   http://www.theguardian.com/world/2014/dec/14/-sp-ebola-diary-burials-go-on-christmas-is-cancelled-in-sierra-leone. Accessed 14 Dec 2014

Boseley S (2014b) Sierra Leone to use scare tactics campaign in Freetown to curb Ebola. The Guardian.   http://www.theguardian.com/world/2014/dec/16/sierra-leone-scare-tactics-free-town-curb-ebola. Accessed 16 Dec 2014

Bowden D (2014) Sierra Leone braced for more Ebola cases. Sky News. http://news.sky.com/story/1393826/sierra-leone-braced-for-more-ebola-cases. Accessed 18 Dec 2014

Branswell H (2014) Canada imposes Ebola quarantine on 'high-risk' travellers. The Star. http://www.thestar.com/news/canada/2014/11/10/canada_imposes_ebola_quarantine_on_highrisk_travellers.html. Accessed 12 Nov 2014

Byrne C (2014) Sending love to soldiers deployed in support of Operation United Assistance. Clarksville   Online.   http://www.clarksvilleonline.com/2014/12/12/sending-love-soldiers-deployed-support-operation-united-assistance/. Accessed 12 Dec 2014

Caldwell M (2014) German Ebola treatment center officially opened in Liberia. DW. http://www.dw.de/german-ebola-treatment-center-officially-opened-in-liberia/a-18149209. Accessed 23 Dec 2014

California Department of Industrial Relations (2014) Cal/OSHA updates its guidance for protecting workers in inpatient health care settings from Ebola. 14 Nov 2014

Carroll C (2014) Most US troops in Liberia could soon be home. Stars and Stripes. http://www.stripes.com/news/most-us-troops-in-liberia-could-soon-be-home-1.317134. Accessed 3 Dec 2014

Caulderwood K (2014) Many Ebola donations have yet to be delivered, watchdog group says. International Business Times. http://www.ibtimes.com/many-ebola-donations-have-yet-be-delivered-watchdog-group-says-1743476. Accessed 9 Dec 2014

CBC News (2014) Ebola outbreak: male survivors told to abstain from sex for 3 months. CBC News.   http://www.cbc.ca/news/health/ebola-outbreak-male-survivors-told-to-abstain-from-sex-for-3-months-1.2853427. Accessed 28 Nov 2014

CBS Baltimore (2014) Funeral planned for Md. doctor who died from Ebola. CBS Baltimore. http://baltimore.cbslocal.com/2014/11/20/funeral-planned-for-md-doctor-who-died-from-ebola/. Accessed 20 Nov 2014

CBS DC (2014) Nurse exposed to Ebola discharged from NIH. CBS DC. http://washington.cbslocal.com/2014/12/19/patient-exposed-to-ebola-discharged-from-nih/. Accessed 20 Dec 2014

CBS Philly (2014) Del. Senator travels to Liberia to see American response to Ebola outbreak. CBS Philly. http://philadelphia.cbslocal.com/2014/12/20/del-senator-travels-to-liberia-to-see-american-response-to-ebola-outbreak/. Accessed 20 Dec 2014

Centers for Disease Control and Prevention (2014a) CDC is increasing supply of Ebola specific PPE for U.S. hospitals. Infection Control Today. http://www.infectioncontroltoday.com/news/2014/11/cdc-is-increasing-supply-of-ebolaspecific-ppe-for-us-hospitals.aspx. Accessed 7 Nov 2014

Centers for Disease Control and Prevention (2014b) Enhanced airport entry screening to begin for travelers to the United States from Mali. 16 Nov 2014

Chang C (2014) Jihadists send 'vial of Ebola' to newspaper. New York Post. http://nypost.com/2014/11/10/jihadist-group-sends-newspaper-vial-of-ebola-virus/. Accessed 11 Nov 2014

Chaon A (2014) Rural Sierra Leone waits for help as Ebola does its worst. Medical Express. http://medicalxpress.com/news/2014-11-rural-sierra-leone-ebola-worst.html. Accessed 9 Nov 2014

Clarke S (2014) SES to beam Ebola channel. Television Business International. http://tbivision.com/news/2014/11/ses-beam-ebola-channel/354271/. Accessed 10 Nov 2014

Clottey P (2014) UN Ebola response team establishing office in Mali. VOA News. http://www.voanews.com/content/un-ebola-response-team-establising-office-in-mali/2531082.html. Accessed 23 Nov 2014

Committee to Protect Journalists (2014) In Sierra Leone, journalist imprisoned after criticizing president. 4 Nov 2014

Conteh P (2014) Update on Ebola in Sierra Leone by the Ebola Czar, Palo Conteh. Awareness Times. http://news.sl/drwebsite/publish/article_200526803.shtml. Accessed 4 Dec 2014

Cooper H, Tavernise S (2014) Health officials reassess strategy to combat Ebola in Liberia. New York Times. http://www.nytimes.com/2014/11/13/world/africa/officials-consider-scaling-back-of-ebola-centers-in-liberia.html?_r=0. Accessed 13 Nov 2014

Cowell A (2014) Ebola patient is moved to London, and 2 others are rested in Britain. New York Times. http://www.nytimes.com/2014/12/31/world/europe/ebola-virus-britain.html?_r=0. Accessed 30 Dec 2014

Cullen P (2014) Irish burial experts help control Ebola outbreak in Sierra Leone. The Irish Times. http://www.irishtimes.com/news/world/africa/irish-burial-experts-help-control-ebola-outbreak-in-sierra-leone-1.2013521. Accessed 25 Nov 2014

Daily Times (2014) China plans 1,000 more staff to fight Ebola in Africa. The Daily Times. http://www.dailytimes.com.pk/foreign/05-Nov-2014/china-plans-1-000-more-staff-to-fight-ebola-in-africa. Accessed 5 Nov 2014

Daniel S (2014) Mali scrambles to contain Ebola after new confirmed death. AFP, Yahoo News. http://news.yahoo.com/mali-suffers-ebola-case-death-nurse-224857619.html. Accessed 12 Nov 2014

Deahl M (2014) Ebola: 'We relieve pain and distress, but in all honesty we rarely save.' The Guardian. http://www.theguardian.com/global-development/2014/dec/23/ebola-british-doctor-sierra-leone. Accessed 23 Dec 2014

Diarra ST (2014) Fear lingers in Mali despite no new Ebola cases. USA Today. http://www.usatoday.com/story/news/world/2014/12/24/mali-ebola-fears-linger/20645875/. Accessed 25 Dec 2014

Doucleff M (2014) Endless Ebola epidemic? That's the 'risk we face now,' CDC says. NPR. http://www.npr.org/blogs/goatsandsoda/2014/12/15/370446566/endless-ebola-endemic-thats-the-risk-we-face-now-cdc-says. Accessed 16 Dec 2014

Eiklor R (2014) Reporter explains his trip to Africa. Spectrum News, TWC News. http://buffalo.twcnews.com/content/news/783802/reporter-explains-his-trip-to-africa/. Accessed 9 Nov 2014

Evening Edinburgh News (2014) Scottish Ebola nurse named as Pauline Cafferkey. Evening Edinburgh News. http://www.edinburghnews.scotsman.com/news/health/scottish-ebola-nurse-named-as-pauline-cafferkey-1-3646288. Accessed 30 Dec 2014

Eversley M (2014) Photographer documenting Ebola dies of apparent heart attack. USA Today. http://www.usatoday.com/story/news/nation/2014/12/11/michel-du-cille/20284429/. Accessed 12 Dec 2014

Farge E (2014a) "Dramatic improvement" in Ebola outlook in Liberia – U.S. general. Reuters. http://in.reuters.com/article/2014/11/24/health-ebola-liberia-idINL6N0TE3HZ20141124. Accessed 24 Nov 2014

Farge E (2014b) Health teams scour Sierra Leone capital in Ebola drive. Reuters. http://www.reuters.com/article/2014/12/17/us-health-ebola-leone-idUSKBN0JV0SI20141217. Reuters. Accessed 17 Dec 2014

Farge E (2014c) Ebola response in rural Sierra Leone not yet rapid enough. Reuters. http://www.reuters.com/article/2014/12/21/us-health-ebola-leone-idUSKBN0JZ0KE20141221. Accessed 21 Dec 2014

Farge E (2014d) Exhausted Sierra Leone medics battle Ebola in the 'red zone.' Reuters. http://www.reuters.com/article/2014/12/23/us-health-ebola-leone-idUSKBN0K119E20141223. Accessed 23 Dec 2014

Ferris S (2014) 114 hospital workers cleared of Ebola in NYC. The Hill. http://thehill.com/policy/healthcare/225836-114-hospital-workers-cleared-of-ebola-in-nyc. Accessed 3 Dec 2014

Finley JC (2014) Suspicious package referencing Ebola sent to U.S. Embassy in New Zealand. UPI. http://www.upi.com/Top_News/World-News/2014/11/12/Suspicious-package-referencing-Ebola-sent-to-US-Embassy-in-New-Zealand/4281415797519/. Accessed 12 Nov 2014

Finnan D (2014) Combating Ebola at Sierra Leone's Freetown port. RFI. http://www.english.rfi.fr/africa/20141106-combating-ebola-sierra-leones-freetown-port. Accessed 6 Nov 2014

Fitzgerald T (2014) Schools defend decision to take pupils to west Africa after Ebola fears raised by surgeon dad. Manchester Evening News. http://www.manchestereveningnews.co.uk/news/greater-manchester-news/schools-defend-decision-take-pupils-8209119. Accessed 1 Dec 2014

Fox M (2014) Could Christmas worsen Ebola's spread? NBC News. http://www.nbcnews.com/storyline/ebola-virus-outbreak/could-christmas-worsen-ebolas-spread-n270471. Accessed 19 Dec 2014

Fox News (2014) Surgeon who contracted Ebola virus in Sierra Leone dies at Nebraska hospital. Fox News. http://www.foxnews.com/health/2014/11/17/surgeon-who-contracted-ebola-virus-in-sierra-leone-dies-at-nebraska-hospital/. Accessed 17 Nov 2014

France 24 (2014) France extends Ebola passenger screenings to flights from Mali. France 24, AFP, Reuters. http://www.france24.com/en/20141115-france-extends-ebola-passenger-screenings-cover-flights-mali/. Accessed 15 Nov 2014

Frankfurter Allgemeine (2014) Ebola patient discharged as cured. Frankfurter Allgemeine. http://www.faz.net/aktuell/rhein-main/frankfurt-ebola-patient-als-geheilt-entlassen-13302595.html. Accessed 22 Jun 2017

Gale J, Kitamura M (2014) West Africa short 75 percent of needed beds for Ebola. Business Week. http://www.businessweek.com/news/2014-11-04/west-africa-short-75-percent-of-needed-beds-for-ebola. Accessed 4 Nov 2014

Gallagher J (2014a) Ebola are cases levelling off? BBC. http://www.bbc.com/news/health-29847058. Accessed 1 Nov 2014

Gallagher J (2014b) Ebola outbreak MSF says new Liberia tactics needed. BBC. http://www.bbc.com/news/health-29991092. Accessed 10 Nov 2014

Gayle D (2014) Mali battles to control Ebola after Imam from neighbouring Guinea who didn't know he had disease infected two nurses before dying. The Daily Mail. http://www.dailymail.co.uk/news/article-2834286/Mali-battles-control-Ebola-Imam-neighbouring-Guinea-didn-t-know-disease-infected-two-nurses-dying.html. Accessed 14 Nov 2014

Gbenda TS (2014) Sierra Leone news: as quarantined homes grumble over food supply… EduNations intervenes. Awareness Times. http://news.sl/drwebsite/publish/article_200526769.shtml. Accessed 28 Nov 2014

Giahyue JH (2014) Liberia suspends Ebola curfew to allow New Year's Eve worship. Reuters. http://in.reuters.com/article/2014/12/31/health-ebola-liberia-idINKBN0K90KU20141231. Accessed 31 Dec 2014

Gill R (2014) Air passengers being traced after nurse contracts Ebola. Buying Business Travel. http://buyingbusinesstravel.com/news/3023572-air-passengers-being-traced-after-nurse-catches-ebola. Accessed 30 Dec 2014

Gorman (2014) CDC worker monitored for possible Ebola exposure in lab error. Reuters. http://www.reuters.com/article/2014/12/25/us-health-ebola-usa-idUSKBN0K21BQ20141225. Accessed 25 Dec 2014

Grady D, McNeil DG Jr (2014) CDC Ebola error in lab may have exposed technician to virus. New York Times. http://www.nytimes.com/2014/12/25/health/cdc-ebola-error-in-lab-may-have-exposed-technician-to-virus.html?_r=0. Accessed 31 Dec 2014

Graef A (2014) CDC reports lab error led to possible Ebola exposure. UPI. http://www.upi.com/Top_News/US/2014/12/25/CDC-reports-lab-error-led-to-possible-Ebola-exposure/4741419530501/. Accessed 25 Dec 2014

Guensburg C (2014) Guinea fights to reduce Ebola risks to miners. VOA News. http://www.voanews.com/content/guinea-fights-to-reduce-ebola-risks-to-miners/2557615.html. Accessed 13 Dec 2014

Haglage A (2014a) Fighting Ebola and starvation in Sierra Leone. The Daily Beast. http://www.thedailybeast.com/articles/2014/11/05/fighting-ebola-and-starvation-in-sierra-leone.html. Accessed 5 Nov 2014

Haglage A (2014b) The photojournalist who stared down Ebola. The Daily Beast. http://www.thedailybeast.com/articles/2014/11/08/the-photojournalist-who-stared-down-ebola.html. Accessed 9 Nov 2014

Haglage A (2014c) The American Ebola rescue plan hinges on one company. Meet Phoenix. The Daily Beast. http://www.thedailybeast.com/articles/2014/11/22/meet-the-rescue-pilots-of-ebola-air.html. Accessed 22 Nov 2014

Harding A (2014a) On the frontline in Sierra Leone as Ebola virus spreads. BBC. http://www.bbc.com/news/world-africa-29888067. Accessed 4 Nov 2014

Harding A (2014b) Sierra Leone foreign Ebola relief operation criticized. BBC. http://www.bbc.com/news/world-africa-30267600. Accessed 30 Nov 2014

Heckle H (2014) Spanish woman cured of Ebola moves to normal room. Associated Press. https://www.apnews.com/6f475e1a0d4841d7bf77341fcb3a082a. Accessed 14 Jun 2017

Heilprin J (2014) WHO says Liberia, Guinea meeting Ebola targets. Associated Press, Yahoo News. https://news.yahoo.com/says-liberia-guinea-meeting-ebola-targets-145318860.html. Accessed 1 Dec 2014

Hinshaw D (2014) U.S. buys up Ebola gear, leaving little for Africa. The Wall Street Journal. http://online.wsj.com/articles/u-s-buys-up-ebola-gear-leaving-little-for-africa-1416875059. Accessed 24 Nov 2014

Hladky GB (2014) Connecticut hospital costs for Ebola planning top $5 million. Hartford Courant. http://www.courant.com/politics/capitol-watch/hc-connecticut-hospital-costs-for-ebola-planning-top-5-million-20141201-story.html. Accessed 1 Dec 2014

Holloway L (2014) 18,000 nurses plan to strike over Ebola preparedness. The Root. http://www.theroot.com/articles/culture/2014/11/_18_000_nurses_plan_to_strike_over_ebola_preparedness_at_kaiser_permanente.html. Accessed 9 Nov 2014

IANS (2014a) Ebola in India: 24 new thermal scanners to be arranged at international airports. IANS, The Health Site. http://www.thehealthsite.com/news/ebola-in-india-24-new-thermal-scanners-to-be-arranged-at-international-airports/. Accessed 20 Nov 2014

IANS (2014b) Taiwans suspected Ebola case turns out to be a hoax. IANS, Free Press Journal. http://freepressjournal.in/taiwans-suspected-ebola-case-turns-out-to-be-a-hoax/. Accessed 6 Dec 2014

IANS (2014c) Latest Ebola news: New Zealand sends 82 volunteers to fight the Ebola crisis. IANS, The Health Site. http://www.thehealthsite.com/news/latest-ebola-news-new-zealand-sends-82-volunteers-to-fight-the-ebola-crisis/. Accessed 7 Dec 2014

Ide W (2014) VOA exclusive: Guangzhou hotel serves as China's Ebola quarantine. VOA News. http://www.voanews.com/content/voa-exclusive-hotel-in-guangzhou-serves-as-chinas-loose-ebola-quarantine/2533378.html. Accessed 25 Nov 2014

Jamaica Observer (2014) Ebola centre nearly ready in Jamaica. Nation News. http://www.nation-news.com/nationnews/news/59386/ebola-centre-nearly-ready-jamaica. Accessed 16 Nov 2014

Jasper C, Bennett S (2014) Ebola-zone airline capacity to outside world declines up to 81%. Business Week. http://www.businessweek.com/news/2014-12-15/ebola-zone-airline-capacity-to-outside-world-declines-up-to-81-percent. Accessed 15 Dec 2014

Johnson S (2014) Ebola case confirmed in Glasgow. The Telegraph. http://www.telegraph.co.uk/news/uknews/scotland/11316757/Ebola-case-confirmed-in-Glasgow.html. Accessed 12 Jul 2017

Kamara JA (2014) Sierra Leone news: Magbente discharges first Ebola survivors. Awareness Times. http://news.sl/drwebsite/publish/article_200526910.shtml. Accessed 18 Dec 2014

Kamara A, Collins J (2014) Radio educates Sierra Leone amid Ebola lockdown. USA Today. http://www.usatoday.com/story/news/world/2014/11/29/ebola-sierra-leone-radio-schools/19334935/. Accessed 30 Nov 2014

Karimi F (2014) Ebola outbreak: clinical drug trials to start next month as death toll mounts. CNN. http://www.cnn.com/2014/11/13/health/west-africa-ebola/index.html?hpt=hp_t2. Accessed 13 Nov 2014

Karmo H (2014) Liberia: fake death certificate sparks Ebola outbreak leading to eight cases. AllAfrica. http://allafrica.com/stories/201411271573.html. Accessed 28 Nov 2014

Kilmarx PH, Clarke KR, Dietz PM et al (2014) Ebola virus disease in health care workers—Sierra Leone, 2014. MMWR Morb Mortal Wkly Rep 63:1168–1171

Kim EK (2014) US Ebola survivors meet on TODAY, give thanks for 'angel' Kent Brantly, 'little things,' and family. Today. http://www.today.com/health/us-ebola-survivors-meet-today-show-give-thanks-angel-kent-1D80318755. Accessed 28 Nov 2014

KSN (2014) Kansas National Guard to deploy to West Africa for Ebola. KSN. http://ksn.com/2014/11/16/kansas-national-guard-to-deploy-to-west-africa-for-ebola/. Accessed 16 Nov 2014

Landauro I (2014) UN employee with Ebola evacuated to France for treatment. The Wall Street Journal. http://online.wsj.com/articles/u-n-employee-with-ebola-evacuated-to-france-for-treatment-1414891739. Accessed 2 Nov 2014

Larner T (2014) Passenger Ebola checks at UK airports, including Birmingham, nears 1,000. The Birmingham Mail. http://www.birminghammail.co.uk/news/health/passenger-ebola-checks-uk-airports-8362158. Accessed 30 Dec 2014

Laurent O (2014) Behind Time's person of the year Ebola fighters cover. Time. http://time.com/time-person-of-the-year-cover-photographs/. Accessed 10 Dec 2014

Leadership (2014a) Liberia's economy to shrink this year due to Ebola – minister. Leadership. http://leadership.ng/news/391294/liberias-economy-shrink-year-due-ebola-minister. Accessed 21 Nov 2014

Leadership (2014b) FG begins training of 250 volunteers to contain Ebola in Liberia, Guinea, Sierra Leone. Leadership. http://leadership.ng/news/392442/fg-begins-training-250-volunteers-contain-ebola-liberia-guinea-sierra-leone. Accessed 1 Dec 2014

Lederer EM (2014) Sierra Leone seeing 80–100 new Ebola cases daily. Associated Press, ABC News. http://abcnews.go.com/US/wireStory/sierra-leone-80-100-ebola-cases-daily-27394068. Accessed 6 Dec 2014

Ledgerwood JE, DeZure AD, Stanley DA et al (2017) Chimpanzee adenovirus vector Ebola vaccine. N Engl J Med 376:928–938

Long C, Peltz J (2014) Dr Craig Spencer to be released from hospital after beating Ebola but no sex for three months. Associated Press, News.com.au. http://www.news.com.au/world/north-america/dr-craig-spencer-to-be-released-from-hospital-after-beating-ebola-but-no-sex-for-three-months/story-fnh81jut-1227119996083. Accessed 11 Nov 2014

Lowe JJ, Gibbs SG, Schwedhelm SS et al (2014) Nebraska biocontainment unit perspective on disposal of Ebola medical waste. Am J Infect Control 42:1256–1257

Lupkin S (2014a) Last person completes Ebola monitoring in Texas. ABC News. http://abcnews.go.com/Health/person-completes-ebola-monitoring-texas/story?id=26742640. Accessed 7 Nov 2014

Lupkin S (2014b) Dr. Craig Spencer leaves New York hospital Ebola-free. ABC News. http://abcnews.go.com/Health/dr-craig-spencer-leaving-york-hospital-ebola-free/story?id=26831620. Accessed 18 Jun 2017

Marcelo P (2014) Massachusetts doctor cured of Ebola returning to Liberia. ABC News. http://abcnews.go.com/Health/wireStory/massachusetts-doctor-cured-ebola-returning-liberia-27636716. Accessed 16 Dec 2014

Martin J (2014) Patient who may have Ebola arrives in Atlanta. ABC News. http://abcnews.go.com/Health/wireStory/patient-ebola-arrives-atlanta-27359762. Accessed 4 Dec 2014

Martinez L, Mohney G (2014) Ebola patients wife will pay for evacuation to Nebraska. ABC News. http://abcnews.go.com/Health/ebola-patients-wife-pay-evacuation-nebraska/story?id=26939023. Accessed 16 Nov 2014

Mathis-Lilley B (2014) Kaci Hickox still doesn't have Ebola, might move out of Maine. The Slatest. http://www.slate.com/blogs/the_slatest/2014/11/10/kaci_hickox_ebola_nurse_likely_not_infected_may_leave_state.html. Accessed 10 Nov 2014

Mazumdar T (2014) Journey through the Ebola heartland in Sierra Leone and Guinea. BBC. http://www.bbc.com/news/world-africa-30160666. Accessed 23 Nov 2014

McLaughlin EC (2014) Ebola fighters are Time's 'Person of the Year.' CNN. http://www.cnn.com/2014/12/10/world/time-person-of-the-year/. Accessed 10 Dec 2014

McNeil DG Jr (2014) Contest seeks novel tools for the fight against Ebola. New York Times. http://www.nytimes.com/2014/12/13/health/ebola-contest-brings-ideas-for-cooling-suits-and-virus-repellents.html?_r=0. Accessed 12 Dec 2014

McNeil DG Jr, Höijenov K (2014) Quick response and old fashioned detective work thwart Ebola in Mali. New York Times. http://www.nytimes.com/2014/11/11/health/quick-response-and-old-fashioned-detective-work-thwart-ebola-in-mali.html?_r=0. Accessed 10 Nov 2014

Médecins Sans Frontières (2014a) Ebola: international response slow and uneven. 1 Dec 2014

Médecins Sans Frontières (2014b) Ebola: a day in the life of a chlorine sprayer. 16 Dec 2014

Medhora S (2014) Ebola: 17 Australian health workers deployed to Sierra Leone. The Guardian. http://www.theguardian.com/world/2014/nov/28/ebola-17-australian-health-workers-deployed-to-sierra-leone. Accessed 28 Nov 2014

MENAFN (2014) Ebola scare: Mali nurse faces stones from neighbors. MENAFN. http://www.menafn.com/1094017228/Ebola-scare-Malinurse-faces-stones-from-neighbors. Accessed 20 Nov 2014

MENAFN, AFP (2014) S. Leone nurses strike over Ebola hazard pay amid lockdown. MENAFN, AFP. http://www.menafn.com/1094056164/SLeone-nurses-strike-over-Ebola-hazard-pay-amid-lockdown. Accessed 27 Dec 2014

Miles T (2014a) Change of Ebola pace may be reflected in burial practices. Reuters. http://in.reuters.com/article/2014/11/07/health-ebola-burials-idINL6N0SX4A820141107. Accessed 7 Nov 2014

Miles T (2014b) Mali due to declare 108 Ebola free after quarantine. Reuters. http://www.reuters.com/article/2014/11/10/us-health-ebola-mali-idUSKCN0IU1E320141110. Accessed 10 Nov 2014

Miles T (2014c) Refile-Update 1 – WHO says Sierra Leone's Ebola prognosis is "very good." Reuters. http://www.reuters.com/article/2014/12/01/health-ebola-who-idUSL6N0TL3JA20141201. Accessed 1 Dec 2014

Monnier O (2014) Ebola in Mali 'under control' if no case next week, MSF says. Business Week. http://www.businessweek.com/news/2014-11-08/ebola-in-mali-under-control-if-no-case-next-week-msf-says. Accessed 9 Nov 2014

Morning Edition (2014a) U.N. team strives to reach Ebola emergency response goals. NPR. http://www.npr.org/2014/12/03/368143597/u-n-team-strives-to-reach-ebola-emergency-response-goals. Accessed 3 Dec 2014

Morning Edition (2014b) With Ebola cases down, officials worry Liberians aren't worried enough. NPR. http://www.npr.org/2014/12/08/369276253/with-ebola-cases-down-officials-worry-liberians-arent-worried-enough. Accessed 8 Dec 2014

Myall S (2014) Ebola: chilling trip inside the new treatment centre where British medics are fighting killer virus. The Mirror. http://www.mirror.co.uk/news/world-news/ebola-chilling-trip-inside-new-4565864. Accessed 5 Nov 2014

Nathanson K (2014) 'Perhaps I can do food': how one woman makes a difference against Ebola. NBC News. http://www.nbcnews.com/storyline/ebola-virus-outbreak/perhaps-i-can-do-food-how-one-woman-makes-difference-n271106. Accessed 21 Dec 2014

NBC DFW (2014) County officials say Ebola response cost $384,000. NBC DFW. http://www.nbcdfw.com/news/local/County-Officials-Say-Ebola-Response-Cost-384000-284773071.html. Accessed 4 Dec 2014

NBC News (2014a) 'You look great': President George W. Bush visits nurse who beat Ebola. NBC News. http://www.nbcnews.com/storyline/ebola-virus-outbreak/you-look-great-president-george-w-bush-visits-nurse-who-n244091. Accessed 7 Nov 2014

NBC News (2014b) Ebola-stricken surgeon Dr. Martin Salia arrives in U.S. NBC News. http://www.nbcnews.com/storyline/ebola-virus-outbreak/ebola-stricken-surgeon-dr-martin-salia-arrives-u-s-n249246. Accessed 21 Jun 2017

NBC News (2014c) How to spend 21 days in Ebola quarantine: foosball, WiFi for troops. NBC News. http://www.nbcnews.com/storyline/ebola-virus-outbreak/how-spend-21-days-ebola-quarantine-foosball-wifi-troops-n253666. Accessed 23 Nov 2014

NBC News (2014d) Cost for Dallas to care for Ebola nurse Nina Pham's dog was $27K: city. NBC News. http://www.nbcnews.com/storyline/ebola-virus-outbreak/cost-dallas-care-ebola-nurse-nina-phams-dog-was-27k-n261601. Accessed 4 Dec 2014

NBC News (2014e) CDC worker 'remains well' after possible Ebola exposure at lab. NBC News. http://www.nbcnews.com/storyline/ebola-virus-outbreak/cdc-worker-remains-well-after-possible-ebola-exposure-lab-n275326. Accessed 26 Dec 2014

Neergaard L (2014) Liberia's president tells Congress help needed to stamp out Ebola, prevent future outbreaks. Associated Press, The Star Tribune. http://www.startribune.com/lifestyle/health/285375461.html. Accessed 11 Dec 2014

Neporent L (2014) 'Post-Ebola Syndrome' persists after virus is cured, doctor says. ABC News. http://abcnews.go.com/Health/post-ebola-syndrome-persists-virus-cured-doctor/story?id=26657931. Accessed 3 Nov 2014

New Zealand Herald (2014) Ebola scare sparks Parliament lockdown. New Zealand Herald. http://www.nzherald.co.nz/nz/news/article.cfm?c_id=1&objectid=11356742. Accessed 11 Nov 2014

Newmyer T (2014) So long Ebola Czar. Ron Klain is heading back to the private sector. Fortune. http://fortune.com/2014/12/06/so-long-ebola-czar/. Accessed 6 Dec 2014

News & Observer (2014) NC Ebola hotline has new phone number. News & Observer. http://www.newsobserver.com/2014/11/12/4315903/nc-ebola-hotline-has-new-phone.html. Accessed 12 Nov 2014

News Ghana (2014) Mali records 2 more suspected Ebola deaths. News Ghana. http://www.spyghana.com/mali-records-2-more-suspected-ebola-deaths/. Accessed 15 Nov 2014

News OK (2014) 7th doctor dies of Ebola in Sierra Leone. News OK. http://newsok.com/article/feed/761514. Accessed 18 Nov 2014

Novelli M (2014) There's no Ebola in the Gambia – but it's killing tourism there. The Conversation. http://theconversation.com/theres-no-ebola-in-the-gambia-but-its-killing-tourism-there-35567. Accessed 17 Dec 2014

NU.nl (2014) Naval ship *Karel Doorman* provides aid for Ebola in Guinea. NU.nl. http://www.nu.nl/ebola/3962423/marineschip-karel-doorman-lost-hulpgoederen-ebola-in-guinee.html. Accessed 12 Jul 2017

Nuckols B (2014) Doctor who died of Ebola hailed as hero. Associated Press, ABC News. http://abcnews.go.com/US/wireStory/funeral-md-set-surgeon-died-ebola-27247791?page=2. Accessed 30 Nov 2014

O'Carroll L (2014a) Fresh Ebola outbreak in Sierra Leone raises fears of new infection chain. The Guardian. http://www.theguardian.com/world/2014/nov/04/ebola-outbreak-sierra-leone. Accessed 4 Nov 2014

O'Carroll L (2014b) Sierra Leone's Ebola orphans face a situation 'worse than war.' The Guardian. http://www.theguardian.com/global-development/2014/nov/07/sierra-leone-ebola-orphans-parents-worse-than-war. Accessed 7 Nov 2014

O'Connor N (2014) Cabinet to send 'limited number' of Irish troops to West Africa to fight Ebola. Yahoo News. https://uk.news.yahoo.com/ireland-sending-small-number-troops-fight-ebola-sierra-133300281.html#u83W3dl. Accessed 11 Nov 2014

Osayande A (2014) Nigeria: special insurance cover for Ebola volunteers. AllAfrica. http://allafrica.com/stories/201412031355.html. Accessed 3 Dec 2014

Palmer KM (2014) The US is stockpiling Ebola survivors' plasma to treat future patients. Wired. http://www.wired.com/2014/11/feds-stockpiling-ebola-survivors-plasma-treat-future-patients/. Accessed 24 Nov 2014

Park A (2014) Here's how to remove Ebola waste from a hospital. Time. https://time.com/3614010/heres-how-to-remove-ebola-waste-from-a-hospital/. Accessed 3 Dec 2014

Pattison L (2014) Sierra Leone: showing solidarity as Ebola hits new districts. International Federation of the Red Cross and Red Crescent Societies. http://www.ifrc.org/en/news-and-media/news-stories/africa/sierra-leone/sierra-leone--showing-solidarity-as-ebola-hits-new-districts-67804/. Accessed 19 Dec 2014

Paye-Layleh J (2014a) 100-bed Ebola treatment unit opens in Liberia. Associated Press, CP 24. http://www.cp24.com/world/100-bed-ebola-treatment-unit-opens-in-liberia-1.2095482. Accessed 10 Nov 2014

Paye-Layleh J (2014b) Liberia hopes for no new Ebola cases by new year. Associated Press, The Tribune. http://www.sanluisobispo.com/2014/11/27/3370613/germany-unveils-dedicated-ebola.html. Accessed 27 Nov 2014

Paye-Layleh J (2014c) Liberia reports dozens of new Ebola cases on border. Associated Press, Military Times. http://www.militarytimes.com/story/military/2014/12/30/liberia-ebola/21041231/. Accessed 30 Dec 2014

Paye-Layleh J, Corder M (2014) UN peacekeeper in Liberia tests positive for Ebola. ABC News. http://abcnews.go.com/International/wireStory/peacekeeper-liberia-tests-positive-ebola-27383914. Accessed 5 Dec 2014

Paye-Layleh J, Dilorenzo S (2014) Ebola-hit nations' economies 'crippled.' Associated Press, IOL. http://www.iol.co.za/news/africa/ebola-hit-nations-economies-crippled-1.1789681#.VH3Nnbd0ziw. Accessed 2 Dec 2014

Paye-Layleh J, Roy-Macaulay C (2014) Chinese-built Ebola center dedicated in Liberia as another Sierra Leonean doctor infected. Associated Press, The Republic. http://www.therepublic.com/view/story/63cbaab6748142d7aad47d07f887262c/AF--Ebola-West-Africa. Accessed 25 Nov 2014

Payne S (2014) Ebola: Spanish aid worker sent for tests at Madrid hospital after needlestick injury in Mali. International Business Times. http://www.ibtimes.co.uk/ebola-spanish-aid-worker-sent-tests-madrid-hospital-after-needlestick-injury-mali-1475956. Accessed 21 Nov 2014

Pengelly M (2014) 'Ebola czar' defends CDC procedures in light of technician's potential exposure. The Guardian. http://www.theguardian.com/world/2014/dec/28/ebola-czar-defends-cdc-procedures-potential-exposure. Accessed 28 Dec 2014

Perring R (2014) 100 people tested for Ebola in hospitals across England. Express. http://www.express.co.uk/news/uk/539586/Ebola-Britain-test-100-people-hospital-England. Accessed 24 Nov 2014

Poudel A (2014) Liberia returnees asked to abstain from sex. My Republica. http://www.myrepublica.com/portal/index.php?action=news_details&news_id=87057. Accessed 21 Nov 2014

PR Newswire (2014) EU boosts anti-Ebola aid after Commissioners mission to worst-hit countries. Star Africa. http://en.starafrica.com/news/eu-boosts-anti-ebola-aid-after-commissioners-mission-to-worst-hit-countries.html. Accessed 17 Nov 2014

Press Association (2014a) UK sets up three new Ebola labs. Press Association, Yahoo News. https://uk.news.yahoo.com/uk-sets-three-ebola-labs-142422282.html#c7I1p64. Accessed 2 Nov 2014

Press Association (2014b) Ebola case nurse being discharged. The Independent. http://www.independent.ie/world-news/ebola-case-nurse-being-discharged-30720474.html. Accessed 5 Nov 2014

PTI (2014a) 'No-Ebola certificate' must to enter India from affected countries. PTI, The Times of India. http://timesofindia.indiatimes.com/india/No-Ebola-certificate-must-to-enter-India-from-affected-countries/articleshow/45308821.cms. Accessed 28 Nov 2014

PTI (2014b) China to test its Ebola vaccine on humans. PTI, The India Express. http://indianexpress.com/article/world/asia/china-to-test-its-ebola-vaccine-on-humans/. Accessed 25 Dec 2014

Reuters (2014a) Shipping lines apply Ebola clause to fend off virus risks. Reuters, The Daily Mail. http://www.dailymail.co.uk/wires/reuters/article-2820424/Shipping-lines-apply-Ebola-clause-fend-virus-risks.html. Accessed 4 Nov 2014

Reuters (2014b) Man recovering from Ebola quarantined at Delhi airport. Reuters, The Times of India. http://timesofindia.indiatimes.com/india/Man-recovering-from-Ebola-quarantined-at-Delhi-airport/articleshow/45194610.cms? Accessed 18 Nov 2014

Reuters (2014c) Sierra Leone to pay families of health workers who die of Ebola. Reuters, KFGO. http://kfgo.com/news/articles/2014/nov/11/sierra-leone-to-pay-families-of-health-workers-who-die-of-ebola/. Accessed 11 Nov 2014

Reuters (2014d) Liberia won't extend Ebola state of emergency, says president. Reuters. http://in.reuters.com/article/2014/11/13/health-ebola-liberia-idINKCN0IX1Q720141113. Accessed 13 Nov 2014

Reuters (2014e) Mali tries to trace 343 contacts in second Ebola wave. Reuters. http://www.reuters.com/article/2014/11/14/us-health-ebola-mali-idUSKCN0IY19A20141114. Accessed 14 Nov 2014

Reuters (2014f) Senegal reopens air, sea borders with Ebola-hit nations – report. Reuters. http://news.trust.org//item/20141114232639-stakm/?source=fiTheWire. Accessed 16 Jun 2017

Reuters (2014g) Chinese team arrives in Liberia to staff Ebola clinic. Reuters. http://www.reuters.com/article/2014/11/15/us-health-ebola-liberia-china-idUSKCN0IZ0RU20141115. Accessed 15 Nov 2014

Reuters (2014h) U.N. Ebola mission chief in Guinea dies of natural causes. Reuters, Fox News. http://www.foxnews.com/health/2014/11/17/un-ebola-mission-chief-in-guinea-dies-natural-causes/. Accessed 17 Nov 2014

Reuters (2014i) Doctor who treated source of second Mali Ebola outbreak dies. Reuters, Fox News. http://www.foxnews.com/health/2014/11/21/doctor-who-treated-source-second-mali-ebola-outbreak-dies/. Accessed 21 Nov 2014

Reuters (2014j) Cuban doctor with Ebola flies out of Sierra Leone. Reuters, WHTC. http://whtc.com/news/articles/2014/nov/20/cuban-doctor-with-ebola-flies-out-of-sierra-leone/. Accessed 20 Nov 2014

Reuters (2014k) US to allow people from Ebola-hit nations to stay temporarily. Reuters, Today. http://www.todayonline.com/world/americas/us-allow-people-ebola-hit-nations-stay-temporarily. Accessed 20 Nov 2014

Reuters (2014l) Mali records new Ebola case linked to dead nurse. Reuters. http://www.reuters.com/article/2014/11/22/us-health-ebola-mali-idUSKCN0J60EI20141122. Accessed 22 Nov 2014

Reuters (2014m) UN worker leaves French hospital after Ebola recovery. Reuters. http://in.reuters.com/article/2014/11/23/health-ebola-france-idINL6N0TD0CL20141123. Accessed 24 Nov 2014

Reuters (2014n) Italian Ebola patient due to be flown home: health ministry. Reuters, The Daily Star. http://www.dailystar.com.lb/News/World/2014/Nov-24/278711-italian-ebola-patient-due-to-be-flown-home-health-ministry.ashx#ixzz3JzQ8ebt8. Accessed 24 Nov 2014

Reuters (2014o) South Korea to fly medical workers to Europe if infected fighting Ebola. Reuters. http://www.reuters.com/article/2014/11/26/us-health-ebola-southkorea-idUSKCN0JA0L920141126. Accessed 26 Nov 2014

Reuters (2014p) Cuban doctor with Ebola improving in Geneva hospital. Reuters. http://in.reuters.com/article/2014/11/28/health-ebola-cuba-idINL2N0TI12R20141128. Accessed 28 Nov 2014

Reuters (2014q) No more Ebola cases in Mali after patient cured: president. Reuters, NBC News. http://www.nbcnews.com/storyline/ebola-virus-outbreak/no-more-ebola-cases-mali-after-patient-cured-president-n258136. Accessed 30 Nov 2014

Reuters (2014r) American possibly exposed to Ebola being transferred to Atlanta hospital. Reuters. http://www.reuters.com/article/2014/12/03/us-health-ebola-usa-emory-idUSKCN0JH2P320141203. Accessed 3 Dec 2014

Reuters (2014s) Sierra Leone overtakes Liberia in number of Ebola cases: WHO. Reuters, Medical Daily. http://www.medicaldaily.com/sierra-leone-overtakes-liberia-number-ebola-cases-who-313458. Accessed 8 Dec 2014

Reuters (2014t) U.S. agency offers legal immunity to Ebola vaccine makers. Reuters. http://in.reuters.com/article/2014/12/09/us-health-ebola-vaccine-idINKBN0JN1S920141209. Accessed 9 Dec 2014

Reuters (2014u) Mali: no Ebola cases, ministry says. Reuters, New York Times. http://www.nytimes.com/2014/12/12/world/africa/mali-no-ebola-cases-ministry-says.html?_r=0. Accessed 11 Dec 2014

Reuters (2014v) Ebola vaccine trial halted temporarily for checks after joint pains – Geneva hospital. Reuters. http://in.reuters.com/article/2014/12/11/health-ebola-vaccine-idINKBN-0JP1G820141211. Accessed 11 Dec 2014

Reuters (2014w) Mali ends last quarantines, could be Ebola-free next month. Reuters. http://www.reuters.com/article/2014/12/16/us-health-ebola-mali-idUSKBN0JU1NR20141216. Accessed 16 Dec 2014

Reuters (2014x) Hundreds swarm around Sierra Leone Ebola victim, take cell phones images. Reuters. http://www.reuters.com/video/2014/12/19/hundreds-swarm-around-sierra-leone-ebola?videoId=349272617. Accessed 19 Dec 2014

Reuters (2014y) Tekmira to supply Ebola treatment for studies in West Africa. Reuters, CNBC. http://www.cnbc.com/id/102289277#. Accessed 22 Dec 2014

Reuters (2014z) Ebola-hit Sierra Leone marks sombre Christmas at home after ban on public festivities. Reuters, Radio Australia. http://www.radioaustralia.net.au/international/2014-12-26/ebola-hit-sierra-leone-marks-sombre-christmas-at-home-after-ban-on-public-festivities/1402099. Accessed 25 Dec 2014

RFI (2014) Suspected Ebola case reported on French Indian island Réunion. RFI. http://www.english.rfi.fr/africa/20141214-suspected-ebola-case-reported-french-indian-island-reunion. Accessed 14 Dec 2014

Rihouay F, Bennett S (2014) Mali reports five Ebola cases, with sixth possible. Business Week. http://www.businessweek.com/news/2014-11-13/staff-member-at-clinic-in-mali-isolated-for-suspected-ebola. Accessed 14 Nov 2014

Robinson J (2014) Sierra Leone struggling in fight against Ebola because so many doctors and nurses have left to find jobs in Britain, report claims. The Daily Mail. http://www.dailymail.co.uk/news/article-2878800/Sierra-Leone-struggling-fight-against-Ebola-doctors-nurses-left-jobs-Britain-report-claims.html. Accessed 18 Dec 2014

Romero A (2014) Quarantine isle ready for Ebola. The Philippine Star. http://www.philstar.com/headlines/2014/11/05/1388215/quarantine-isle-ready-ebola. Accessed 4 Nov 2014

Roy-Macaulay C (2014a) Ebola kills Sierra Leone doctor, UN doubles staff. ABC News. http://abcnews.go.com/Health/wireStory/sierra-leone-doctor-dies-ebola-26649996. Accessed 3 Nov 2014

Roy-Macaulay C (2014b) Another Sierra Leonean doctor infected with Ebola. Associated Press, Bioscience Technology. http://www.biosciencetechnology.com/news/2014/11/another-sierra-leonean-doctor-infected-ebola. Accessed 11 Nov 2014

Roy-Macaulay C (2014c) 11th Sierra Leonean doctor infected with Ebola. Associated Press, 10 TV. http://www.10tv.com/content/stories/apexchange/2014/12/03/af-ebola-west-africa.html. Accessed 3 Dec 2014

Roy-Macaulay C (2014d) 2 more Sierra Leonean doctors die of Ebola. Associated Press, The San Diego Union-Tribune. http://www.sandiegouniontribune.com/. Accessed 3 Jul 2017

Roy-Macaulay C (2014e) 10th Sierra Leonean doctor dies from Ebola. Associated Press, ABC News. http://abcnews.go.com/Health/wireStory/10th-sierra-leonean-doctor-dies-ebola-27424222. Accessed 7 Dec 2014

Roy-Macaulay C (2014f) Junior doctors in Sierra Leone on strike to demand better care for those infected with Ebola. Associated Press, U.S. News & World Report. http://www.usnews.com/news/world/articles/2014/12/08/who-sierra-leone-has-recorded-most-ebola-cases. Accessed 8 Dec 2014

Roy-Macaulay C (2014g) Sierra Leone to search for Ebola cases in capital. Associated Press, Sioux City Journal. http://siouxcityjournal.com/news/world/africa/sierra-leone-to-search-for-ebola-cases-in-capital/article_15cca1f3-edc2-5bc5-b354-16e02a32ddd9.html. Accessed 16 Dec 2014

Roy-Macaulay C, Diallo B (2014) Ebola: 11th Sierra Leone doctor dies, fire destroys supplies. Associated Press, Yahoo News. http://news.yahoo.com/11th-sierra-leonean-doctor-dies-ebola-102726636.html. Accessed 18 Dec 2014

Roy-Macaulay C, Schemm P (2014) Sierra Leone official: Ebola may have reached peak. Associated Press, ABC News. http://abcnews.go.com/Health/wireStory/sierra-leone-official-ebola-worst-27199617?page=2. Accessed 26 Nov 2014

RT (2014) 'Ebola spread risk too serious': Morocco refuses to host Africa football cup. RT. http://rt.com/news/203595-african-cup-ebola-morocco/. Accessed 9 Nov 2014

Sabin L (2014) Sierra Leone bans community Christmas and New Year celebrations to halt Ebola spread. The Independent. http://www.independent.co.uk/news/world/africa/sierra-leone-bans-community-christmas-and-new-year-celebrations-to-halt-ebola-spread-9922674.html. Accessed 13 Dec 2014

Samba A (2014) Sierra Leone news: Kailahun registers new Ebola case after 11 days. Awareness Times. http://news.sl/drwebsite/publish/article_200526862.shtml. Accessed 11 Dec 2014

Scalese R (2014) MGH patient initially tests negative for Ebola, positive for malaria. Boston.com. https://www.boston.com/news/local-news/2014/12/02/mgh-patient-initially-tests-negative-for-ebola-positive-for-malaria. Accessed 2 Jul 2017

Scalese R, Tedesco A (2014) Patient with suspected Ebola virus being treated at Boston's Mass. General hospital. Boston.com. http://www.boston.com/news/local/massachusetts/2014/12/02/suspected-ebola-patient-being-treated-boston-hospital/kjQngynamiuqmmLOi3lrVN/story.html. Accessed 3 Dec 2014

Schneider C (2014) Egleston building Ebola isolation unit for children. WSB Radio, The Atlanta Journal-Constitution. http://www.wsbradio.com/news/news/local/egleston-building-ebola-isolation-unit-for-childre/nh2ZX/. Accessed 6 Nov 2014

Schnirring L (2014a) Liberia ends Ebola emergency Mali cluster grows. Center for Infectious Disease Research and Policy. http://www.cidrap.umn.edu/news-perspective/2014/11/liberia-ends-ebola-emergency-mali-cluster-grows. Accessed 14 Nov 2014

Schnirring L (2014b) Mali Ebola transmission chain snares two more. Center for Infectious Disease Research and Policy. http://www.cidrap.umn.edu/news-perspective/2014/11/mali-ebola-transmission-chain-snares-two-more. Accessed 25 Nov 2014

Schubert KK (2014) Critically ill Sierra Leone doctor with Ebola now in U.S. Reuters. http://www.reuters.com/article/2014/11/15/us-health-ebola-usa-surgeon-idUSKCN0IZ0DY20141115. Accessed 15 Nov 2014

Seck HH (2014) Marines wrap up Ebola response mission in Liberia. Marine Corps Times. http://www.marinecorpstimes.com/story/military/careers/marine-corps/2014/12/04/marines-conclude-ebola-response-mission/19884829/. Accessed 6 Dec 2014

Sieff K (2014a) Can a U.S. military Ebola treatment center slow Ebola in one hard-hit city? The Washington Post. http://www.washingtonpost.com/world/africa/can-a-us-military-ebola-treatment-center-slow-ebola-in-one-hard-hit-city/2014/11/01/afb7b058-60fd-11e4-9f3a-7e28799e0549_story.html. Accessed 2 Nov 2014

Sieff K (2014b) A doctor's mistaken Ebola test: 'We were celebrating. Then everything fell apart.' The Washington Post. http://www.washingtonpost.com/world/a-doctors-mistaken-ebola-test-we-were-celebrating--then-everything-fell-apart/2014/11/16/946a84da-6dd5-11e4-a2c2-478179fd0489_story.html. Accessed 16 Nov 2014

Sieff K (2014c) Six months after Ebola appeared Sierra Leone still lacks beds for patients. The Washington Post. http://www.washingtonpost.com/world/africa/six-months-after-ebola-appeared-sierra-leone-still-lacks-beds-for-patients/2014/11/19/6101aa7d-ee68-4370-b2e5-899afc09fb02_story.html. Accessed 20 Nov 2014

Sieff K (2014d) Sierra Leone physician who treated doctor with Maryland ties is diagnosed with Ebola. The Washington Post. http://www.washingtonpost.com/world/sierra-leone-physician-who-treated-martin-salia-diagnosed-with-ebola/2014/11/27/af1fbd54-7627-11e4-a755-e32227229e7b_story.html. Accessed 28 Nov 2014

Sierra Express Media (2014) Koinadugu District vows to eradicate Ebola within 45 days. Sierra Express Media. http://www.sierraexpressmedia.com/?p=72148. Accessed 15 Dec 2014

Sifferlin A (2014) Ebola-Stricken families to receive cash payments. Time. http://time.com/3642240/ebola-cash-payments/. Accessed 19 Dec 2014

Sklar DL (2014) Ebola takes center stage at Rose Parade. My News LA. http://mynewsla.com/life/2014/12/27/ebola-takes-center-stage-rose-parade/. Accessed 27 Dec 2014

Sky News (2014) UN chief arrives in Guinea on Ebola tour. Sky News. http://www.skynews.com.au/news/top-stories/2014/12/21/un-chief-arrives-in-guinea-on-ebola-tour.html. Accessed 20 Dec 2014

Smith CS (2014a) Liberia: Ebola sweeps entire family leaves household of 15 stranded. AllAfrica. http://allafrica.com/stories/201412030913.html. Accessed 2 Dec 2014

Smith N (2014b) Thousands of Kaiser Permanente nurses to begin two day strike. ABC 7 News. http://abc7news.com/news/thousands-of-kaiser-nurses-to-begin-two-day-strike/389992/. Accessed 11 Nov 2014

Spickernell S (2014) Ebola outbreak in West Africa: spike in Sierra Leone infections suggests epidemic is far from being over. City A.M. http://www.cityam.com/1415704153/ebola-outbreak-west-africa-has-virus-stopped-spreading-spike-new-cases-sierra-leone. Accessed 11 Nov 2014

Steenhuysen J (2014) Exclusive: U.S. Ebola researchers plead for access to virus samples. Reuters. http://www.reuters.com/article/us-health-ebola-usa-research-exclusive-idUSK-BN0IP1DZ20141105. Accessed 16 Jun 2017

Stobbe M (2014) CDC official says a worst-case scenario estimate of West African Ebola cases will not happen. Associated Press, U.S. News & World Report. https://www.usnews.com/news/us/articles/2014/11/19/cdc-chief-drops-worst-case-ebola-estimate. Accessed 22 Jun 2017

Stobbe M, Roy-Macaulay C (2014) Surgeon with Ebola coming to US for care. Yahoo News. http://news.yahoo.com/surgeon-ebola-coming-us-care-111635455.html. Accessed 14 Nov 2014

Straits Times (2014) Thai police health officials hunting man from Sierra Leone amid Ebola fears. The Straits Times, The Nation, Asia News Network. http://www.straitstimes.com/news/asia/south-east-asia/story/thai-police-health-officials-hunting-man-sierra-leone-amid-ebola-fea. Accessed 25 Nov 2014

Stuart T (2014) 357 people in New York City are on Ebola watch. The Village Voice. https://www.villagevoice.com/2014/11/06/357-people-in-new-york-city-are-on-ebola-watch/. Accessed 15 Jun 2017

Summers A, Nyenswah TG, Montgomery JM et al (2014) Challenges in responding to the Ebola epidemic – four rural counties, Liberia, August–November 2014. MMWR Morb Mortal Wkly Rep 63:1202–1204

Sun LH (2014a) Ebola cases plummet in Liberian hot spot as aid groups gain community trust. The Washington Post. http://www.washingtonpost.com/national/health-science/ebola-cases-plummet-in-liberian-hot-spot-as-aid-groups-gain-community-trust/2014/11/14/5b2efc18-6b88-11e4-a31c-77759fc1eacc_story.html. Accessed 14 Nov 2014

Sun LH (2014b) Cost to treat Ebola in the U.S.: $1.16 million for 2 patients. The Washington Post. https://www.washingtonpost.com/news/post-nation/wp/2014/11/18/cost-to-treat-ebola-in-the-u-s-1-16-million-for-2-patients/?utm_term=.51ab2dba3df5. Accessed 21 Jun 2017

Sun LH (2014c) U.S. designates 35 hospitals to treat Ebola patients. The Washington Post. http://www.washingtonpost.com/national/health-science/us-designates-35-hospitals-to-prepare-for-future-ebola-patients/2014/12/02/d3213c18-7a1a-11e4-b821-503cc7efed9e_story.html. Accessed 2 Dec 2014

Sun LH, Achenbach J (2014) CDC reports potential Ebola exposure in Atlanta lab. The Washington Post. http://www.washingtonpost.com/national/health-science/cdc-reports-potential-ebola-exposure-in-atlanta-lab/2014/12/24/f1a9f26c-8b8e-11e4-8ff4-fb93129c9c8b_story.html. Accessed 24 Dec 2014

Sylvers E (2014) Italian doctor tests positive for Ebola in Sierra Leone. The Wall Street Journal. http://online.wsj.com/articles/italian-doctor-tests-positive-for-ebola-in-sierra-leone-1416832350. Accessed 24 Nov 2014

Szabo L (2014a) New York doctor is free of Ebola. USA Today. http://www.usatoday.com/story/news/nation/2014/11/10/new-york-doctor-ebola-free/18822421/. Accessed 10 Nov 2014

Szabo L (2014b) Airport screenings haven't turned up any Ebola patients. USA Today. http://www.usatoday.com/story/news/nation/2014/12/09/ebola-airport-screening/20148019/. Accessed 10 Dec 2014

Taylor E (2014) German doctors use experimental heart drug in treating Ebola patient. Reuters. http://in.reuters.com/article/2014/11/05/health-ebola-germany-idINL6N0SV4L120141105. Accessed 5 Nov 2014

Telegraph (2014) Ebola patient transferred to London's Royal Free Hospital. The Telegraph. http://www.telegraph.co.uk/news/uknews/scotland/11316994/Ebola-patient-transferred-to-Londons-Royal-Free-Hospital.html. Accessed 12 Jul 2017

The News (2014) World Bank proposes global epidemic fund in wake of Ebola. The News. http://thenewsnigeria.com.ng/2014/11/18/world-bank-proposes-global-epidemic-fund-in-wake-of-ebola/. Accessed 18 Nov 2014

Thomas AR (2014) Another British health worker from Sierra Leone is Ebola positive. The Sierra Leone Telegraph. http://www.thesierraleonetelegraph.com/another-british-health-worker-from-sierra-leone-is-ebola-positive/. Accessed 5 Oct 2017

Trenchard T (2014a) Survivors cope with new Ebola after-effects. Al Jazeera. http://www.aljazeera.com/news/africa/2014/12/survivors-cope-with-new-ebola-after-effects-2014121573521561384.html. Accessed 15 Dec 2014

Trenchard T (2014b) Sierra Leone's 'special forces' Ebola nurses. Al Jazeera. http://www.aljazeera.com/indepth/features/2014/12/sierra-leone-special-forces-ebola-nurses-20141217885310914.html. Accessed 19 Dec 2014

Trotta D (2014) Update 2 – Cuban doctor in Sierra Leone tests positive for Ebola. Reuters. http://www.reuters.com/article/2014/11/19/health-ebola-cuba-idUSL2N0T909K20141119. Accessed 19 Nov 2014

Tyson J (2014) What does the dry season mean for the Ebola response? Devex. https://www.devex.com/news/what-does-the-dry-season-mean-for-the-ebola-response-85092. Accessed 15 Dec 2014

United Nations (2014) Most intense Ebola transmission in West Africa reported in western Sierra Leone – UN. 31 Dec 2014

VOA News (2014a) Liberia sets December 25 goal: no new Ebola cases. VOA News. http://www.voanews.com/content/liberia-sets-december-25-goal-no-new-ebola-cases/2522437.html. Accessed 16 Nov 2014

VOA News (2014b) Trial of 15-minute Ebola test to take place in Guinea. VOA News. http://www.voanews.com/content/trial-of-15-minute-ebola-diagnosis-test-to-take-place-in-guinea/2537970.html. Accessed 28 Nov 2014

VOA News (2014c) Sierra Leone educates on safe Ebola burials. VOA News. http://www.voanews.com/content/sierra-leone-educates-on-safe-burials/2568099.html. Accessed 21 Dec 2014

Vogel L (2014) Call for Ebola medics falls on deaf ears: MSF. Médicins Sans Frontières, CMAJ. http://www.cmaj.ca/content/early/2014/11/03/cmaj.109-4934.full.pdf. Accessed 15 Jun 2017

Von Drehle D, Baker A (2014) The Ebola fighters. Time. http://time.com/time-person-of-the-year-ebola-fighters/. Accessed 5 Jul 2017

WAND (2014) Illinois suspends Ebola hotline as interest fades. WAND. http://www.wandtv.com/story/27479111/illinois-suspends-ebola-hotline-as-interest-fades. Accessed 25 Nov 2014

Ward J (2014) Exclusive: MI5 fears Islamic State Ebola 'bomb.' The Daily Star. http://www.daily-star.co.uk/news/latest-news/410596/MI5-fears-Islamic-State-infected-Ebola-attack. Accessed 15 Nov 2014

Warner G (2014) Guarding the Ebola border. NPR. http://www.npr.org/blogs/money/2014/11/18/364144837/guarding-the-ebola-border. Accessed 18 Nov 2014

Watt H (2014) Only eleven Ebola patients in British hospital in Sierra Leone. The Telegraph. http://www.telegraph.co.uk/news/worldnews/ebola/11256447/Only-eleven-Ebola-patients-in-British-hospital-in-Sierra-Leone.html. Accessed 27 Nov 2014

Weekend Edition (2014) In Liberia, Ebola shifts from cities to villages. NPR. http://www.npr.
org/2014/11/30/367544593/in-liberia-ebola-shifts-from-cities-to-villages. Accessed 30 Nov
2014

Williams W (2014) Liberia village becomes a new Ebola epicenter. ABC News. http://abcnews.
go.com/International/wireStory/liberia-village-ebola-epicenter-26802843. Accessed 10 Nov
2014

World Health Organization (2014a) Ebola response roadmap situation report. 5 Nov 2014

World Health Organization (2014b) Ebola response roadmap situation report update. 7 Nov 2014

World Health Organization (2014c) Field situation: How to conduct safe and dignified burial of a
patient who has died from suspected or confirmed Ebola virus disease

World Health Organization (2014d) Mali case, Ebola imported from Guinea. 10 Nov 2014

World Health Organization (2014e) Ebola response roadmap situation report. 12 Nov 2014

World Health Organization (2014f) Mali confirms its second fatal case of Ebola virus disease. 12
Nov 2014

World Health Organization (2014g) Ebola response roadmap situation report update. 14 Nov 2014

World Health Organization (2014h) Ebola response roadmap situation report. 19 Nov 2014

World Health Organization (2014i) Ebola response roadmap situation report update. 21 Nov 2014

World Health Organization (2014j) Ebola response roadmap situation report. 26 Nov 2014

World Health Organization (2014k) WHO congratulates Spain on ending Ebola transmission. 2
Dec 2014

World Health Organization (2014l) Ebola response roadmap situation report. 3 Dec 2014

World Health Organization (2014m) Ebola response roadmap situation report. 10 Dec 2014

World Health Organization (2014n) Ebola response roadmap situation report. 17 Dec 2014

World Health Organization (2014o) Ebola response roadmap situation report. 24 Dec 2014

World Health Organization (2014p) Ebola response roadmap situation report. 31 Dec 2014

Worzi A (2014a) Liberia: U.S. builds third Ebola treatment center in Bassa. AllAfrica. http://
allafrica.com/stories/201411242012.html. Accessed 23 Nov 2014

Worzi A (2014b) Liberia: young life opens camp for Ebola survivors. AllAfrica, Daily Observer.
http://allafrica.com/stories/201412091314.html. Accessed 8 Dec 2014

WTAM (2014) Northeast Ohio declared Ebola free. WTAM. http://www.wtam.com/articles/wtam-
local-news-122520/northeast-ohio-declared-ebola-free-12938529/. Accessed 5 Nov 2014

Zoroya G (2014a) U.S. uniformed officers to treat Ebola patients in Liberia. USA Today. http://
www.usatoday.com/story/news/world/2014/11/05/ebola-americans-military-treatment-public-
health-service/18538273/. Accessed 15 Jun 2017

Zoroya G (2014b) U.S. military will build fewer Ebola clinics in Liberia. USA Today. http://
www.usatoday.com/story/news/world/2014/11/18/ebola-us-military-clinics-usaid/19233583/.
Accessed 18 Nov 2014

Zoroya G (2014c) U.S. officers mourn losing their 1st Ebola patient. USA Today. http://
www.usatoday.com/story/news/world/2014/11/22/ebola-us-public-health-service-patient-
dies/19396309/. Accessed 22 Nov 2014

Zoroya G (2014d) Nurse's death that shook U.S. clinic in Liberia proves not to be Ebola case.
USA Today. http://www.usatoday.com/story/news/world/2014/11/25/us-public-health-service-
monrovia-ebola-clinic-update/70076888/. Accessed 26 Nov 2014

Zoroya G (2014e) They survived Ebola only to become social outcasts. USA Today. https://www.
usatoday.com/story/news/world/2014/12/13/ebola-survivors-stigma-immunity-liberia-monro-
via/20251081. Accessed 14 Dec 2014

Chapter 7
Simmering to the End (January 2015–June 2016)

Abstract By January 2015, the Ebola outbreak was clearly in decline. Liberia and Guinea both had falling caseloads. Sierra Leone had high case levels at the start of 2015, but soon these too began to fall. On March 5, 2015, Liberia released its last known Ebola patient. In mid-March 2015, Sierra Leone launched a new 3-day, nationwide lockdown to find and contain the last few cases. Things looked very positive. But then, in a pattern that would repeat itself in the coming months, a new case suddenly emerged in Liberia. The virus began to show an extraordinary ability to reemerge from undetected chains of transmission. It also became clear that the semen of survivors remained infectious long after the survivors had recovered. In October 2015, a frightening new twist occurred when a UK Ebola survivor developed Ebola-related meningitis almost 9 months after she had recovered from the disease. Despite numerous setbacks and flare-ups, the West African Ebola outbreak was declared officially over on January 14, 2016. Sadly, the very next day – January 15, 2016 – a new Ebola case was detected in Sierra Leone. New cases then began to emerge in Guinea and Liberia. Another round of containment and contact tracing commenced. Finally, by June 9, 2016, all of the new cases had resolved and the 2013–2016 outbreak came to an end.

7.1 Day-by-Day Outbreak Entries (January 2015–June 2016)

January 1, 2015 (Thursday)
President of Sierra Leone Ernest Bai Koroma called on the nation to begin a week of fasting and prayer to end the Ebola outbreak (Reuters 2015a). He also acknowledged that the restrictions imposed by Ebola are a significant hardship for the country:

> *I know what we are being asked to do is very difficult; we are a people that have built our humanity on hugging each other, on shaking hands, on caring for the sick and showing communal empathy by participating in funeral activities. But today the Ebola devil of illness and death hides in the innocent clothing of our culture to get us.* (Reuters 2015a)

© Springer International Publishing AG, part of Springer Nature 2018
S. G. Bullard, *A Day-by-Day Chronicle of the 2013-2016 Ebola Outbreak*,
https://doi.org/10.1007/978-3-319-76565-5_7

All of the passengers on Pauline Cafferkey's Heathrow to Glasgow flight have been traced. The NHS in Scotland has requested that eight passengers monitor their temperature for 20 days and report any symptoms. These are the passengers who sat in the area immediately around Cafferkey. They include people who sat two rows in front and two rows behind the infected nurse (Booth 2015).

January 2, 2015 (Friday)

Unconfirmed reports suggest that Muslim fighters for the Islamic State (i.e., ISIS) in Mosul, Iraq, may have contracted Ebola (Daily Mail 2015; Strum 2015). The WHO is trying to investigate, but UN workers are banned from ISIS territory. If the rumors are true, and at present they are considered very unlikely, it is unclear how the disease could have reached the area. Some ISIS fighters have been recruited from West Africa, so they could have brought the disease to Iraq with them (Daily Mail 2015). ISIS members may also have become infected while preparing for a biological terror attack.

A South Korean medical worker may have been exposed to Ebola while collecting a blood sample in Sierra Leone. The worker will be transported to Germany for observation (IANS 2015a).

The infected 50-year-old Italian doctor [Fabrizio Pulvirenti] being treated at Rome's Spallanzani Institute has recovered from Ebola (AFP 2015a, p). He was evacuated from Sierra Leone in mid-November 2014.

Gambia Bird Airlines has suspended all flights effective immediately. It will reimburse passengers with existing bookings. All flights have been suspended, not just those to Ebola-affected areas. The company did not explain why its flights have been canceled, but the West African airline has been heavily impacted by the Ebola outbreak (Gill 2015).

January 3, 2015 (Saturday)

Pauline Cafferkey is now in critical condition. Her condition has been deteriorating over the last 2 days (BBC 2015a).

The Hastings Treatment Center in Sierra Leone released its thirteenth batch of Ebola survivors today. Among them is a 2-month-old baby, one of the youngest Ebola survivors known. At the release ceremony, survivors were given a package of food and supplies and ~$60 to help them return home. To date, the Hastings Treatment Center has released about 400 survivors (Awoko 2015a).

The South Korean medic exposed to Ebola has been airlifted to Charite hospital in Berlin, Germany. The healthcare worker was working with a delirious Ebola patient when the patient jerked and a blood-filled syringe pierced the medic's gloves (Associated Press 2015a).

January 4, 2015 (Sunday)

Sierra Leone has extended the Ebola lockdown of the northern Tonkolili District for an additional 2 weeks (AFP 2015b). Ebola screenings will also be adjusted at Freetown International Airport (APA 2015a). The change comes after an airport worker contracted Ebola and exposed another person to the virus. Employees will now have their temperatures taken at the entrance to the airport and the entrance to the terminal (APA 2015a).

A US healthcare worker who suffered a high-risk Ebola exposure in Sierra Leone has been transferred to the Biocontainment Unit at Nebraska Medicine in Omaha for observation (Silva 2015).

January 5, 2015 (Monday)
Nine counties in southeast Liberia have reported no new Ebola cases for the last 21 days (Dixon 2015). Lofa County in northern Liberia has reported no new cases for over 40 days (Dixon 2015). Not all of the news from Liberia is good, however. Every mother in the village of Joeblow has died from Ebola (Knapton 2015). A total of 14 mothers have died, leaving 15 children orphaned (Knapton 2015).

With the falling number of Ebola cases, the Liberian government has decided it is time for students to return to school. Liberian schools will reopen on February 2, 2015 (Reuters 2015b).

British nurse Pauline Cafferkey remains in critical condition, but her condition has stabilized (Gallagher 2015).

All supplies of the experimental Ebola drug ZMapp are exhausted. More antibodies for the drug are being grown in genetically modified tobacco plants and it is hoped more of the drug will be available soon. So far during the outbreak, seven people have been treated with ZMapp. Five of them have survived and two have died (Boseley 2015a).

UNICEF, in conjunction with the Paul G. Allen Family Foundation, is launching an app in West Africa entitled #ISurvivedEbola. The goal is to reduce the stigma of Ebola and help survivors adjust back into their communities. Ebola survivors in Guinea, Sierra Leone, and Liberia will be given smartphones to document their stories and share tips about how to cope with returning home (Reuters 2015c).

The United States will stop screening travelers from Mali starting Tuesday, January 6, 2015 (Caldwell 2015).

January 6, 2015 (Tuesday)
House-to-house searches for Ebola victims continue in Sierra Leone. Daniel Bob Jones is the leader of a search team working in the Freetown slums of Bonga Town and Crab Town. He says there is plenty of space available in Ebola clinics now. Even so, his team has a hard time convincing people there is enough room available to care for all of the victims (Dunn 2015a).

Medical workers at the hospital in Makeni, Sierra Leone, have ended their strike. The government has met the worker's demands and promises to pay their hazard pay (O'Carroll 2015a).

Clinical trials of the antiviral drug brincidofovir have stared at the ELWA-3 Ebola center in Monrovia, Liberia (ABC News 2015a).

The United Kingdom has tightened its screening procedures for healthcare workers returning from West Africa. Any worker who had contact with Ebola patients and reports feeling ill will be isolated and assessed. The move comes after the confusion surrounding the arrival of infected nurse Pauline Cafferkey. Cafferkey felt sick at Heathrow airport and requested multiple temperature screenings. Even so, she was still allowed to travel from London to Glasgow (Merrifield 2015).

The WHO says there are no Ebola cases in Iraq (Outbreak News Today 2015a). The claims that ISIS fighters were infected with the disease were only rumors.

There are currently 2542 US troops helping with the Ebola outbreak in West Africa (Tilghman 2015a).

January 7, 2015 (Wednesday)

Total cases: 20,747 (541 new)   Fatalities: 8235 (330 new)
                                 (World Health Organization 2015a)

A new Ebola treatment center and laboratory will open tomorrow in Kono District, Sierra Leone (Samba 2015a).

The Australian Ebola clinic at the Hastings Airfield near Freetown, Sierra Leone, has released its first Ebola survivor, 11-year-old Aminata Bangura. The staff plans to have survivors leave handprints on one of the clinic's walls. Aminata's print is the first. So far, the clinic has admitted 37 patients. It opened in December 2014 (Yenko 2015).

Over 100 burial teams in Sierra Leone are being funded by the United Kingdom. A member of Red Cross Burial Team 9 in Freetown says the teams try to support the customs of Ebola victims. If the victim's relatives provide a coffin, the body is buried in the coffin. If the family wants the deceased dressed in special clothes, the team dresses them as requested. The goal is to let families know their loved one is respected and is being given a dignified funeral (Mazumdar 2015a).

January 8, 2015 (Thursday)

Officials in Sierra Leone think Operation *Western Area Surge* is being very successful. They have decided to extend it for another 2 weeks. So far, the campaign has identified 941 suspected Ebola cases, 243 of whom have tested positive for the disease (APA 2015b).

Pujehun District in Sierra Leone has been declared Ebola-free. The district has gone 42 days without a new Ebola case. The first confirmed case occurred in the district on August 8, 2014. The last occurred on November 26, 2014. There have been 31 confirmed cases and 24 deaths in the district. Pujehun District is the first district in Sierra Leone to become Ebola-free (AllAfrica 2015a).

With the number of Ebola cases falling, the Liberian Football Federation has restarted competitive soccer matches in Liberia. Games were stopped in late July 2014 due to the outbreak (Baber 2015).

Workers at the crematorium in Boys Town, Liberia, face significant stigma. Cremation is disliked in Liberia and residents often ridicule or threaten the workers. Out of fear of attack, the 30 or so workers live at the crematorium. They have trouble obtaining food because locals do not want them visiting the markets (Andrews 2015).

Coming Attractions Bridal & Formal in Tallmadge, Ohio, will permanently close at the end of January 2015. Infected nurse Amber Vinson visited the store in October 2014 just before she was diagnosed with Ebola. The store had to temporarily close and the owners lost an estimated $100,000. The losses were due to a viral illness, so they were not covered by the store's insurance policy (Associated Press 2015b).

January 9, 2015 (Friday)
Operation *Stop Ebola* has been launched in two communities outside of Monrovia, Liberia. Ebola cases are still occurring in Clara Town and New Kru Town, possibly because the residents are not aggressively following anti-Ebola protocols. The goal of the operation is to increase Ebola awareness in the communities through fliers, brochures, and public addresses (Fahngon 2015).

Schools in Sierra Leone remain closed and will not be reopened until the number of Ebola cases falls. Officials hope classes will start by the end of March 2015. If schools do not reopen by May 2015, the entire school year will have been lost due to the outbreak (Kamara 2015a).

MSF has opened a new Ebola treatment center in Kissy, Sierra Leone, on the outskirts of Freetown. The facility is on the grounds of Methodist Boys High School. The center has 20 beds, but will expand to 80 beds. It will focus on treating pregnant women (PRN 2015a).

The number of tourists visiting Sierra Leone has dramatically fallen. In January 2014, 1532 tourists arrived at Lungi airport. In November 2014, only 191 arrived (Awoko 2015b).

The WHO has concluded that two Ebola vaccines, one made by GlaxoSmithKline the other by Merck and NewLink, have acceptable safety profiles. Additional trials of these vaccines will soon begin with West Africa volunteers (Cheng 2015a).

January 10, 2015 (Saturday)
Kailahun District in Sierra Leone has gone 27 days without a new Ebola case (O'Carroll 2015b).

January 11, 2015 (Sunday)
Ebola often causes a skin rash. Sometimes this rash is extremely dramatic. American doctor, Dr. Joel Selanikio, describes the condition of 16-year-old Hawa whom he treated in Lunsar, Sierra Leone:

> *I pulled away her blanket and I found that rather than just having a rash, her entire body surface was peeling off in thick pieces revealing very red, painful-looking skin underneath.*
>
> *Honestly, every person around that bed literally gasped when they saw what she looked like. It was like a burn victim. I've honestly never seen anything like it, except in a burn victim.* (Weekend Edition 2015)

The Ebola outbreak is significantly affecting family budgets in Sierra Leone. A market woman says a fish used to cost $2.33; now one costs $3.51. The income of one taxi driver, a victim of the now decimated tourist industry, has been cut in half. He currently lives on about $8.50 per day (Dunn 2015b).

With fewer Ebola cases occurring in Liberia, a 20-man Liberian ambulance team has been transferred to Sierra Leone (Brooks C 2015a).

Pauline Cafferkey is being treated with blood plasma from Ebola survivor William Pooley (Daily Record 2015).

January 12, 2015 (Monday)
Some communities in Sierra Leone are enforcing their own anti-Ebola regulations. Pa Alimamy Bongo, the section chief of Rokupa in the east end of Freetown, says his community imposes a $20–50 fine for shaking hands. They also have a $100 fine for failing to report a sick family member or for allowing a visitor to stay in a person's house without pre-approval from a community elder (World Bulletin 2015).

Infected British nurse, Pauline Cafferkey is no longer critically ill and is showing signs of improvement (BBC 2015b).

January 13, 2015 (Tuesday)
A male Red Cross nurse has died from Ebola in Kenema, Sierra Leone (ABC News 2015b).

The 163-member Chinese medical team started working in Liberia on December 23, 2014. So far they have treated 67 patients. These include 5 confirmed and 45 suspected Ebola patients (Xinhua News Agency 2015a).

The CDC laboratory worker who was exposed to live Ebola samples in Atlanta has not developed Ebola (Stobbe 2015). Similarly, the patient who arrived at the Nebraska treatment center during the first week of January 2015 has not developed Ebola (Associated Press 2015c).

January 14, 2015 (Wednesday)

Total cases: 21,296 (549 new)   Fatalities: 8429 (194 new)
                            (World Health Organization 2015b)

A mob in Dar es Salaam, Guinea, killed two police officers they thought were spreading Ebola. The incident began when three police officers and a driver gave a sedative to a sick local healer. The healer died soon afterward and the villagers assumed the death was related to the injection. In response, the villagers attacked the officers with machetes and clubs and set fire to their bodies. Two of the officers died; the third was injured (AFP 2015c).

President of Sierra Leone Ernest Bai Koroma predicts that Sierra Leone will have no new Ebola cases by the end of March 2015. He also thinks the country will be Ebola-free by May 2015 (ABC News 2015c).

Twelve of Liberia's 15 counties have had no Ebola cases in the last 7 days (APA 2015c).

The World Bank says the Ebola outbreak is having a major impact on household finances in Liberia. About 60% of women and 40% of men are currently out of work. To make up for lost income, 80% of families have sold assets, slaughtered livestock, borrowed money, or spent savings (DeCapua 2015).

An Ebola scare has occurred in Killeen, Texas. Yesterday ~730 h, the body of a 24-year-old US soldier was found on the doorstep of his off-base apartment (Vanden Brook and Locker 2015; KVUE and KCEN 2015). The soldier had recently returned from Liberia and was self-monitoring for Ebola symptoms. A pool of vomit was found near his body (Vanden Brook and Locker 2015). Despite the major concern about Ebola, preliminary Ebola tests have been negative (Vanden Brook and Locker 2015; KVUE and KCEN 2015).

All players arriving in Equatorial Guinea for the Africa Cup of Nations soccer tournament will be tested for Ebola. Anyone displaying symptoms or refusing to be tested will be quarantined for 21 days (Reuters 2015d)

Emory University Hospital says it has collected 18 units of plasma from Ebola survivors (Fox 2015a).

January 15, 2015 (Thursday)
Ebola caseloads are significantly declining in West Africa. Last week, Sierra Leone and Guinea had the lowest numbers of new Ebola cases since August 2014 (BBC 2015c). Liberia had the lowest number since June 2014 (BBC 2015c). Health officials are generally optimistic, but numerous Ebola hotspots remain (Associated Press 2015d).

Officials in Guinea plan to reopen schools on January 19, 2015 (BBC 2015c). The schools have been closed for 5 months due to the outbreak.

The WHO published 14 articles today that discuss the origin, course, and challenges of the Ebola outbreak (World Health Organization 2015c).

January 16, 2015 (Friday)
In Sierra Leone, medical workers appear to be having success treating Ebola patients with convalescent plasma. A professor familiar with the trials says 35 of 40 Ebola patients (87.5%) treated with convalescent plasma have recovered (Samba 2015b).

Two people in The Gambia have been charged with smuggling two people from Sierra Leone into The Gambia (Kanteh 2015).

Two healthcare workers who may have been exposed to Ebola are being transported to the United Kingdom for observation. One is a female Australian nurse whose PPE was damaged while she was working in Sierra Leone. The other had contact with a person who died from Ebola (Parker and Miller 2015).

January 17, 2015 (Saturday)
For the first time since it opened, there are no Ebola patients at the ELWA-3 treatment center in Monrovia, Liberia (PRN 2015b).

Between January 1 and 5, 2015, 156 children under the age of 5 were buried in King Tom Cemetery, Sierra Leone. Most are thought to be Ebola victims (Wintercross 2015).

January 18, 2015 (Sunday)
Mali is now officially Ebola-free. It has been 42 days since the last Ebola case in the country (Stout 2015).

The crematorium in Monrovia, Liberia, is no longer in operation. Its services are no longer needed because there are fewer cases in the country and most of the recent Liberian Ebola victims are being buried. Seven barrels at the crematorium contain the ashes and charred bones of Ebola victims. A piece of paper on each barrel records the dates the bodies inside it were incinerated. Unfortunately, the identity of the victims is unknown. Officials say they will dispose the unidentified remains in a dignified manner, possibly in the form of a memorial (Giahyue 2015a).

Many of the US-built Ebola centers in Liberia opened too late to be of much help with the outbreak. For example, the clinic in Tubmanburg has only treated 46 patients since it opened on November 18, 2014. Three of the seven centers in Monrovia will temporarily close. A few of the others are being used to store food and supplies (Sieff 2015a).

January 19, 2015 (Monday)
Schools in Guinea reopened today. Many people are excited about classes restarting, but others worry about the possibility of exposing students to Ebola. Some parents kept their children home. In Conakry, school employees took the temperature of every arriving student. Only children with normal readings were allowed to enter school buildings (Diallo 2015a).

Volunteers are going house-to-house in the town of Tombo, Sierra Leone, to spread Ebola awareness and identify hidden patients (Awareness Times 2015a).

In Newark, New Jersey, today, a female healthcare worker traveling from Sierra Leone began vomiting on United Airlines Flight 45 (Strunsky 2015). She was removed from the plane and taken to Hackensack University Medical Center. She is being tested for Ebola. Flight 45 originated in Brussels (Strunsky 2015). The removal of the woman was dramatic and stressful for the other passengers. Five responders in hazmat suits boarded the plane (Saker 2015). Everyone was asked to fill out cards with their contact information so they could be reached by health officials. At one point, a team member asked a passenger to stop photographing the incident (Saker 2015).

Aeroflot Flight 2455 was quarantined for 4 h at Moscow's Sheremetyevo airport today because a female passenger was suspected of having Ebola. The flight was traveling from Paris, France, to Moscow, Russia. The traveler was removed from the plane and given a temporary visa so she could receive treatment in the city (RT 2015).

A South Korean medical worker has been discharged from the hospital in Berlin, Germany. The worker had been under observation since January 4, 2015. They were drawing blood from an Ebola patient in Sierra Leone when they suffered a needlestick injury. The worker has not developed Ebola (Korea Times 2015).

January 20, 2015 (Tuesday)
Attendance at Guinean schools was generally poor yesterday. Many students stayed home. One class that normally has 50 students had only 5 attendees. Some classes were empty (Kamara 2015e).

Three priests were beaten up in the village of Kabak, Guinea, today. The priests were spraying insecticide, but the villagers thought they were spreading Ebola (Iyengar 2015).

Accurate numbers remain elusive, but it is thought that there may be up to 10,000 Ebola orphans in West Africa (Mazibuko 2015).

The World Bank believes the economic impact of Ebola on West Africa may be lower than initially estimated. It was thought that the outbreak would cause $25 B in losses. It now appears that the three most heavily affected countries may have "only" suffered $1.6 B in losses (Reuters 2015e).

January 21, 2015 (Wednesday)

Total cases: 21,724 (428 new)   Fatalities: 8641 (212 new)
                        (World Health Organization 2015d)

As Ebola case numbers decline, the halving time for cases has reached 1.4 weeks in Guinea, 2.0 weeks Liberia, and 2.7 weeks in Sierra Leone (World Health Organization 2015d).

Officials in Sierra Leone are becoming more optimistic about the effectiveness of their Ebola-fighting efforts. Krio language posters in Freetown read "Togeda we go stop ebola." In colloquial English this means "together we will stop Ebola" (Farge and Fofana 2015).

Sierra Leone plans to reopen schools in March 2015. To help protect returning students, teachers will be trained to take the students temperatures and chlorinated water will be provided for hand-washing. The head of the UK's Sierra Leone Ebola task force recommends an official risk assessment be conducted before schools are allowed to reopen (Reuters 2015f).

Jackson K.P. Naimah, a Liberian physician assistant at the ELWA-3 Ebola Management Center in Paynesville, Liberia, says treating Ebola patients is a heart-rending emotional rollercoaster. When patients survive it makes him extremely happy. When they die he gets depressed. It is difficult for Naimah to relax because his friends often avoid him out of fear of Ebola (Médecins Sans Frontières 2015a).

January 22, 2015 (Thursday)
Ciatta Bishop, the head of Liberia's National Ebola Burial Team, says that so far during the outbreak, more than 2800 bodies have been collected in Liberia (Xinhua and NAN 2015).

Kailahun District in Sierra Leone has gone 42 days without a new Ebola case (Samba 2015c). [On January 10, 2015, it was reported that the district had gone 27 days without a new Ebola case]

Sierra Leone will stop providing Ebola hazard pay for healthcare workers at the end of March 2015. Workers have been receiving up to $118 a week in hazard pay (Siddiqui 2015).

Clinical trials of ZMapp will begin in Liberia in about 3 weeks (Pollack 2015).

The University of Nebraska's Biocontainment Unit has released a patient who had been under observation since early January 2015. The patient had suffered a high-risk Ebola exposure, but did not develop Ebola (Reuters 2015g).

About 20 soldiers from Fort Bragg have completed their quarantine period and will be reunited with their families today (WRAL 2015).

January 23, 2015 (Friday)
Liberia says there are only five active Ebola cases left in the country (Reuters 2015h). Three of the patients are in Monrovia, the other two in Bomi and Grand Cape Mount counties (Reuters 2015h). Due to the drop in cases, the mobilization orders for about 350 US reservists have been canceled (Tilghman 2015b). About 2300 US troops are currently deployed in West Africa as part of Operation *United Assistance* (Tilghman 2015b).

With Ebola cases declining, Sierra Leone's president has announced that all district quarantines will be lifted as of today. There will no longer be any travel restrictions between districts and business hours will be extended on Saturdays (AFP 2015d).

GlaxoSmithKline's Ebola vaccine will start large-scale phase III clinical trials in Liberia. Up to 30,000 people will take part in the study. One third of the participants will receive the trial vaccine. The vaccine doses are expected to arrive in Liberia today (Outbreak News Today 2015b).

January 24, 2015 (Saturday)
Infected British nurse Pauline Cafferkey has recovered from Ebola and been released from the hospital (Jenkins 2015).

Researchers are concerned that the falling number of Ebola cases will make it difficult to conduct field trials of the GlaxoSmithKline Ebola vaccine in Liberia. The researchers are considering moving some of the vaccine trials to Sierra Leone where Ebola cases are more common (Hirschler 2015).

January 25, 2015 (Sunday)
Recovered Spanish nurse María Teresa Romero Ramos has adopted a puppy named "Alma" (Couzens 2015). Ramos's previous dog "Excalibur" was put down when Ramos became infected with Ebola. Officials were worried that the dog could carry the disease.

January 26, 2015 (Monday)
The Ebola treatment unit in Foya, Liberia, has closed. Foya was one of the hardest hit areas during the outbreak, so the closure of the Foya treatment center is highly symbolic (AFP 2015e).

MSF says there are only about 50 Ebola patients in its eight facilities in Guinea, Liberia, and Sierra Leone (PRN 2015b).

Oxfam has called for a Marshall Plan-type recovery program for Ebola-affected countries in West Africa. The Marshall Plan was the highly successful economic recovery program launched after World War II to rebuild devastated European countries. Officials worry that without significant support, West African countries could suffer economic and social collapse (BBC 2015d).

Senegal has reopened its land border with Guinea (Reuters 2015i).

January 27, 2015 (Tuesday)
Officials are generally optimistic about the downward trend in Ebola cases, but are well aware that all case needs to be contained so the disease does not reemerge. Emmanuel d'Harcourt, senior health director for the International Rescue

Committee, said that a similar situation occurred in mid-May 2014. Cases appeared to be on the decline, then hidden cases suddenly emerged and the epidemic exploded (Lewis 2015).

In many parts of West Africa, the "Ebola handshake," which consists of bumping elbows, hitting arms, or knocking shoes, is the new normal (Connolly 2015).

January 28, 2015 (Wednesday)

Total cases: 22,092 (368 new)   Fatalities: 8810 (169 new)
                                 (World Health Organization 2015e)

There were 99 confirmed Ebola cases last week in Guinea, Liberia, and Sierra Leone [presumably many of the 368 new cases cited in today's situation report are suspected cases]. This is the first week since the week of June 29, 2014 that there were less than 100 new cases. Unfortunately, Mali Prefecture in Guinea has reported its first Ebola case (World Health Organization 2015e).

The capacity of the ELWA-3 Ebola treatment center in Monrovia, Liberia, has been reduced from 120 to 60 beds. The higher capacity is no longer needed. At the height of the outbreak, ELWA-3 was one of the largest and most active treatment centers. From its opening on August 17, 2014, to December 31, 2014, ELWA-3 admitted 1826 patients. Of these, 1225 tested positive for Ebola. Seven hundred twenty-seven of the confirmed Ebola cases died; 498 survived (Dosso 2015).

Preliminary test results of the GlaxoSmithKline Ebola vaccine yield a mixed picture of the vaccine's effectiveness. On the positive side, the vaccine seems well tolerated by humans; only 2 out of 59 test subjects developed short-lived fevers. Inoculated subjects also developed some immune response. On the negative side, the immune response was lower than what was seen in trials with macaques (Rampling et al. 2015).

January 29, 2015 (Thursday)
Researchers believe that the Ebola virus circulating in Guinea has mutated. This is not unexpected given that viruses evolve very rapidly. The yet-to-be-answered question, however, is whether the mutations will allow the virus to spread more quickly. Of special concern is the possibility that the mutations could allow for some infected people to remain asymptomatic. If so, a seemingly well victim could act as an Ebola carrier. Dr. Anavaj Sakuntabhai says that several asymptomatic patients have already been seen (Mazumdar 2015b).

A patient with Ebola-like symptoms has been isolated in California. They have been transferred from Mercy General Hospital in Sacramento to the University of California at Davis Medical Center. UC Davis has a specialized ward available for Ebola patients. Little information has been released about the patient, but officials think it is unlikely the person actually has the disease (Bernstein 2015).

January 30, 2015 (Friday)
Liberia is hoping to be Ebola-free by the end of February 2015 (AllAfrica 2015b). Liberian schools will reopen on February 16, 2015 (Giahyue 2015b). Initially the

government had planned to open schools on February 2, but they decided to delay the opening so students and parents could have more time to prepare (Giahyue 2015b).

January 31, 2015 (Saturday)

As Liberia prepares to reopen its schools, there are concerns about students returning to school buildings that were used as Ebola treatment centers. For example, Nathaniel V. Massaquoi Elementary School in Monrovia was used as a holding center for suspected Ebola cases. Many patients died there before they could be transferred to other facilities. The government promises to decontaminate the school before it is reopened, but parents remain wary. This problem is not unique to Liberia. Many schools in Guinea and Sierra Leone were used as treatment centers (Sieff 2015b).

A British military nurse in Sierra Leone has suffered a needlestick injury while treating an infected Ebola patient. The nurse has been transported to the Royal Free Hospital in London and will be kept under observation for 21 days (Ward 2015).

The drug company Chimerix has discontinued clinical trials of its drug brincidofovir in Liberia. Phase II trials of brincidofovir were underway, but because of the falling case numbers, Chimerix has decided to withdraw from the efficacy trials. The company has also stopped planning for future randomize drug trials (Kroll 2015).

February 1, 2015 (Sunday)

A model developed at the University of Georgia suggests that the Ebola outbreak in Liberia could be over between March and June 2015 (Banton 2015).

February 2, 2015 (Monday)

Large-scale Ebola vaccine trials have begun in Liberia. The goal is to inoculate 30,000 individuals, including healthcare workers, with two different vaccines (BBC 2015e). Presumably, some individuals will get one vaccine and some will get the other.

A second British healthcare worker has been transported to the Royal Free Hospital in London following a needlestick injury in Sierra Leone (BBC 2015f). This comes after a similar incident on January 31, 2015. Though similar, the incidents appear to be unrelated.

The US Air Force is completing work on 25 air transportable isolation modules for patients with infectious diseases. The modules should be ready by April 2015. Each module can fit up to four patients and can be carried by a C-17 or C-130 (Schogol 2015).

February 3, 2015 (Tuesday)

Ebola aid payments continue to fall far short of pledged levels. A total of $2.89 B has been pledged, but so far only $1.09 B has been delivered (Schlanger 2015).

February 4, 2015 (Wednesday)

Total cases: 22,495 (403 new)   Fatalities: 8981 (171 new)
                                 (World Health Organization 2015f)

Liberia plans to close four Ebola treatment units in and around Monrovia. The Island Clinic and the Unity Conference Center Ebola treatment unit have already closed, with Unity closing on February 1, 2015. Two Ebola treatment units at the Ministry of Defense will close on February 25, 2015 (Sendolo 2015a).

A new Ebola case has been detected in Margibi County, Liberia. This is troubling because the county has not has any cases for almost a month. Officials say the sick patient's wife brought the patient to Margibi County from Monrovia (Brooks C 2015b).

Schools in Sierra Leone will reopen on March 30, 2015 (Johnson 2015a).

The US Department of State will allow adult family members to return to the US embassy in Freetown, Sierra Leone (U.S. Department of State 2015). The agency ordered all non-employed dependents out of Sierra Leone on August 14, 2014.

Preliminary field results suggest the drug favipiravir can reduce Ebola mortality. Trials of the drug took place at two sites in Guinea using 69 patients. The fatality rate for patients with moderate blood levels of Ebola was significantly lower in treated versus untreated patients – 15% mortality compared to 30% mortality. For ethical reasons, this was not a traditional controlled study where some patients received the drugs and others did not. Data for the untreated group came from patients who had been treated earlier at a MSF facility in Guéckédou, Guinea (Fink 2015a).

Doctors think post-Ebola syndrome may affect about half of West African Ebola survivors. It is unclear what causes the syndrome, but it may be a type of autoimmune response that makes the immune system become hyperstimulated. Symptoms are varied, but vision is often affected. Significant eye pain and blindness can occur. Doctors point out that given the severity of Ebola, it may not be surprising that the disease causes long-term effects in patients. For example, some Lassa fever survivors suffer nerve damage and hearing loss (Farge 2015a).

After an internal review, the CDC believes that the Ebola samples that were accidentally transferred to a BSL-2 lab on December 22, 2014, were likely dead (Steenhuysen 2015). This does not change the severity of the mishap, but it suggests that the exposed technicians were not at risk of developing Ebola.

It is thought that British nurse Pauline Cafferkey became infected because she wore a visor instead of goggles while working with Ebola patients. Both types of PPE effectively protect healthcare workers while they are being worn, but there are differences in the way they are removed. These differences (not explicitly described) are thought to have led to Cafferkey's infection (BBC 2015g).

The United Kingdom has announced that a new medal will be awarded to medical workers and military personnel who helped with the West African Ebola outbreak (Watt 2015).

February 5, 2015 (Thursday)
After a consistent downward trend in the number of Ebola cases, Liberia, Sierra Leone, and Guinea all had a slight uptick in cases during the past week. There were a total of 124 new confirmed cases in the three countries last week. The week before, there had been 99 new cases (Zoroya 2015a).

UN officials think the majority of Ebola flare-ups are being caused by improper burials. Some residents continue to bury their dead secretly using dangerous traditional burial practices. Given the strong social and religious feelings people have about funeral rites, preventing such burials is very difficult (Reuters 2015j).

The US military mission to Liberia is winding down. There are currently about 1300 US troops in the country. The numbers will drop through March 2015. Once the majority of troops are gone, a small 100-person force will remain in the country to deal with additional contingencies. The cost of the US deployment has been about $900 M (Zoroya 2015b).

February 6, 2015 (Friday)
Guinea is seeing an increase in active Ebola cases. There are currently 53 confirmed cases in the country. Officials think the new cases are being discovered because healthcare workers are starting to visit parts of the country that were previously inaccessible (Reuters 2015k).

The US State Department has awarded the Phoenix Air Group a new contract to transport Ebola cases. Phoenix Air Group has ferried US Ebola victims from West Africa to treatment centers in the United States. The new contract calls for the company to remain on standby to respond to additional Ebola cases. It also asks the company to train government workers in infectious transportation management (Sickles 2015).

February 7, 2015 (Saturday)
Ebola is especially dangerous to the very young. The mortality rate for children under 5 is ≥80%. Additionally, 21 pregnant women are known to have survived Ebola, but their fetuses almost never survived (K 2015).

Due to the apparent effectiveness of the drug favipiravir, Guinea plans to make wider use of the drug at Ebola treatment centers (HNGN 2015).

February 8, 2015 (Sunday)
Two Ebola burial workers were attacked by a mob in Forecariah, Guinea (AFP 2015f). It is unclear why the attack occurred.

February 9, 2015 (Monday)
A violent protest erupted in Conakry, Guinea today. The incident began after an imam was arrested for holding a funeral for a person thought to have died from Ebola. Protestors set up barricades and burned tires. They then attacked police with sticks and stones. Police responded with tear gas and baton charges. About 12 people were wounded in the clashes. Protestors insist the person died from natural causes and did not have Ebola (AFP 2015g).

The Gambia has lifted all of its travel bans to Ebola-affected countries (AllAfrica 2015c).

February 10, 2015 (Tuesday)
As healthcare workers move deeper into remote sections of Guinea, they are encountering resistance from residents. Negative rumors about healthcare workers persist in the rural areas. Some think workers are spreading Ebola. Others think workers are harvesting organs at Ebola treatment centers. To avoid conflict, the Red Cross keeps a low profile in rural Guinea and sometimes drives cars without Red Cross emblems (Hussain 2015).

Sierra Leone is trying to solve the problem of "ghostworkers." A ghostworker is someone who fraudulently collects money from the government for work associated with the Ebola outbreak. Several types of ghosts exist. A ghost can be a fictitious name that is added to a list of Ebola workers. A ghost can also be a real Ebola worker who lists their name several times to receive extra pay. It is unclear how many ghostworkers there currently are in Sierra Leone. There may have been around 6000 at the end of 2014 (Farge 2015b).

February 11, 2015 (Wednesday)

Total cases: 22,894 (399 new)   Fatalities: 9177 (196 new)
                        (World Health Organization 2015g)

President Obama has announced that he is withdrawing almost all US troops from West Africa. A token force of 100 troops will be left behind to deal with contingencies (Shear and Davis 2015). This official statement confirms previous reports about US troop withdrawal.

Today's WHO situation report shows a dramatic increase in Ebola cases in Guinea. There were 65 new confirmed cases in Guinea last week, compared to 39 the week before (World Health Organization 2015f, g). Most of the new cases were in Conakry and in Forecariah Prefecture. Caseloads in Sierra Leone and Liberia were more or less steady, with 76 and 3 new confirmed cases, respectively (World Health Organization 2015g).

February 12, 2015 (Thursday)
Prescott et al. (2015) describe the ability of Ebola to remain viable in an infected corpse. Infected cynomolgus macaques were euthanized when they were close to death. Samples from their bodies were collected over a 10-week period. Viable virus particles were detected for up to 7 days after death. Ebola viral RNA was found in blood and saliva for up to 3 weeks (Prescott et al. 2015).

The World Bank will provide 10,500 tons of corn and rice seed to West African farmers. Officials are very worried about food production in Ebola-affected areas. Many farmers have died or abandoned their fields. The seed will cost $15 M and will be made available so farmers can prepare for the April planting season (IBNS 2015).

February 13, 2015 (Friday)
About 12,000 schools are now open in Guinea. Attendance is running at about 85% (AFP 2015h).

A crowd attacked an Ebola transit center in Faranah, Guinea, today and set fire to a MSF vehicle. The incident was sparked when a Red Cross team tried to disinfect a school (Reuters 2015l). It is unclear what specifically led to the attack, but persistent rumors in the area say that healthcare workers are spreading Ebola, not fighting it.

ZMapp is being shipped to Africa for clinical trials. The drug is difficult to make, but enough has been produced for field testing to begin (Fox 2015b).

February 14, 2015 (Saturday)
Sierra Leone has imposed a mini-quarantine on the Freetown community of Aberdeen. There have been five new Ebola cases in the area recently. Some of the victims are fishermen who returned from sea with Ebola-like symptoms (Associated Press 2015e).

The National Audit Office of Sierra Leone says there have been significant problems with the dispersal of Ebola funds (Reuters 2015m; Thomas 2015). Almost one-third of the $20 M earmarked for Ebola efforts are unaccounted for. Money was often paid without receipts or invoices. Thus, it is impossible to determine how the money was spent or if it was spent appropriately (Reuters 2015m).

UNICEF workers visited the village of Komendeh Luyama, Sierra Leone, today. The community of 1200 has been hard-hit by Ebola. Forty-two people in Komendeh Luyama have contacted Ebola, 31 of them have died. The disease arrived in the village on October 10, 2014. Initially, people denied the existence of Ebola, but then realized its dangers. Community leaders moved fast to contain the virus. Quarantine sites were established in three homes. The first house was the home of the initial victim. The second house held people who had handled the corpse of the first victim. The third house held people who had visited the first victim's house. Community leaders banned movement into and out of the village and made sure people followed good hygiene practices like hand-washing (James 2015).

The Sierra Leone Association of Journalists has launched a campaign to increase Ebola awareness. People are encouraged to wear yellow ribbons as a symbol of their commitment to fight Ebola (APA 2015d).

February 15, 2015 (Sunday)
No significant Ebola-related events were reported today. This is the first day since July 9, 2014, that no reportable events occurred. For the remainder of the text, no entry will be included for days without notable events.

February 16, 2015 (Monday)
Schools have reopened in Liberia (DiLorenzo 2015; Paye-Layleh 2015a). Most schools are functioning normally, but some remain closed because they do not have running water for hand-washing. Not everyone thinks the schools are safe and some parents kept their children home (DiLorenzo 2015).

F. Zeela Zaizay, a registered nurse and Map International team leader, says people in Liberia have started to abandon some Ebola-fighting practices. For example, some residents are moving dead people back to their home villages for burial (McKenna 2015).

The Liberian Red Cross has released a song entitled "Let Us Live Together Again." It is intended to reduce the stigma of Ebola survivors and encourage tolerance and support for survivors (RTT News 2015).

A female British Red Cross worker has been evacuated from Kono, Sierra Leone. On Saturday, February 14, 2015, she was splashed in the eye with body fluids while she was removing her PPE. A Swiss Air rescue plane transported her to the United Kingdom (Brown 2015).

February 17, 2015 (Tuesday)
Ebola training in Freetown, Sierra Leone, includes role-playing in a mock hospital with Ebola survivors playing the part of victims. The goal is to introduce healthcare workers to the environment of an Ebola treatment center. The mock patients exhibit the symptoms of Ebola victims. Environmental conditions are also simulated. For example, needles and sharps are accidentally left on the ground (De Vries 2015).

February 18, 2015 (Wednesday)

Total cases: 23,253 (359 new)   Fatalities: 9380 (203 new)
                                 (World Health Organization 2015h)

During the week ending February 15, 2015, there were 45 unsafe burials in Sierra Leone and 39 in Guinea (World Health Organization 2015h).

Residents of Port Loko District, Sierra Leone, may be hiding patients or avoiding clinics. In response, officials have launched a 2-week, door-to-door Ebola campaign in the district. Teams say people are cooperating (Johnson 2015b).

February 19, 2015 (Thursday)
Quarantined families in Sierra Leone are having a hard time obtaining food. One family has been isolated since January 9, 2015. They have received only one food package which was delivered at the start of their isolation. Currently, the family only has rice to eat and even that is running low. Other residents are aware of the problem. Consequently, some people hide in the forest rather than risk quarantine. The food delivery system for quarantined families is long and convoluted. It begins when a contact tracer provides the names of people needing food to a supervisor. The supervisor then sends the list to government nutritionists. The list is then passed to the district medical officer. Finally, NGOs are contacted to deliver food to the families (Maxmen 2015). Given the large number of links in this chain, it is not surprising that errors and omissions occur.

Ismail Ould Cheikh Ahmed, the head of UNMEER, believes the worst of the Ebola outbreak is over (Marteh 2015).

Osterholm et al. (2015) conclude that airborne transmission of Ebola can probably occur, at least in some situations. The authors reviewed all of the current data on Ebola transmission. They find that most transmission events occur through direct contact. However, it also seems that Ebola can sometimes spread through the air via aerosols and droplets (Osterholm et al. 2015).

Ghana has lifted its ban on international conferences. The country had banned international meetings to prevent the spread of Ebola (Ghana Business News 2015).

February 20, 2015 (Friday)
The WHO has approved a rapid Ebola-detection test. The ReEBOV Antigen Rapid Test works within 15 min. It is made by Corgenix. The test is not perfect, but it can correctly identify 92% of infected Ebola victims. It can also correctly rule out infection in 85% of uninfected people. Officials have high hopes for the test. Traditional Ebola tests can take days to return results. The new test should help medical workers quickly separate Ebola patients from other patients (Boseley 2015b).

MSF has closed the Kailahun Ebola treatment center in Sierra Leone. Kailahun District has gone 66 days without a new Ebola case (Kamara 2015c). At one point, the Kailahun center was one of the most active Ebola treatment units. Its closure is highly symbolic of the recent advances made against the disease.

Liberia will reopen its land borders on Sunday, February 22, 2015. The country will also lift its nationwide 0000–0600 h curfew (Executive Mansion 2015).

February 21, 2015 (Saturday)
Eight healthcare workers from the S.D. Cooper Hospital in Monrovia, Liberia, have been placed under observation after coming into contact with an Ebola victim. A female patient had been transferred to S.D. Cooper from a different hospital. She had Ebola, but the staff at S.D. Copper did not know it. They worked with her before they were aware she was Ebola-positive. Despite this set back, the number of Ebola cases in Liberia remains very low. There are only eight confirmed Ebola cases in the country (Paye-Layleh 2015b).

Unfounded Ebola fears continue to crop up around the world. On February 20, 2015, a man died in Quebec, Canada, after returning from West Africa. News sources (and presumably officials) speculated that he might have died from Ebola. However, the man had returned from Burkina Faso – a country with no known Ebola cases (QMI 2015). It is therefore extremely unlikely that he had the disease.

February 22, 2015 (Sunday)
An Australian nurse working in Sierra Leone has been transferred to the United Kingdom for observation. The nurse suffered an unspecified, low-risk incident involving Ebola (AAP 2015).

February 23, 2015 (Monday)
Liberians are overjoyed that the Ebola curfew has been lifted. People stayed out into the early morning hours. Many say they finally feel free. Retailers are also excited. The end of the curfew gives customers more time to shop and visit restaurants and bars (AFP 2015i).

A Sierra Leone orphanage has been quarantined after a staff member developed Ebola. Augustine Baker collapsed during a meeting. Tests confirmed he has Ebola. The 33 orphans at the facility are now under observation (BBC 2015h).

February 24, 2015 (Tuesday)
The number of Ebola cases in Sierra Leone is rising. Dr. Felicity Fitzgerald says the admissions board at the Connaught Hospital Ebola Isolation Unit is now full. She also says there were three times more new cases during the past week than there were the week before. There are now 65 confirmed Ebola cases in Freetown (Fitzgerald 2015).

Liberia has placed Gaygbah Town and the surrounding villages under quarantine. Four new Ebola cases have recently occurred in the area. The new cases started on February 4, 2015, when a woman brought her infected husband to a local clinic from Monrovia. The man died and several community members were infected (Baysah 2015).

February 25, 2015 (Wednesday)

Total cases: 23,729 (476 new)   Fatalities: 9604 (224 new)
(World Health Organization 2015i)

Because of the risk posed by convalescent semen, some male Ebola survivors are placing themselves into self-imposed quarantine. The WHO recommends male survivors abstain from sex for at least 90 days after recovery. To help make sure they comply with these recommendations, some men have chosen to isolate themselves from their wives and girlfriends (Shryock and Bavier 2015).

Augustine Baker, a staff member who worked with Ebola orphans in Sierra Leone, has died from Ebola (BBC 2015i). His loss is deeply felt by Sierra Leone Ebola-fighters.

In Liberia, about 20% of the people who had stopped working because of the outbreak have returned to work (AllAfrica 2015d).

February 26, 2015 (Thursday)
The 101st Airborne Division cased its colors at a ceremony in Monrovia, Liberia, today. This symbolically marks the end of Operation *United Assistance*. It officially ends US troop deployments to West Africa (AFP 2015j; Hoskins 2015). Liberian President Ellen Johnson Sirleaf thanked the United States for its help with the crisis and expressed the profound gratitude of the Liberian people (Biddle 2015).

Paolo Conteh, Sierra Leone's Ebola Czar, is dismayed at the rising number of Ebola cases in Sierra Leone. There have been double digit increases in new cases during 3 days of the past week. He believes the increases are due to lax enforcement of anti-Ebola protocols. He is especially concerned about unsafe burials that are occurring in the western part of the country (Sierra Leone Times 2015).

MSF says there has been a general drop in fatality rates at its West African Ebola clinics. The current mortality rate is about 52%. Last March it was 62%. It is unclear what is causing the drop. Patients could be arriving at clinics with lower viral loads than before. If so, this could be because patients are seeking treatment sooner (although data suggests this is not the case), or because people are taking more safety precautions and having less exposure to Ebola. It is also possible that the active Ebola strain may have mutated to become less lethal (McNeil 2015).

A total of 2592 blood serum samples are being shipped from Sierra Leone to South Africa for future Ebola research. South Africa has the only BSL-4 laboratory in Africa (Xinhua News Agency 2015b).

The FDA has approved Corgenix Medical Corp's ReEBOV Antigen Rapid Test for emergency use. The test takes 15 min to complete and is conducted by placing a drop of blood onto a paper test strip (Reuters 2015n). The WHO approved the use of the test on February 20, 2015.

February 27, 2015 (Friday)
A fishing village just outside Makeni, Sierra Leone, has been quarantined after a sudden spike in Ebola cases. The flare-up started when a sick man fled quarantine in Freetown and came to the village. A local healer treated him using traditional methods. The sick man died about a day after he arrived. Numerous people have since been infected. The deceased man's father has died, as has the traditional healer who performed the man's burial. Bill Boyes, spokesman for the International Medical Corps in Makeni, says before the spike, things had been quiet at the Makeni treatment center. Then on Sunday, February 22, 2015, ambulances started to arrive. There are now 31 confirmed Ebola patients at the facility (O'Carroll 2015c).

The WHO says an independent advisory body will decide in August 2015 whether to recommend mass Ebola vaccination in West Africa. The decision will be based on the results of the ongoing field trials of vaccine candidates (Nebehay 2015).

February 28, 2015 (Saturday)
Due to the recent uptick in Sierra Leone Ebola cases, President Ernest Bai Koroma has reinstated some Ebola restrictions. The rules include limiting the number of passengers taxis can carry, banning nighttime boat launches, and reinforcing health checkpoints. In terms of the taxi regulations, two people may ride in a taxi car; four people may ride in a taxi van (The Star 2015).

The Vice President of Sierra Leone, Samuel Sam-Sumana, has quarantined himself after one of his bodyguards died from Ebola (The Star 2015).

A clinical trial of ZMapp has begun in Liberia (Reuters 2015o).

March 2, 2015 (Monday)
Liberia has gone 7 days without a new confirmed Ebola case (AllAfrica 2015e; BBC 2015j). At present, there are two confirmed cases in the country and 116 people under surveillance (AllAfrica 2015e). Officials stress the need for caution, but these numbers suggest that Liberia is well on its way to becoming Ebola-free.

Testing errors in Guinea led to several Ebola-positive patients being accidentally released from treatment centers. Dr. Sakoba Keita, Guinea's anti-Ebola coordinator, confirms that in January and February 2015 at least 23 botched blood tests led to four Ebola-positive patients being released. Two of these patients have died. The errors took place in Conakry and Coyah. In some cases, diagnostic blood samples were accidentally placed in test tubes with the blood-thinning agent heparin (Farge 2015c).

A committee of Sierra Leone's Parliament has ordered the arrest of the country's National Ebola Response Center coordinator, Steven Ngaojia. Ngaojia apparently took part in the misappropriation of Ebola funds (Samba 2015d).

March 4, 2015 (Wednesday)

Total cases: 23,969 (240 new)   Fatalities: 9807 (203 new)
                                 (World Health Organization 2015j)

Liberia will discharge its last Ebola patient tomorrow. The patient is being treated at the Chinese Ebola Treatment Unit in Paynesville. Liberia's Assistant Health Minister, Tolbert Nyenswah, says a ceremony will be held to mark the occasion (APA 2015e).

The recent rise in Ebola cases in Sierra Leone has some residents questioning the wisdom of reopening schools. Schools are scheduled to reopen on March 30, 2015, but this may be delayed until case levels fall (Naija247 2015).

A new estimate by Street Child of Sierra Leone says there may be 12,000 Ebola orphans in Sierra Leone (O'Carroll 2015d).

Facing Ebola as a healthcare worker is extremely difficult. Dr. Monica Rull, a volunteer medical coordinator, says medical organizations like MSF understand that some workers will not be able to deal with the pressure of working with such a dangerous disease. Protocols are in place to allow these workers to leave graciously (Ravelo 2015).

March 5, 2015 (Thursday)
Liberia has released its last Ebola patient, 58-year-old English teacher Beatrice Yardolo (Associated Press 2015f, Williams 2015c). Yardolo was admitted to the Chinese-run Ebola Center in Paynesville on February 18, 2015 (Associated Press 2015f). To make sure she has really recovered from the disease, she was given three separate Ebola tests. All were negative. There are presently 102 contacts under observation in Liberia. Once the country has gone 42 days without a new case, Liberia will be considered Ebola-free (Williams 2015c).

In contrast to Liberia's success, Sierra Leone is suffering a setback in its fight against Ebola. Dr. James Meiring, working with the International Medical Corps in Sierra Leone, says there has recently been an increase in Ebola cases in the country. In his ward, there are currently 21 confirmed Ebola patients and 27 high-risk contacts under observation (Lancaster Guardian 2015).

With case levels dropping, the Canadian Red Cross has ended its campaign to recruit Canadian healthcare workers to fight Ebola in West Africa (Lunn 2015).

March 6, 2015 (Friday)
Ebola survivors in Sierra Leone have requested free follow-up medical care for lingering Ebola-related medical problems, including post-Ebola syndrome (Kamara 2015b).

March 7, 2015 (Saturday)

The crematorium used to incinerate Liberian Ebola victims has been dismantled. Over the course of the outbreak, an estimated 3000 people were cremated in Liberia. Nineteen barrels containing the ashes of Ebola victims will be buried on a 25 acre plot bought by the government [the Disco Hill cemetery]. Local religious leaders held a ceremony at the crematorium's site today to mark the end of its use (Paye-Layleh 2015c).

Officials in West Africa, especially in Liberia, are reminding people to stay vigilant against Ebola. Even a single case can reignite the epidemic. Officials stress that Ebola-fighting efforts must continue until no active cases remain in West Africa (Frankel 2015).

The WHO has begun large-scale testing of Merck's VSV-EBOV Ebola vaccine in Guinea (Cheng 2015b).

March 9, 2015 (Monday)

Drums holding the ashes of Ebola victims have begun to be transferred from Liberia's crematorium to the cemetery on Disco Hill. Relatives of the deceased dressed in mourning attire watched the proceedings (Williams 2015d).

More precise casualty figures have been released for the Liberian Ebola outbreak. Officials say 6097 total deaths (from Ebola and non-Ebola causes) were recorded in the country between March 2014 and February 2015. Of those, 2711 were cremated and 3386 were interred by burial teams. Oral swabs for Ebola tests were collected from 70.6% of the bodies (Gortor 2015a).

March 10, 2015 (Tuesday)

About 60 US troops have completed their 3-week Ebola quarantine at Fort Bragg, North Carolina (WNCN 2015).

March 11, 2015 (Wednesday)

Total cases: 24,282 (313 new)   Fatalities: 9976 (169 new)
                             (World Health Organization 2015k)

A female British military healthcare worker [Anna Cross] has contracted Ebola while working in Sierra Leone. She is currently being treated in the Kerry Town Ebola Treatment Unit (BBC 2015k).

Today is Decoration Day in Liberia. It is a holiday similar to Memorial Day in the United States and is a time when people visit the graves of loved ones. Today's Decoration Day is a rather somber occasion for families whose loved ones were cremated. There is no grave for them to visit. In a country where burial is the cultural norm, the lack of a grave can cause significant psychological stress for surviving family members (MacDougall 2015; Muchler and Collins 2015).

March 12, 2015 (Thursday)

The official death toll from the Ebola outbreak has passed 10,000. There have been 10,004 confirmed or suspected deaths in Sierra Leone, Liberia, and Guinea (Al Jazeera 2015a).

The infected UK healthcare worker [Anna Cross] has been evacuated to Britain. Two close contacts have also been evacuated to the United Kingdom and will be monitored. All three patients are being treated at the Royal Free Hospital in London. Two other workers who had some contact with the infected patient are being monitored in Sierra Leone (Whitman 2015).

Liberia says Ebola victims will not be officially mourned until the country is declared Ebola-free. Officials think it would be premature to hold a ceremony before the outbreak is officially over (Butty 2015a).

Dr. Nancy Snyderman has quit her position at NBC News (Farberov 2015). She had been severely criticized for breaking quarantine in October 2014.

March 13, 2015 (Friday)

A male US healthcare worker has contracted Ebola in Sierra Leone (Sifferlin 2015a; Sweeney 2015). The patient is a clinician who was working for the US charity Partners in Health (Sweeney 2015). He is currently in serious condition and has been transferred to the NIH site in Bethesda, Maryland, for treatment (Sifferlin 2015a).

The remaining two healthcare workers who had contact with the most recent British patient have been transported from Sierra Leone to the United Kingdom. They were taken to the Royal Victoria Infirmary in Newcastle (BBC 2015l).

March 14, 2015 (Saturday)

Ten Americans who may have had contact with the latest US Ebola patient are being flown from Sierra Leone to the United States for observation. All of the new patients work for Partners in Health. It is unclear where all of the people will be taken, but it is reported that at least one will go to Emory University Hospital and four will go to the Nebraska Medical Center (Reuters 2015p).

March 15, 2015 (Sunday)

Eight of the 11 Americans exposed to Ebola in Sierra Leone (including the clinician with Ebola) have returned the United States. The three others will return Monday (Cohen 2015).

March 16, 2015 (Monday)

The American Ebola patient being treated at the NIH is now in critical condition. On Sunday night, one of the patients being monitored in Nebraska started exhibiting Ebola-like symptoms. They were isolated, but the symptoms resolved today and the patient has tested negative for Ebola (Associated Press 2015g).

Data from Kailahun District in Sierra Leone provide an empirical assessment of Ebola's impact. The first Ebola case was recorded in the district on May 25, 2014. The district was declared Ebola-free on January 22, 2015. During that time [242 days], more than 300 people died from Ebola. There are now 182 Ebola widows in the district and 620 children who lost parents or guardians to the disease. Of the survivors, 186 exhibit symptoms of post-Ebola syndrome (Kamara 2015d).

March 17, 2015 (Tuesday)

Guinea is suffering a significant setback in its fight against Ebola. Recently, 21 new Ebola cases were found in a single day. Three Guinean doctors have also been infected. Spokeswoman for UNMEER, Fatoumata Lejeune-Kaba, says it appears that people are not following anti-Ebola protocols (Samb and Farge 2015).

A total of 15 American healthcare workers have returned to the United States after being exposed to the most recent American Ebola patient. All of the returnees work for Partners in Health. It is unclear how so many people became exposed from a single patient (Fox 2015c).

March 18, 2015 (Wednesday)

Total cases: 24,701 (419 new)   Fatalities: 10,194 (218 new)
                              (World Health Organization 2015l)

During the week ending March 15, 2015, there were 95 new confirmed Ebola cases in Guinea and 55 in Sierra Leone. There were no new cases in Liberia, continuing Liberia's move toward becoming Ebola-free (World Health Organization 2015l).

Sierra Leone Ebola Czar Major Paolo Conteh says the King Tom Cemetery is now full. Future Ebola burials will need to take place at the Waterloo cemetery (Awoko 2015c).

Results from an opinion poll in Britain suggest that healthcare workers returning from West Africa face significant stigma at home. Only 36% of respondents say they would be willing to speak to a newly returned worker face-to-face. However, 78% say they admire the healthcare workers for their service (British Red Cross 2015a).

March 19, 2015 (Thursday)

Sierra Leone will implement another nationwide lockdown to try to stop the Ebola outbreak (BBC 2015m). The lockdown will last for 3 days and will be in effect from 0600 h March 27 to 1800 h March 29, 2015. It will be similar to the nationwide lockdown held in September 2014 (Williams 2015a). It is hoped that the new lockdown will allow officials to identify the remaining Ebola cases in the country and slow or stop the outbreak (BBC 2015m).

March 20, 2015 (Friday)

A new Ebola case has been confirmed in Liberia (Reuters 2015q). The new patient is a woman [Ruth Tugbah] who was diagnosed at the MSF center in Redemption Hospital (The Samaya 2015). The patient came from the Caldwell community near Monrovia (Rueters 2015q). This is a significant setback for Liberia. The country has been moving toward being declared Ebola-free. Liberia's last confirmed case was released from treatment on March 5, 2015.

The families of Liberian healthcare workers who died fighting Ebola are receiving $5000 benefit checks. So far, 11 families have received the benefits (Associated Press 2015h).

March 21, 2015 (Saturday)
Liberian officials are investigating the country's new Ebola case. It is unclear how the woman became infected. She has no clear links with past patients and has not traveled recently (Associated Press 2015i).

Forty-two Ghanaian healthcare workers who worked with Ebola patients in Sierra Leone have been placed in 21-day quarantine in the Ivory Coast (Starr FM Online 2015). They will not return to Ghana until they finish their quarantine.

March 23, 2015 (Monday)
Officials say the latest Liberian Ebola patient is doing well. It is still unclear how she was infected. The woman [Ruth Tugbah] is apparently a food seller. Speculation on the street is that she caught the disease from handling infected money (Spy Ghana 2015).

Sixty-three troops from the US 36th Engineer Brigade finished their quarantine period and were reunited with their families at the Starker Physical Fitness Center at Fort Hood, Texas, today (Thayer 2015).

A man has been jailed in Britain for claiming to have Ebola. The man entered Diana, Princess of Wales Hospital, coughed on a receptionist, said he had Ebola, and claimed his wife had died from the disease. He was sentenced to 14 months in prison. The man has a history of making false statements to officials and businesses (Lister 2015).

March 24, 2015 (Tuesday)
More information has become available about the most recent Liberian Ebola patient. She is Ruth Tugbah, a 44-year-old street vendor. She lives in a house with 52 other people and recently sold food to a school with 1900 students (Fink 2015b). Given these demographic parameters, officials are very worried that new Ebola cases will appear. Indeed, the woman's 18-year-old daughter, Beneta Kun, developed a fever and weakness today and has been admitted to an Ebola treatment center (Fink 2015b). It is not clear if Beneta has Ebola. About 80 people who had contact with Tugbah are under surveillance (Sendolo 2015b). Tugbah's boyfriend seems to be an Ebola survivor. Health officials are testing his semen to see if he may have inadvertently passed the disease to Tugbah through sex (Paye-Layleh 2015d). [By May 2015 investigators had determined that Tugbah had most likely been infected through sexual contact with an Ebola survivor (Christie et al. 2015). This was exceptionally troubling because the survivor had developed Ebola 199 days before having sex with Tugbah. The case added considerable evidence to the idea that Ebola could remain infective in semen long after a survivor had recovered from the disease (Christie et al. 2015)]

Troops and medics from the 14th Combat Support Hospital at Fort Benning, Georgia, are preparing to deploy to Liberia (WLTZ 2015).

March 25, 2015 (Wednesday)

Total cases: 24,907 (206 new)   Fatalities: 10,326 (132 new)
(World Health Organization 2015m)

MSF has shut the ELWA-3 Ebola treatment center in Monrovia, Liberia. At its peak, ELWA-3 had 250 beds and was one of the largest treatment centers in West Africa. It was also one of the most active. ELWA-3 opened in mid-August 2014. It admitted a total of 1917 patients. Of these, 1234 were confirmed Ebola cases. Eight hundred one patients died at the facility (AllAfrica 2015f).

Phase III trials of the Merck and NewLink Genetics Ebola vaccine have started in Guinea. The trial will vaccinate 10,000 participants using a ring vaccination strategy. In ring vaccination, a "ring" of contacts is vaccinated around an infected person. It is hoped results from the trials will be available by July 2015 (Sifferlin 2015b) [at July 31, 2015, WHO news release stated the trial started on March 23, 2015 (World Health Organization 2015n)].

March 26, 2015 (Thursday)
Residents in Sierra Leone are preparing for the country's 3-day lockdown. Ebola Czar Paolo Conteh has reminded the country's healthcare workers that Ebola hazard pay will end on March 31, 2015 (Awoko 2015d).

The American Ebola patient being treated at the NIH has improved. The patient is now in serious condition (Associated Press 2015j).

March 27, 2015 (Friday)
Sierra Leone's 3-day, nationwide lockdown has started (AFP and Reuters 2015a). During the lockdown, all residents must stay indoors and remain off of the streets. There is a 2-h exemption this evening for Muslims going to prayer and a 5-h exemption on Sunday, March 29, 2015, for Christians going to church (BBC 2015n). Early reports indicate that residents are largely complying with the stay-at-home order (AFP and Reuters 2015a). During the lockdown, 25,650 personnel in three-man teams will visit households to discuss Ebola and locate unidentified victims (Xinhua 2015a). Each team will include a healthcare worker, a social mobilizer, and a local resident (Xinhua 2015a).

Guinea has deployed security forces to its border with Sierra Leone. The move is aimed at stopping people from entering Guinea. Civilians are fleeing Sierra Leone to avoid the Ebola lockdown (Roy-Macaulay and Diallo 2015).

Liberian Ebola victim Ruth Tugbah has died (Toweh 2015). Unconfirmed reports suggest that there are two additional Ebola cases in the country, Tugbah's 18-year-old daughter and a young man from New Kru Town (Berdjis 2015).

Corporal Anna Cross has been released from the Royal Free Hospital in Britain (BBC 2015o). She is the UK military healthcare worker who was infected in Sierra Leone and evacuated to the United Kingdom on March 12, 2015. She is now Ebola-free. Corporal Cross was the first Ebola patient treated with the experimental Ebola drug MIL 77. It is unclear what role, if any, the drug played in her survival. Corporal Cross lost 22 lb while she was sick (BBC 2015o). Corporal Cross was diagnosed in Sierra Leone by a military doctor and initially isolated in the Ebola treatment center where she worked. She says it was ironic to be treating patients in the center 1 day, only to be sitting with them as a patient the next (Sky News 2015a).

Kenya Airways is expected to resume flights to Liberia on Monday, March 30, 2015 (AllAfrica 2015g).

March 28, 2015 (Saturday)
Unrest has developed in parts of Sierra Leone due to the 3-day lockdown. The government had warned citizens that they needed to stockpile supplies ahead of the lockdown, but some poor residents have already run out of food. Food distribution points have been established, but delivery is not always smooth. Soldiers at one distribution site used tear gas to break up an unruly crowd (Olu-Mammah and Fofana 2015).

March 29, 2015 (Sunday)
Guinean President Alpha Condé has declared a 45-day health emergency for five prefectures in the west of the country. The affected areas include Forecariah, Coyah, Dubreka, Boffa, and Kindia Prefectures. A major focus of the emergency will be to ensure that the dead are safely buried. All burials will be monitored by Red Cross workers or security forces, and all bodies will be tested for Ebola. Additionally, only close family members will be allowed to attend funeral services (Diallo 2015b).

March 30, 2015 (Monday)
The 3-day, nationwide lockdown in Sierra Leone has ended. The effort is believed to have been effective. At least 40 bodies were discovered and 172 sick people were transported to hospitals. As the shops reopen, there have been some runs on supplies. For example, one bakery in Freetown ran out of bread within 3 h of opening (MENAFN and AFP 2015a).

Guinea has closed its border with Sierra Leone. The closure was unexpected and caught many people off guard (Diallo 2015c).

Due to the risk posed by convalescent semen, the Liberian government is requesting all Ebola survivors to abstain from sex or use condoms. It is unclear how long people should do this, but the government says people should use these practices longer than the 3 months recommended by the WHO (South China Morning Post 2015).

Fourth grader Grace Winnie explains how Liberian students wash their hands. She says students at her school rub their palms together ten times, wash between the fingers and thumb five times, and then scrub around their nails (Irwin 2015).

The latest US Ebola patient continues to improve. The patient is now in fair condition (MENAFN and AFP 2015b).

April 1, 2015 (Wednesday)

Total cases: 25,213 (306 new)   Fatalities: 10,460 (134 new)
(World Health Organization 2015o)

Ten of the suspected cases identified during Sierra Leone's 3-day lockdown have tested positive for Ebola (CBS News 2015). As case numbers fall, Sierra Leone will begin to reduce the number of Ebola healthcare workers in the country (Fofana 2015a). The last Cuban healthcare workers left Sierra Leone today (AFP 2015k). Schools in Sierra Leone are scheduled to reopen on April 14, 2015 (Fofana 2015a).

The five US healthcare workers who were being monitored for Ebola in Nebraska have been released. None developed the disease (Reuters 2015r).

Emory University Hospital continues to collect and store convalescent blood plasma (Emory Medicine 2015).

Since March 2014, Ghana has tested 140 people for Ebola (Ghanaian Times 2015). All have been negative.

April 3, 2015 (Friday)

Levine et al. (2015) have developed a score-based system for clinically determining whether a suspect patient has Ebola. Points are assigned for each symptom exhibited by a patient. The higher the score, the more likely it is the patient has Ebola. The six factors most closely associated with having Ebola are having had contact with a sick person, diarrhea, anorexia, muscle pain, difficulty swallowing, and lack of abdominal pain. Data came from an assessment of 382 patients treated at the Bong Ebola Treatment Unit in Liberia (Levine et al. 2015).

April 4, 2015 (Saturday)

A 9-month-old boy has died from Ebola in Kailahun District, Sierra Leone. This is the first Ebola case in Kailahun in almost 4 months (Fofana 2015b; O'Carroll 2015e).

April 7, 2015 (Tuesday)

Officials say the reports of a 9-month-old boy dying from Ebola in Kailahun District, Sierra Leone, were wrong. The child died from other causes and did not have Ebola (Reuters 2015s).

In Freetown, Sierra Leone, 13 people were arrested for conducting an unsafe burial. A tip led police to a group of people with a coffin containing the body of a 50-year-old man. The group did not have a burial certificate. The body was given to an official burial team for proper internment (Xinhua 2015b).

Residents of Giah Town, Liberia, blocked the road leading to the Disco Hill Ebola cemetery. The residents say the government still owes them $25,000 for the land. The land was purchased in December 2014, but so far, the government has only paid half of the agreed-upon price (Weedee-Conway 2015).

The most recent US Ebola patient continues to improve. The patient is now in good condition (Fox 2015d).

The World Federation of Science Journalist has developed an online Ebola course. The class is designed to help journalists better report about the disease (Sci Dev Net 2015).

April 8, 2015 (Wednesday)

Total cases: 25,550 (337 new)   Fatalities: 10,587 (127 new)
(World Health Organization 2015p)

There were 30 new confirmed Ebola cases in West Africa during the past week. This is the lowest weekly total since the third week of May 2014 (World Health Organization 2015p).

MSF Head of Mission Jose Hulsenbek says the agency has treated a total of 4962 Ebola patients in Guinea, Liberia, and Sierra Leone. Of these, 2329 have survived. Over the same period, 28 MSF staff members contracted Ebola, 14 of them died (Milton 2015).

April 9, 2015 (Thursday)
Half of all new Ebola cases are currently coming from two districts on the Sierra Leone-Guinea border (News24 2015a)

The most recent US Ebola patient has recovered and been released from the NIH facility in Maryland (Sifferlin 2015c). The patient began treatment at the site on March 13, 2015.

April 10, 2015 (Friday)
As case numbers fall, the WHO believes the risk of Ebola spreading out of West Africa is diminishing (Mundasad 2015).

April 11, 2015 (Saturday)
Officials say only 28 confirmed Ebola patients were treated in the 11 US-built Ebola treatment centers in Liberia. While this appears to be a very small number, Jeremy Konyndyk of the US Agency for International Development thinks the US approach was the correct one. At the time US aid was committed, models were predicting very high levels of Ebola infection in West Africa. It was important for facilities to be in place if large numbers of victims needed treatment. So far, the US response to the West African Ebola outbreak has cost $1.4 B (Onishi 2015).

April 14, 2015 (Tuesday)
Schools in Sierra Leone have reopened (Butty 2015b; Jabati 2015). All students have their temperatures taken before they are allowed to enter school buildings. To help with this, 65,000 thermometers were distributed to the country's 9000 schools. Cleaning supplies were also distributed (Butty 2015b).

Since October 2014, New Jersey has screened 1408 passengers arriving from West Africa for Ebola. Of these, 642 were monitored for 21-day quarantine periods. Twenty-one were sent to hospitals for additional screening. None of the quarantined individuals developed Ebola. By mid-March 2015, the state had spent $2.6 M on its Ebola response (O'Brien 2015).

April 15, 2015 (Wednesday)

Total cases: 25,826 (276 new)   Fatalities: 10,704 (117 new)
                              (World Health Organization 2015q)

Traces of Ebola have been found in the semen of an Ebola survivor 175 days (i.e., 6 months) after his blood tested negative for the disease. The WHO now requests that survivors practice safe sex until it can be determined how long convalescent semen remains infectious (AFP 2015l).

April 16, 2015 (Thursday)
The quarantine of the Kroo Bay community in Sierra Leone has been lifted. An Ebola case was detected in the slum 21 days earlier. Officials quarantined the area to prevent the spread of the disease. No one else in the community became infected (Turay 2015).

April 17, 2015 (Friday)
Liberia, Sierra Leone, and Guinea have requested an $8 B Marshall Plan to help rebuild the region's economy and assist with Ebola prevention (AFP 2015m).

April 18, 2015 (Saturday)
Protesting Liberian healthcare workers blocked the entrance to the ELWA-3 Ebola treatment center. The workers say the government has not paid their Ebola hazard pay (Sky News 2015b).

April 19, 2015 (Sunday)
Zimbabwe has banned the repatriation of bodies from West Africa. The country is concerned that deceased Zimbabwe citizens could have died from Ebola or been in close proximity to the bodies Ebola victims (AllAfrica 2015h).

April 20, 2015 (Monday)
The *New York Times* has won two Pulitzer prizes for its coverage of the West African Ebola outbreak. The first prize went to the *New York Times* staff for excellence in international reporting. The second prize went to freelance photojournalist Daniel Berehulak for feature photography (Wulfhorst 2015).

April 21, 2015 (Tuesday)
The UK's Royal Fleet Auxiliary ship *Argus* has been awarded an Admiralty Board Letter of Commendation for its work in West Africa. This is an exceptionally rare award. The last time it was issued was in 1939 at the beginning of World War II (Mitchell 2015).

Guinea has reopened its border with Liberia (Gortor 2015b).

April 22, 2015 (Wednesday)

Total cases: 26,079 (253 new)   Fatalities: 10,823 (119 new)
(World Health Organization 2015r)

Eleven people have been given life sentences for the murder of the Ebola team in Womey, Guinea, in September 2014 (Reuters 2015t).

April 23, 2015 (Thursday)
US regulators have issued a global recall for a 10-min Ebola test produced by LuSys Laboratories, Inc. Officials say the test has not been cleared for sale and that it has not been demonstrated to be accurate (AFP 2015n).

Five US troops contracted malaria while they were deployed in West Africa (Kime 2015).

April 25, 2015 (Saturday)

An unexpected consequence of the Ebola outbreak in Sierra Leone has been an increase in the risk of rabies. During the epidemic, many dog owners worried that their dogs could carry Ebola. So they freed them. This has caused the dog population in the country to increase and has led to an increase in the incidence of rabies (VOA News 2015a).

April 28, 2015 (Tuesday)

MSF has turned over control of the ELWA-3 Ebola treatment center to the Liberian Ministry of Health (AllAfrica 2015i). The center currently has a 30-bed capacity (AllAfrica 2015i). Assuming no new cases develop, Liberia will be declared Ebola-free on May 9, 2015 (Heritage Liberia 2015).

The WHO will try to identify and isolate all remaining West African Ebola cases by the end of May 2015 (Cheng 2015c).

April 29, 2015 (Wednesday)

Total cases: 26,312 (233 new)   Fatalities: 10,899 (76 new)
(World Health Organization 2015s)

Peter Jan Graaff has been appointed the Special Representative for UNMEER. He visited Sierra Leone today (United Nations 2015).

April 30, 2015 (Thursday)

The United States has closed one of its Ebola treatment centers in Liberia. With its closing, only six of the US-built facilities remain open (VOA News 2015b).

Post-Ebola Syndrome appears to be very common among Ebola survivors. In Monrovia, Liberia, almost 40% of 1000 survivors have developed eye disorders. Uveitis – an inflammation of the eye that causes blurred vision – is the most commonly reported problem. Without treatment, uveitis can lead to blindness. Officials worry that many survivors will not receive the care they need before irreversible eye damage has occurred. American survivor Ian Crozier also has severe eye problems (McKay 2015).

May 4, 2015 (Monday)

UNMEER says its goal is to end Ebola before the start of the rainy season, approximately at the beginning of June (GNA 2015).

In Sierra Leone, 600 staff members of the Police Training School Ebola Treatment Centre at Hastings were presented with Certificates of Merit and Appreciation for their work during the outbreak. The holding and treatment center admitted 575 patients while it was open between December 18, 2014 and April 15, 2015 (AllAfrica 2015j).

Given the decreasing number of Ebola cases in Liberia, the CDC has altered its recommendations for US citizens traveling to the country. The agency no longer recommends avoiding nonessential travel to Liberia. The CDC does recommend that travelers use enhanced precautions while they are in Liberia (Centers for Disease Control and Prevention 2015a).

May 6, 2015 (Wednesday)

Total cases: 26,628 (316 new)   Fatalities: 11,020 (121 new)
                                (World Health Organization 2015t)

There were 18 new confirmed Ebola cases during the week ending May 3, 2015. Nine were in Guinea; nine were in Sierra Leone (World Health Organization 2015t).

Of 1100 Liberians households surveyed in December 2014, 93% say they first learned about Ebola from the radio and 98% changed one personal behavior in response to the outbreak (such as increasing hand-washing). However, 33% thought Ebola could be spread by mosquitoes and 26% thought it could be prevented by bathing in hot water or salt water (Waylaun 2015).

May 7, 2015 (Thursday)
Varkey et al. (2015) describe the effect Ebola has had on Dr. Ian Crozier's eyes and vision. About 2 months after Dr. Crozier was released from Emory University Hospital, he developed severe eye problems, mainly with his left eye (Grady 2015; Varkey et al. 2015). He experienced intense pain, decreased visual acuity, and increased eye pressure. When tested, Ebola virus was found in the aqueous humor of his eyes, but not on the surface of his eyes or in his tears (Varkey et al. 2015). His vision is normally 20/15. Five days after the onset of symptoms, the acuity of the left eye had dropped to 20/60. It eventually dropped to 20/400. After treatment, his visual acuity returned to 20/15 (Varkey et al. 2015). Another striking feature of Dr. Crozier's eye pathology is that the color of his left eye has changed from blue to green. It is unclear if this is a permanent change (Grady 2015). Dr. Crozier has also been suffering joint and muscle pain, fatigue, and hearing loss (Grady 2015).

May 8, 2015 (Friday)
Many of Guinea's traditional healers have stopped treating patients due to the Ebola outbreak. This has imposed significant economic hardship on the healers. If they do not practice, they do not earn an income. Consequently, some have turned to begging (Diallo 2015).

May 9, 2015 (Saturday)
Liberia is now officially Ebola-free (World Health Organization 2015u). It has been 42 days – two incubation periods – since the last known Ebola case in the country. Liberian President Ellen Johnson Sirleaf says Liberians should celebrate, but they should also remain mindful and vigilant (Fink 2015c). The White House has congratulated Liberia for becoming Ebola-free (Levine 2015).

May 11, 2015 (Monday)
Liberians are celebrating the end of the Ebola outbreak. The government has declared today a public holiday and people are celebrating in the streets. Many are carrying or wearing signs saying Liberia is Ebola-free (Associated Press et al. 2015).

In Sierra Leone, Red Cross burial volunteer Abdul Karim Conte has been burying five to ten bodies a day. He sometimes dreams about the victims and worries their spirits are angry with him (International Federation of Red Cross and Red Crescent Societies 2015).

Canada will resume processing the visa applications of Liberian residents. Canada stopped processing Liberian applications at the end of October 2014 (Canadian Press 2015).

May 12, 2015 (Tuesday)

A male nurse [Stefano Marongiu] has tested positive for Ebola in Sardinia, Italy (AGI 2015; Sky News 2015c). The nurse had been working for an Italian NGO in Sierra Leone. He developed symptoms Sunday, May 10, 2015. He has been isolated in the Hospital of Sassari and will be transferred to Rome via a specially equipped plane for treatment in Lazzaro Spallanzani Hospital (AGI 2015).

The end of the Liberian Ebola outbreak is having some unintended consequences. Because of the outbreak, many Liberians are now afraid to visit medical clinics (Fox 2015e). As a result, people are not being treated for common illnesses like malaria. Officials worry that this will lead to significant morbidity and mortality in the country (Fox 2015e). It is also believed that too few data were collected from vaccine trials to assess the effectiveness of the experimental Ebola vaccines being tested in Liberia (Reuters 2015u).

China has closed its Ebola treatment unit in Liberia and has turned the facility over to the Liberian Government (AllAfrica 2015k)

West African radio stations and disk jockeys are being recognized for their help in fighting Ebola. Radio broadcasts provided residents with critical information about the disease (Conteh 2015).

May 13, 2015 (Wednesday)

Total cases: 26,759 (131 new)   Fatalities: 11,080 (60 new)
(World Health Organization 2015v)

The WHO has released more information about the new Italian Ebola patient. The patient [Stefano Marongiu] had been working in Sierra Leone and flew from Freetown to Rome via Casablanca, Morocco, on May 7, 2015. He began to develop symptoms on May 10, 2015 and was isolated. He has been transferred to a treatment facility in Rome. Those who had contact with the patient are under surveillance (World Health Organization 2015w).

There were nine new confirmed Ebola cases during the week ending May 10, 2015. This is the lowest weekly number of Ebola cases this year (World Health Organization 2015v).

Kenya has lifted its travel ban on Liberia. However, Kenya will continue to screen passengers coming from Liberia until the entire outbreak has ended (Okafor 2015).

May 15, 2015 (Friday)
Guinea may be seeing an uptick in Ebola cases. Five new cases were identified in the country in past day alone. It is thought that unsafe burials are contributing to the increase in cases (Reuters 2015v).

May 16, 2015 (Saturday)
Thirteen people who had contact with the Italian Ebola victim are now quarantined in Italy (IANS 2015b).

May 19, 2015 (Tuesday)
There has been a spike in Ebola cases in Sierra Leone and Guinea (Reuters 2015w). A total of 36 new cases were identified in the past week. This is almost four times more than the previous week. Many of the 27 new Guinean cases occurred in Forecariah Prefecture (Nossiter 2015; Reuters 2015w).

May 20, 2015 (Wednesday)

Total cases: 26,969 (210 new)   Fatalities: 11,135 (55 new)
(World Health Organization 2015x)

There has been a substantial increase in the number of Ebola cases in West Africa. During the week ending May 17, 2015, 27 new cases were reported in Guinea, compared to 7 the previous week. Most of the new cases are in Dubreka and Forecariah Prefectures. Many of the cases in Dubreka are linked to the funeral of a suspected Ebola victim who was buried in mid-April 2015. However, nine of the Guinean cases have no known origin. This means some chains of transmission remain undetected. In response to the increase in cases, the WHO has deployed a response team to the border of Guinea and Guinea-Bissau (World Health Organization 2015x).

Sierra Leone officials are reminding people to remain vigilant and continue to follow all Ebola-fighting regulations. Ebola Czar Paolo Conteh told a cautionary tale about a man who recently fled quarantine in Freetown. The infected man was located after a week and was returned to isolation. However, because of his escape, 52 additional people are now under quarantine. At present, a total of 578 people are under quarantine in Sierra Leone (Johnson and Larson 2015).

May 21, 2015 (Thursday)
Liberia plans to erect a national memorial for Ebola victims (VOA News 2015c).

May 22, 2015 (Friday)
Some families in Guinea are transporting the bodies of Ebola victims in public taxis. Police Captain Claude Onivogui says families are dressing up the bodies of Ebola victims and positioning them upright between other passengers so they look like they are alive. It is believed that this is being done so the dead can be brought to their home villages for traditional burial (Associated Press 2015k).

Now that Liberia is Ebola-free, food sellers are requesting that the country lift its ban on bushmeat (AllAfrica 2015l).

A threatening package was sent to former British MP George Galloway's West Yorkshire office. Inside the package were a handkerchief and a note. The note said the handkerchief was infected with Ebola. Tests detected no Ebola (Yorkshire Post 2015).

May 24, 2015 (Sunday)
Mohamed Sesay is the only survivor of an eight-person laboratory unit in Sierra Leone. Sesay was working in the Lassa fever laboratory at the Kenema Government Hospital when the Ebola outbreak struck. As the outbreak exploded, he and his colleagues tested an ever-increasing number of blood samples for Ebola. Over time each team member, including Sesay, contracted Ebola. All of the others died, leaving Sesay as the only survivor of the group (World Health Organization 2015y).

May 25, 2015 (Monday)
Six Guineans have been arrested for transporting a corpse in a taxi. The body was propped upright between three people and dressed in a T-shirt, jeans, and sunglasses. The deception was discovered when the "passenger" remained motionless during a checkpoint inspection (BBC 2015p).

May 26, 2015 (Tuesday)
More people were hospitalized in Dallas, Texas, during to the Ebola outbreak than previously reported. In addition to Amber Vinson and Nina Pham, 12 other people were hospitalized with Ebola-like symptoms, including 9 healthcare workers. All tested negative for Ebola and were released (Jacobson 2015).

May 27, 2015 (Wednesday)

Total cases: 27,049 (80 new)   Fatalities: 11,149 (14 new)
(World Health Organization 2015z)

May 29, 2015 (Friday)
An angry crowd attacked a police station and public buildings in the village of Kamsar, Guinea, today. The attack started when aid workers tried to identify a woman who was thought to have had contact with an Ebola patient (Brice 2015).

June 1, 2015 (Monday)
UN Ebola chief Dr. David Nabarro is optimistic about the course of Sierra Leone's Ebola fight. He says a great deal of progress is being made and it will probably only be a couple of weeks before the outbreak in Sierra Leone is over (Al Jazeera 2015b).

Sierra Leone's Chiefdom of Kaffu Bullom is experiencing a surge in Ebola cases. During the past week, six people have died from Ebola in the chiefdom. The spike started when an infected person returned to area from Kambia. The surge is of particular concern because an international airport is located in the chiefdom (Awareness Times 2015b, Bruz 2015).

Sierra Leonean lawmaker Alie Badara has been arrested for conducting an unsafe burial. His father died and Badara washed his corpse and conducted traditional burial rites (AFP 2015o).

June 2, 2015 (Tuesday)
Kenya Airways has resumed flights to Sierra Leone (Ngunze 2015).

June 3, 2015 (Wednesday)

Total cases: 27,181 (132 new)   Fatalities: 11,162 (13 new)
                                (World Health Organization 2015aa)

Ebola activity remains relatively high in West Africa. During the week ending May 31, 2015, 25 new confirmed cases occurred in Guinea and Sierra Leone (World Health Organization 2015aa).

Travelers arriving in the United States from West Africa are still being monitored for Ebola. Virginia says it is currently monitoring 103 travelers (WRIC 2015).

June 4, 2015 (Thursday)
The WHO is worried that the start of the West African rainy season will make field operations and Ebola containment more difficult (BERNAMA 2015).

June 7, 2015 (Sunday)
A 6-day, door-to-door Ebola campaign has started in Boké and Coyah Prefectures, Guinea (World Health Organization 2015ac)

June 8, 2015 (Monday)
Guinea and Sierra Leone have both extended their health emergencies. The continued states of emergency will allow officials to keep anti-Ebola protocols and restrictions in place (Radio Cadena Agramonte 2015).

June 9, 2015 (Tuesday)
UNMEER's headquarters in Accra, Ghana, will close at the end of June 2015 (BBC 2015q). The station was established in September 2014 to help coordinate the international response to the outbreak.

June 10, 2015 (Wednesday)

Total cases: 27,273 (92 new)   Fatalities: 11,173 (11 new)
                               (World Health Organization 2015ab)

The decline in West African Ebola cases appears to have stalled. There were 31 new confirmed cases during the week ending June 7, 2015. Sixteen cases were in Guinea and 15 in Sierra Leone (World Health Organization 2015ab).

The infected Italian nurse, now identified as Stefano Marongiu, has recovered from Ebola and been released from the hospital (AFP 2015p).

June 11, 2015 (Thursday)
Dr. Abdul Kamara is the National Lab Services Manager of the Ministry of Health and Sanitation in Sierra Leone. He says between May 2014 and June 9, 2015, the lab conducted 53,784 Ebola tests. Of these, 45,146 were negative and 8638 were positive (Awoko 2015e).

Britain has finalized the design for a medal for UK workers who helped with the West African Ebola outbreak. The medal's obverse will have a portrait of the Queen designed by Ian Rank-Broadley. The reverse will be designed by John Bergdahl and feature a flame over the Ebola virus. Above the flame will be the words "For Service." Below the flame will be the words "Ebola Epidemic West Africa." More than 3000 medals are expected to be issued. They will be made by the Worcestershire Medal Service in Bromsgrove (Wilson 2015).

June 12, 2015 (Friday)
President of Sierra Leone Ernest Bai Koroma has announced a new 3-week, day-time curfew for Kambia and Port Loko Districts (Reuters 2015w). The curfew will begin immediately and run from 0600 to 1800 h each day. Sierra Leone's health minister says there are currently 22 people in Ebola treatment centers in the country, all in Kambia and Port Loko Districts (Bangkok Post 2015; Reuters 2015w).

June 17, 2015 (Wednesday)

Total cases: 27,341 (68 new)   Fatalities: 11,184 (11 new)
(World Health Organization 2015ac)

The United States has started to scale back airport screening for travelers arriving from Liberia. Liberian passengers still have to enter the United States through one of the five designated airports, but much less actual screening will take place (AllAfrica 2015m).

A 5-year study has started in Liberia to assess the long-term health effects of Ebola (e.g., post-Ebola syndrome). The study will also help determine how long survivors need to abstain from sex after they recover from the disease (Fox 2015f). Six survivors enrolled for the study at JFK hospital in Monrovia today (AFP 2015q).

June 19, 2015 (Friday)
Tekmira Pharmaceuticals will stop testing the TKM-Ebola-Guinea drug in Sierra Leone. It is a bit unclear why the company will stop the tests. The study's lead investigator says the research has reached a statistical endpoint (Ranosa 2015). This could mean the effect size of the drug is small. It could also mean that falling case numbers in Sierra Leone will prevent a large enough sample size from being obtained.

June 22, 2015 (Monday)
Two new Ebola cases have occurred in Freetown, Sierra Leone, in a slum known as Magazine. Freetown's last known case occurred 3 weeks ago. Officials say the first victim is a fisherman who caught the disease from his girlfriend in Port Loko. The second case is a person in the fisherman's home (Reuters 2015x).

Liberian businessman Delino Kollie is distributing cell phones to village chiefs along the Liberia-Guinea border. Kollie is concerned that Ebola could be reintroduced to Liberia from Guinea. He is urging chiefs to contact government officials if they suspect anyone with Ebola has entered their village. Phones will be given to about 20 chiefs (AllAfrica 2015n).

June 23, 2015 (Tuesday)
In Guinea, the disruption and fear caused by the Ebola outbreak caused 74,000 fewer malaria cases to be evaluated by medical workers in 2014 (Plucinski et al. 2015).

June 24, 2015 (Wednesday)

Total cases: 27,479 (138 new)   Fatalities: 11,222 (38 new)
(World Health Organization 2015ad)

There were 12 new confirmed Ebola cases in Guinea during the week ending June 21, 2015. There were eight new cases in Sierra Leone (World Health Organization 2015ad).

Dr. Amadou Talibe, an Ebola Response team worker in Dubreka, Guinea, believes the high mobility of the Guinean people is causing the uptick in Ebola cases (Bah 2015).

June 25, 2015 (Thursday)
Guinea has placed the villages of Sikhourou Koloteya, Tanéné, Bamba, and Tamarasy under 21-day quarantine. All four communities have had Ebola cases in the last few weeks. During the quarantine period, health officials will go door-to-door to provide information about Ebola and look for hidden cases. Sikhourou Koloteya is under quarantined as of today. The other villages will begin their quarantines tomorrow (Reuters 2015y).

Field tests of Corgenix Medical Corp's ReEBOV Ebola test have yielded very positive results. Test samples were assessed with both PCR and the ReEBOV fingerprick test. PCR is considered to be 100% accurate, but is time consuming. The fingerprick test takes only 15 min. The fingerprick test correctly identified all Ebola-positive samples. However, it also indicated that some uninfected samples were Ebola-positive. Thus, the ReEBOV test is considered to have 100% sensitivity and 92% specificity. Researchers are very happy with these results. The new test will allow Ebola cases to be rapidly identified in the field (Williams 2015b).

June 26, 2015 (Friday)
Three doctors and 28 nurses have been quarantined in Freetown, Sierra Leone. The healthcare workers assisted a pregnant, Ebola-positive woman. The woman is the third Ebola case reported from Freetown in the last week (AAP and Reuters 2015).

June 28, 2015 (Sunday)
Sierra Leone will crack down on violators of the country's anti-Ebola laws. Previously, almost all violators (such as those who practiced unsafe burials) were fined. The fines, however, have not stopped people from breaking the laws. Now violators will face 6 months in jail without the option of fines. There are currently 1029 people under quarantine in Sierra Leone (AFP 2015r).

June 30, 2015 (Tuesday)

A new Ebola case has been confirmed in Liberia. A 17-year-old boy [Abraham Memaigar] died on June 28, 2015, in the village of Nedowein near the country's international airport (Doucleff 2015; Reuters 2015z). He had been diagnosed with malaria, but samples taken before his death tested positive for Ebola (Fallah 2015). To see if these results were accurate, his body was exhumed and additional samples were taken. They confirmed the boy died from Ebola (Fallah 2015). This is the first known Ebola case in Liberia since the country was declared Ebola-free on May 9, 2015. Liberian officials are urging citizens to stay calm. They say the victim's corpse has been buried and contact tracing is underway (Doucleff 2015). Nearby homes have been quarantined (Doucleff 2015).

July 1, 2015 (Wednesday)

Total cases: 27,550 (71 new)   Fatalities: 11,235 (13 new)
                 (World Health Organization 2015ae)

Officials have confirmed two more Ebola cases in Liberia (Reuters 2015aa). The Liberian Information Ministry says both of the new cases live in or near the deceased teenager's house (Reuters 2015aa). One of the new patients is 24 years old, the other is 27 (Reuters 2015z). Officials have not yet determined how the initial victim became infected. It does not appear that he had any connections to Guinea or Sierra Leone (AllAfrica 2015o). Liberia's Deputy Health Minister says there are no plans to close Liberia's borders with Guinea or Sierra Leone (David 2015).

There are only seven patients in Ebola treatment centers in Sierra Leone (Awoko 2015f).

July 2, 2015 (Thursday)

About 100 people who had contact with Abraham Memaigar, the most recent Liberian Ebola fatality, are now under surveillance in Liberia (Fallah 2015). Four of these people are considered at high risk of exposure and have been taken to Monrovia for monitoring (Reuters 2015z). Neighbors say that Memaigar shared a meal of dog meat with several people. Three of these people have developed Ebola (Toweh and Giahyue 2015). The villagers think the meat is the source of the infection (Fallah 2015; Toweh and Giahyue 2015).

The CDC says 10,344 people were monitored for Ebola in the United States between November 2014 and March 2015 (Rettner 2015).

Government health officials in the Democratic Republic of the Congo and the WHO are investigating a possible Ebola outbreak in the Democratic Republic of the Congo. On June 26, 2015, six hunters became ill with Ebola-like symptoms in the village of Masambio. Four have since died (Reuters 2015ab). If it is Ebola, it is unclear if these infections are related to the West African outbreak or if they represent a separate disease event.

July 3, 2015 (Friday)
It is still unclear how Abraham Memaigar contracted Ebola. An anonymous villager says that, despite his family's denial, the boy actually did visit Guinea. He may have crossed into Guinea to see relatives when his soccer team traveled to Zorzor, Liberia, for a match (Front Page Africa 2015).

July 4, 2015 (Saturday)
The sick hunters in the Democratic Republic of the Congo have all tested negative for Ebola (Reuters 2015ac).

July 6, 2015 (Monday)
UN Special Envoy David Nabarro says as the outbreak winds down, Ebola flare-ups, like the one currently underway in Liberia, could continue for some time. He also says it is unclear how the recent Liberian Ebola victims became infected. They might have been infected through an undetected train of transmission, they may have caught the disease from a survivor, or they might have been infected from an outside zoonotic source (Boseley 2015c). This last possibility may refer to the dog meat some of the recent victims are reported to have consumed.

July 7, 2015 (Tuesday)
Researchers in Liberia have recovered and tested the remains of the dog linked to the new Liberian Ebola cases. The remains, said to be in bad condition, tested negative for Ebola (Reuters 2015ad).

July 8, 2015 (Wednesday)

Total cases: 27,609 (59 new)   Fatalities: 11,261 (26 new)
                                   (World Health Organization 2015af)

Two more Liberians have tested positive for Ebola. This brings the total number of cases in the county's recent flare-up to five (Schnirring 2015).

Sierra Leone will keep its current curfews in effect until Ebola is eliminated. The curfews are part of Operation *Northern Push*, which is an effort to end Ebola in the country's northwest regions (AFP 2015s).

July 9, 2015 (Thursday)
Genetic analysis of the virus isolated from Abraham Memaigar suggests he may have caught Ebola from a survivor rather than a current Ebola patient. The virus that killed Memaigar is most similar to the strain that was circulating in Liberia in July–August 2014. That strain is genetically different from the strain that is currently circulating in Guinea and Sierra Leone. If the new infection did come from a survivor, it is unclear how. Sexual transmission seems the most likely route, although Ebola can remain active in a several body areas (like the fluids of the eyes) long after a survivor has recovered (Fink 2015d).

July 11, 2015 (Saturday)
Two Ebola patients fled from a treatment center outside Freetown, Sierra Leone, today. The 32-year-old woman and 8-year-old girl were located in the evening and returned to the clinic (AFP 2015t).

July 13, 2015 (Monday)
Meyer et al. (2015) report that an experimental aerosolized Ebola vaccine provides full protection to rhesus macaques.

July 14, 2015 (Tuesday)
A Liberian woman died from Ebola shortly after she was admitted to a hospital in Monrovia (AFP and Reuters 2015b). The victim, Kebbeh Kollie, is the sixth known victim of the new Liberian outbreak (Giahyue 2015c). Kollie was the sister of one of the other five Liberian Ebola cases. Sixteen people are currently under quarantine in the country (Giahyue 2015c).

July 15, 2015 (Wednesday)

Total cases: 27,678 (69 new)   Fatalities: 11,276 (15 new)
                               (World Health Organization 2015ag)

   An International Medical Corps nurse has died from Ebola in Sierra Leone (O'Carroll 2015f).

July 16, 2015 (Thursday)
Due to the increase in Ebola cases in Freetown, Sierra Leone, the 34 Military Hospital will start admitting Ebola patients again (Reuters 2015ae).
   Some Ebola burial teams in Sierra Leone are reportedly extorting bribes to safely bury Ebola victims. Bribes of up to $247 are being requested before burials will be performed. Ebola Czar Paolo Conteh says these reports are being investigated (Reuters 2015ae).
   MSF currently has 92 international and ~1760 native staff on the ground in Liberia, Guinea, and Sierra Leone (Médecins Sans Frontières 2015b).

July 17, 2015 (Friday)
The four remaining Liberian Ebola patients have all recovered. The patients will be discharged with a ceremony on Monday, July 20, 2015 (Associated Press 2015l). Despite this good news, Liberian officials are looking for a male herbalist who fled quarantine in Nimba County (Reuters 2015af). The herbalist was under observation because he had treated Abraham Memaigar (Reuters 2015af).

July 20, 2015 (Monday)
The last four Liberian Ebola patients, two men and two boys, were released from the ELWA-2 clinic in Monrovia today (AFP 2015u). There are now no known Ebola cases in Liberia.

July 22, 2015 (Wednesday)

Total cases: 27,741 (63 new)   Fatalities: 11,284 (8 new)
                                (World Health Organization 2015ah)

There were 26 new confirmed Ebola cases during the week ending July 19, 2015. Twenty-two were in Guinea and four were in Sierra Leone (World Health Organization 2015ah).

July 23, 2015 (Thursday)
The United Kingdom has relaxed its Ebola screening procedures for travelers arriving from West Africa (BBC 2015r). On-site screenings will no longer take place at the Birmingham or Manchester airports or at the Eurostar terminal in St. Pancras. However, travelers arriving at these sites will still be screened over the phone. Normal screening procedures will continue at Heathrow and Gatwick airports where more than 90% of West African travelers enter the UK (BBC 2015r; Gibbons 2015).

July 26, 2015 (Sunday)
Ten of Sierra Leone's 14 districts have reported no new Ebola cases in the last 90 days. Tonkolili District reported one new Ebola case on Saturday. It had been 150 days since Tonkolili's last Ebola case (AFP 2015v).

July 29, 2015 (Wednesday)

Total cases: 27,784 (43 new)   Fatalities: 11,294 (10 new)
                                (World Health Organization 2015ai)

There were seven new confirmed Ebola cases during the week ending July 26, 2015. Four were in Guinea and three were in Sierra Leone. This is the lowest weekly total in over a year (World Health Organization 2015ai).

July 31, 2015 (Friday)
Phase III efficacy trials of the Merck and NewLink Genetics VSV-ZEBOV Ebola vaccine have yielded extraordinarily promising results [the World Health Organization (2015ai) attributed the vaccine to Merck, Sharp & Dohme; Henao-Restrepo et al. (2015) referred to the vaccine as rVSV-ZEBOV] (Henao-Restrepo et al. 2015; Reuters 2015ag; World Health Organization 2015aj). In Guinea, 4123 high-risk individuals were immediately vaccinated after they had contact with a person who was infected with Ebola (Henao-Restrepo et al. 2015). None of them developed the disease. This suggests that the vaccine might be 100% effective at preventing infection (Reuters 2015ag). The results are so promising the WHO released a press statement today entitled "world on the verge of an effective Ebola vaccine" (World Health Organization 2015ai). The statement described the trial and explained the potential significance of the vaccine. It also said that the trial started on March 23, 2015, but was stopped on July 26, 2015, so that all of the participants,

including those in the control group, could be immediately vaccinated (World
Health Organization 2015aj). If the vaccine's efficacy proves to be as high as these
initial results suggest, it could be a game-changer for Ebola treatment and prevention. Widespread use of the vaccine could end the current outbreak and prevent
future Ebola outbreaks.

There are concerns that there could be a new Ebola flare-up in Sierra Leone. A
man died from Ebola in Freetown. He had traveled to the city from Tonkolili to
mark the end of Ramadan. He did not know he was infected and had contact with
numerous people before he died. As a result, 624 people are now under quarantine
(DW 2015).

August 1, 2015 (Saturday)
Despite the positive results of recent Ebola vaccine trials, experts caution that it will
probably be at least several months before a vaccine is available for widespread
general use (VOA News 2015d).

August 2, 2015 (Sunday)
Two new Ebola cases have occurred in Sierra Leone. Both are relatives of the man
who recently died in Freetown (Al Jazeera 2015c).

August 5, 2015 (Wednesday)

Total cases: 27,898 (114 new)   Fatalities: 11,296 (2 new)
                                 (World Health Organization 2015ak)

There were only two new confirmed Ebola cases during the week ending
August 2, 2015: one in Guinea and one in Sierra Leone. This is very good news.
However, the WHO cautions that several high-risk events have recently
occurred in both countries and there will likely be more cases in the near future
(World Health Organization 2015ak).

August 6, 2015 (Thursday)
There are only four known Ebola cases in Sierra Leone. Sierra Leone's Ebola Czar,
Paolo Conteh, is optimistic and believes the end of the outbreak may be near
(Associated Press 2015m).

August 7, 2015 (Friday)
Due to the drop in cases, Sierra Leone's president has decided to end some of the
country's Ebola-fighting regulations. The restrictions on general public gatherings,
attending sports activities, and visiting nightclubs and movie theaters are all immediately lifted. The state of emergency is still in effect (Sierra Leone Telegraph 2015).

August 10, 2015 (Monday)
Residents of Sierra Leone are celebrating the lifting of many of the country's Ebola-
fighting restrictions. Ten of the country's 14 districts have been Ebola-free for over
100 days (O'Carroll 2015g).

August 11, 2015 (Tuesday)
The Kelekula Interim Care Center has closed in Liberia. The center took care of children who had been rejected by their families because of Ebola [it appears that some of the children had Ebola, others were Ebola orphans]. More than 50 children were housed in the facility during the outbreak, five of them died (Karmo 2015).

Two prototypes of a new infectious patient transport module have been unveiled at Dobbins Air Reserve Base, Marietta Georgia. The units, known as Containerized Bio-Containment Systems (CBCS), fit into aircraft and are designed to transport patients with highly infectious diseases (Frampton 2015).

August 12, 2015 (Wednesday)

Total cases: 27,965 (67 new)   Fatalities: 11,298 (2 new)
                         (World Health Organization 2015al)

There were three new confirmed Ebola cases during the week ending August 9, 2015: two in Guinea and one in Sierra Leone (World Health Organization 2015al).

Liberia is expanding its screening of travelers from Sierra Leone and Guinea. Liberia is doing everything it can to prevent the virus from being reintroduced to the country (Mahmud 2015).

August 15, 2015 (Saturday)
Sierra Leone has lifted the quarantine of Massessebeh village. This was the last major quarantine in the country. President Ernest Bai Koroma cut the quarantine ropes himself while the villagers celebrated (News24 2015b).

August 17, 2015 (Monday)
There were no new Ebola cases in Sierra Leone during the past week (Mazumdar 2015c). This is the first time since the beginning of the outbreak this has happened. The WHO says the country is down to its last known chain of Ebola transmission (World Health Organization 2015am). This is very good news, but officials continue to stress that the outbreak is not yet over. Two Ebola patients are being treated in the country, 81 people are under surveillance, and 4 people who are known to have had contact with infected individuals are missing (Mazumdar 2015c).

August 19, 2015 (Wednesday)

Total cases: 27,988 (23 new)   Fatalities: 11,299 (1 new)
                         (World Health Organization 2015an)

Three new Ebola cases were detected in West Africa during the week ending August 16, 2015, all in Guinea (World Health Organization 2015an).

August 24, 2015 (Monday)
Sierra Leone's last known Ebola patient has been released from the hospital (O'Carroll 2015h; Roy-Macaulay 2015). The patient, a woman named Adama Sankoh, contracted the disease from her 23-year-old son last month (O'Carroll

2015h; Roy-Macaulay 2015). Her son died from Ebola. President Ernest Bai Koroma personally presented Sankoh with her certificate of discharge (Roy-Macaulay 2015).

August 25, 2015 (Tuesday)
The 101st Airborne will receive the Joint Meritorious Unit Award for its work fighting Ebola in Liberia (Kenning 2015)

August 26, 2015 (Wednesday)

Total cases: 28,041 (53 new)   Fatalities: 11,302 (3 new)
(World Health Organization 2015ao)

   Three new Ebola cases were detected in Guinea during the week ending August 23, 2015 (World Health Organization 2015ao).

August 27, 2015 (Thursday)
The CDC has released an updated, detailed set of PPE guidelines for US healthcare workers treating Ebola patients (Centers for Disease Control and Prevention 2015b).

August 30, 2015 (Sunday)
Sierra Leone has confirmed a new Ebola death (Reuters 2015ah). A 67-year-old woman died in Kambia District on August 29, 2015. Samples collected from her body confirm she had Ebola (Reuters 2015ah). Twenty high-risk contacts have been isolated and will be vaccinated. This is a significant setback for Sierra Leone (Awoko 2015g). Not only does it represent a new Ebola case in the country, but it also suggests there might be other undetected chains of transmission.

September 2, 2015 (Wednesday)

Total cases: 28,109 (68 new)   Fatalities: 11,305 (3 new)
(World Health Organization 2015ap)

   There were three new confirmed Ebola cases during the week ending August 30, 2015. Two were in Guinea and one was in Sierra Leone (World Health Organization 2015ap).
   In Sierra Leone, 50 people have been quarantined and 200 will be vaccinated as a result of the new Ebola case (Butty 2015c; Regan 2015).

September 3, 2015 (Thursday)
Liberia is Ebola-free after its recent flare-up (AFP 2015w). This is the second time Liberia has reached Ebola-free status. It is hoped that this time the designation will be permanent.

September 8, 2015 (Tuesday)
Three new Ebola cases have been detected in Sella Kafta village in Kambia District, Sierra Leone. All of the new cases are linked to the Ebola victim who died on August 29, 2015 (ABC News 2015d).

September 9, 2015 (Wednesday)

Total cases: 28,183 (74 new)   Fatalities: 11,306 (1 new)
                                (World Health Organization 2015aq)

There were two new confirmed Ebola cases during the week ending September 6, 2015: one in Guinea and one in Sierra Leone (World Health Organization 2015aq).

The WHO says male Ebola survivors should be tested monthly until no active virus remains in their semen (Miles 2015). There are increasing concerns that infectious semen of survivors could cause Ebola flare-ups in West Africa.

September 14, 2015 (Monday)
A 16-year-old girl has died from Ebola in Bombali District, Sierra Leone (Al Jazeera 2015d). It has been 169 days since the district's last Ebola case (Al Jazeera 2015d). Officials think the girl may have become infected through sexual contact with a survivor (Quashie 2015). The girl died on Sunday, but it appears her Ebola-positive status was not detected until today. The village of Robuya has been quarantined and seven high-risk contacts have been isolated (Quashie 2015).

September 15, 2015 (Tuesday)
It remains unclear how the most recent Sierra Leone Ebola fatality became infected. Suspicion remains focused on sexual contact she had with an Ebola survivor. However, Bombali's Ebola Response Coordinator says the survivor in question was discharged in March 2015 (6 months ago), much longer than semen is normally thought to remain infectious (Jerry 2015).

September 16, 2015 (Wednesday)

Total cases: 28,256 (73 new)   Fatalities: 11,306 (0 new)
                                (World Health Organization 2015ar)

There were five new confirmed Ebola cases during the week ending September 13, 2015, all in Sierra Leone. This was the first week in over a year that Guinea did not have a new Ebola case. The last known Guinean case occurred on September 1, 2015, in Conakry (World Health Organization 2015ar). This is also the first week that no confirmed or suspected Ebola deaths occurred, although the situation report does not appear to include the 16-year-old girl who died from Ebola in Sierra Leone on September 13, 2015.

Sierra Leone's GDP is expected to fall by 21.5% in 2015, mostly because of the Ebola outbreak (Sesay 2015).

September 17, 2015 (Thursday)
Sierra Leone is offering $1000 for information on the whereabouts of Kadiatu Sinneh Kamara. Kamara is a 32-year-old niece of the 67-year-old woman who died from Ebola on August 29, 2015 (APA 2015f, states the woman died on August 28). Kamara seems to have gone into hiding and government officials have been unable to locate her.

Currently, one confirmed and one suspected Ebola case are being treated in Guinea (Wild and Camara 2015).

September 18, 2015 (Friday)
The United States will end Ebola screening for travelers from Liberia on Monday, September 21, 2015 (Jansen 2015a). Screening started October 11, 2014.

September 21, 2015 (Monday)
The Guinean government thinks the Ebola outbreak will be over by November 2015 (Wild and Camara 2015).

September 22, 2015 (Tuesday)
Between October 11, 2014 and September 17, 2015, US airports screened 30,982 travelers from West Africa. No Ebola cases were detected (Jansen 2015b). Infected American doctor Dr. Craig Spencer past through airport screening while he was asymptomatic. He developed Ebola symptoms later.

September 23, 2015 (Wednesday)

Total cases: 28,331 (75 new)   Fatalities: 11,310 (4 new)
(World Health Organization 2015as)

There were two new confirmed Ebola cases during the week ending September 20, 2015, both in Guinea (World Health Organization 2015as).

September 25, 2015 (Friday)
Kenya Airways has resumed flights to Liberia and Sierra Leone (Reuters 2015ai).

September 27, 2015 (Sunday)
The last two Sierra Leone Ebola patients have been released from the Mathene Treatment Centre in Makeni (AFP 2015x). The country has started another 42-day countdown. If no new cases are detected, the country will be considered Ebola-free.

September 30, 2015 (Wednesday)

Total cases: 28,424 (93 new)   Fatalities: 11,311 (1 new)
(World Health Organization 2015at)

There were four new confirmed Ebola cases during the week ending September 27, 2015, all in Forecariah, Guinea. One victim is a 10-year-old girl. Two others are traditional healers who treated the girl. The fourth victim is the wife of one of the healers (World Health Organization 2015at)

Nigeria's Arik Air will resume flights to Monrovia, Liberia, starting October 5, 2015 (Aliyu 2015).

October 7, 2015 (Wednesday)

Total cases: 28,457 (33 new)   Fatalities: 11,312 (1 new)
                                   (World Health Organization 2015au)

There were no new confirmed Ebola cases during the week ending October 4, 2015 (World Health Organization 2015au). This is the first time since March 2014 that no new cases were detected during a week (BBC 2015s; World Health Organization 2015au). This is exceptionally good news and suggests the outbreak is nearing its end. There are no contacts currently under observation in Sierra Leone. In Guinea, 509 contacts remain under surveillance (World Health Organization 2015au).

October 9, 2015 (Friday)
Scottish nurse Pauline Cafferkey has suffered an unusual late complication of her Ebola infection (BBC 2015t). She started feeling ill on Tuesday, October 6, 2015, and checked into the Queen Elizabeth University Hospital in Glasgow, Scotland. Ebola virus particles were found in her body (BBC 2015t). This morning, a military aircraft flew her to the Royal Free Hospital in London (Courier 2015). She is currently in serious condition (Courier 2015). People who had close contact with Cafferkey are being monitored (BBC 2015t).

October 10, 2015 (Saturday)
Pauline Cafferkey traveled rather extensively before her recent Ebola relapse. People she had contact with are very concerned that they may have been exposed to Ebola. Cafferkey visited students at Mossneuk Primary School in East Kilbride, Lanarkshire, on October 5, 2015 (Kirby and Cameron 2015). She also attended an awards reception on September 29, 2015, where she met Samantha Cameron, the wife of the British Prime Minister David Cameron (Kirby and Cameron 2015). Health officials stress that there is little risk that people in the community will contract Ebola.

October 11, 2015 (Sunday)
More information is available about Pauline Cafferkey current illness. She began feeling ill the night of October 5, 2015, and went to an out-of-hours GP clinic at New Victoria hospital in Glasgow. The doctor who examined her thought she had a minor illness and sent her home (Brooks 2015a).

October 12, 2015 (Monday)
Fifty-eight people in the United Kingdom who had close contact with Pauline Cafferkey are being monitored for Ebola. They will be under surveillance for 21 days, during which time they will undergo twice daily temperature checks and be asked to restrict their travel. People who had direct contact with Cafferkey's body fluids have been offered the rVSV-ZEBOV vaccine. The vaccine is not yet licensed, but it seems to have been used successfully in field trials in Guinea (Brooks L 2015a).

October 13, 2015 (Tuesday)
Twenty-five people who had close contact with nurse Pauline Cafferkey have elected to take the experimental rVSV-ZEBOV Ebola vaccine. Fifteen people declined the vaccine or could not take it because of existing medical conditions (Bhutia 2015; Brooks L 2015b).

October 14, 2015 (Wednesday)

Total cases: 28,490 (33 new)   Fatalities: 11,312 (0 new)
(World Health Organization 2015av)

Pauline Cafferkey is now in critical condition. She remains isolated at the Royal Free Hospital in London. Doctors have released very little information about her current illness. News reports have described it as a recurrence of her earlier Ebola infection. Commenting on this unexpected situation, Jonathan Ball, professor of molecular virology at the University of Nottingham, says he is not aware of any other case where Ebola has led to life-threatening complications after a person has recovered (Boseley 2015d).

For the second week in a row, there were no new confirmed Ebola cases in West Africa. In Guinea, 150 contacts remain under surveillance (World Health Organization 2015av).

Deen et al. (2015) report that Ebola RNA can remain in the semen of convalescent patients for at least 9 months. Ebola virus RNA was present in the semen of all men tested 2–3 months after the onset of Ebola ($n = 9$ men). It was present in the semen of 65% of men 4–6 months after the onset of disease ($n = 40$ men tested). It was present in the semen of 26% of men 7–9 months after the onset of disease ($n = 43$ men tested). These results suggest that Ebola could be sexually transmitted long after a man has recovered from Ebola. It is not yet clear, however, how easy or difficult it is for sexual contact to actually lead to infection (Deen et al. 2015).

The Chinese corporation, CanSino Biotechnology Inc., will mass produce an Ebola vaccine that was developed by China's Academy of Military Medical Sciences. The company will produce the vaccine at a new facility in Tianjin. The factory is still under construction and should be completed by 2017–2018 (Reuters 2015aj).

October 15, 2015 (Thursday)
Doctors seem to think Pauline Cafferkey is suffering a relapse of Ebola. Dr. Margaret Harris, Communications Officer for the WHO, says that in some survivors it seems that the Ebola virus lies dormant and then begins reproducing again (Cheng 2015d).

October 16, 2015 (Friday)
Two new Ebola cases have been detected in Guinea: one in Forecariah and the other in Conakry (Reuters 2015ak).

October 19, 2015 (Monday)
Pauline Cafferkey's condition has improved. She is now in serious, but stable condition (Clarke-Billings 2015).

October 21, 2015 (Wednesday)
Total Cases: 28,512 (22 new)   Fatalities: 11,313 (1 new) (World Health Organization 2015aw)

Doctors have provided more information about Pauline Cafferkey's recent illness (BBC 2015u). They say she developed meningitis as a result of her Ebola infection. A small amount of virus had remained in her brain after her initial illness and had been slowly replicating. This eventually produced clinical meningitis. Given this unexpected late stage complication, the WHO says physicians should be on the lookout for meningitis in Ebola survivors (BBC 2015u). Fueling these concerns, health officials in Sierra Leone say there have been several unexplained deaths among Ebola survivors (Reuters 2015al). Cafferkey's condition continues to improve (BBC 2015u).

There were three new confirmed Ebola cases in Guinea during the week ending October 18, 2015 (World Health Organization 2015aw).

October 28, 2015 (Wednesday)

Total cases: 28,575 (63 new)   Fatalities: 11,313 (0 new)
                               (World Health Organization 2015ax)

There were three new confirmed Ebola cases during the week ending October 25, 2015, all in Guinea (World Health Organization 2015ax). All three were family members of a woman who died from Ebola. The new patients handled the deceased's woman's body without proper protection (Reuters 2015am).

Burial teams in Sierra Leone continue to conduct safe and dignified burials even though there have been no new Ebola cases in the country for several weeks (Marrier d'Unienville 2015).

October 30, 2015 (Friday)
Empirical data suggest that funerals have been a major source of Ebola infection in West Africa. A poster presented by Mills et al. at the meeting of the American Society of Tropical Medicine and Hygiene reports that of 6403 Ebola victims, 24.5% appear to have been infected while attending a funeral. The percentage of funeral-related infection varies by country. In Sierra Leone, 30.0% of victims were exposed at funerals, in Guinea 23.8%, and in Liberia 14.1% (Susman 2015).

November 1, 2015 (Sunday)
In Guinea, a newborn baby has tested positive for Ebola even though both of his parents are Ebola-negative (APA 2015g). It is unclear if this is a false positive test result. Officials are investigating.

November 4, 2015 (Wednesday)

Total cases: 28,607 (32 new)   Fatalities: 11,314 (1 new)
                               (World Health Organization 2015ay)

There was one new confirmed Ebola case in Guinea during the week ending November 1, 2015. This was the infected newborn reported on November 1, 2015 (World Health Organization 2015ay). No new cases were detected in Sierra Leone.

November 7, 2015 (Saturday)
Sierra Leone is now officially Ebola-free (World Health Organization 2015az). It has been 42 days since the last confirmed Ebola case in the country (Reuters 2015an). Celebrations have been relatively low-key, but elaborate ceremonies are planned (Johnson 2015c). Crowds gathered late Friday night to mark the end of the outbreak (Johnson 2015c)

November 8, 2015 (Sunday)
Residents of Freetown, Sierra Leone, held a candlelight vigil to celebrate the end of the Ebola outbreak (Reuters 2015an).

November 9, 2015 (Monday)
Ten workers at the Queen Elizabeth University Hospital in Glasgow, Scotland, were accidentally exposed to infected Ebola samples. While Pauline Cafferkey was at the facility, at least one of her samples was not labeled high risk. Consequently, the staff did not use appropriate precautions when they handled her samples. The exposed staff members are now under surveillance (Aitken 2015).

Officials in Guinea say some Guinean citizens are prematurely acting as if Ebola is gone. A spokesman for Guinea's Ebola task force says Guineans are not washing their hands as much as before and have resumed shaking hands (Associated Press 2015n).

November 11, 2015 (Wednesday)

Total cases: 28,635 (28 new)   Fatalities: 11,314 (0 new)
(World Health Organization 2015ba)

There were no new confirmed Ebola cases during the week ending November 8, 2015. Guinea is the only Ebola-active country (World Health Organization 2015ba).

November 12, 2015 (Thursday)
Pauline Cafferkey has made a full recovery from her recent attack of Ebola-induced meningitis. She has been transferred from the Royal Free Hospital in London to the Queen Elizabeth University Hospital in Glasgow for follow-up care (BBC 2015v).

November 14, 2015 (Saturday)
The last 68 Ebola contacts have been released from quarantine in Guinea. There are no longer any people in the country known to have had contact with an Ebola victim. Officials are cautiously optimistic that the end of the outbreak may be in sight (Reuters 2015ao).

November 17, 2015 (Tuesday)
Guinea's last known Ebola patient, a baby girl named Nubia, has recovered at a medical facility in Conakry (Reuters 2015ap). Nubia was born on October 27, 2014.

Her infected mother died from Ebola a few hours after she gave birth to Nubia (Zoroya 2015c). Nubia is the first baby born with Ebola known to have survived (Zoroya 2015c). If no new cases occur, Guinea will be considered Ebola-free in 42 days.

November 18, 2015 (Wednesday)

Total cases: 28,634 (−1 new)   Fatalities: 11,314 (0 new)
                                 (World Health Organization 2015bb)

There were no new confirmed Ebola cases during the week ending November 15, 2015 (World Health Organization 2015bb). It is unclear why the total number of Ebola cases was reduced by one.

November 19, 2015 (Thursday)
A 15-year-old-boy named Nathan Gbotoe has been diagnosed with Ebola in Liberia (initial reports indicated he was 10 years old) (Al Jazeera 2015e; Beaubien 2015; Reuters 2015aq). Gbotoe began feeling sick on November 14, 2015 (Beubien 2015). It is unclear how he became infected (Beaubien 2015). Gbotoe is the first Liberian Ebola patient since the country was declared Ebola-free on September 3, 2015.

November 20, 2015 (Friday)
Three new Ebola cases have been identified in Liberia (Cooper and Fink 2015). The new victims are Nathan Gbotoe, his father, and his 8-year-old brother (World Health Organization 2015bc).

November 22, 2015 (Sunday)
A total of 153 contacts are under surveillance in Liberia due to the recent Ebola flare-up (Giahyue 2015d).

November 23, 2015 (Monday)
Nathan Gbotoe has died from Ebola in Paynesville, Liberia (Chan 2015).

November 25, 2015 (Wednesday)

Total cases: 28,637 (3 new)   Fatalities: 11,314 (0 new)
                                (World Health Organization 2015bc)

The three new Ebola cases in today's situation report are all related to the current Liberian flare-up. Nathan Gbotoe's death is not yet included in the fatality data (World Health Organization 2015bc).

November 28, 2015 (Saturday)
Guinea's last known Ebola patient, the baby girl Nubia, has left the hospital (Farge 2015d).

December 2, 2015 (Wednesday)

Total cases: 28,637 (0 new)   Fatalities: 11,315 (1 new)
(World Health Organization 2015bd)

There were no new Ebola cases during the week ending November 29, 2015 (World Health Organization 2015bd).

December 3, 2015 (Thursday)
The last two Liberian Ebola patients, the father and brother of Nathan Gbotoe, have been released from the hospital. Close contacts of the family are still being monitored (AFP 2015y).

December 9, 2015 (Wednesday)

Total cases: 28,637 (0 new)   Fatalities: 11,315 (0 new)
(World Health Organization 2015be)

There were no new Ebola cases during the week ending December 6, 2015 (World Health Organization 2015be).

December 11, 2015 (Friday)
The last Liberian Ebola contacts have ended their surveillance periods (Doctor 2015). None developed Ebola.

The British Red Cross has ended its Ebola outbreak appeal. The appeal started in August 2014 when the agency began to solicit for donations to help with the West African Ebola outbreak. The agency collected $13.3 M during the appeal (British Red Cross 2015b).

December 16, 2015 (Wednesday)

Total cases: 28,640 (3 new)   Fatalities: 11,315 (0 new)
(World Health Organization 2015bf)

There were no new confirmed Ebola cases during the week ending December 13, 2015 (World Health Organization 2015bf).

December 18, 2015 (Friday)
Experts think the recent Liberian Ebola flare-up may have originated with Nathan Gbotoe's mother, Ophelia. Ophelia is an Ebola survivor and was pregnant when Gbotoe became infected (it is unclear at what stage of pregnancy). It is thought that latent Ebola in her system may have become infectious when pregnancy weakened her immune system (Farge and Giahyue 2015).

December 22, 2015 (Tuesday)
Sierra Leone has been removed from the CDC's list of nations subject to enhanced screening for health conditions and diseases (Vaccine News Reports 2015).

December 23, 2015 (Wednesday)

Total cases: 28,637 (−3 new)   Fatalities: 11,315 (0 new)
                             (World Health Organization 2015bg)

There were no new Ebola cases during the week ending December 20, 2015 (World Health Organization 2015bg).

December 29, 2015 (Tuesday)
Guinea is officially Ebola-free (World Health Organization 2015bh). Two 21-day incubation periods have passed since the last known Ebola case occurred in the country. Celebrations are planned, but given Ebola's ability to reemerge, officials are continuing to monitor the situation. Guinea will remain under heightened surveillance for the next 90 days (Du Lac 2015).

There are no known Ebola cases in West Africa.

December 30, 2015 (Wednesday)

Total cases: 28,637 (0 new)   Fatalities: 11,315 (0 new)
                             (World Health Organization 2015bi)

There were no new confirmed Ebola cases during the week ending December 27, 2015 (World Health Organization 2015bi).

January 3, 2016 (Sunday)

Total cases: 28,637 (0 new)   Fatalities: 11,315 (0 new)
                             (World Health Organization 2016a)

There were no new confirmed Ebola cases during the week ending January 3, 2016 (World Health Organization 2016a).

January 6, 2016 (Wednesday)
California will no longer monitor travelers arriving from West Africa for Ebola. Monitoring began on October 12, 2014. Since then ~1300 travelers have been monitored in the state. None developed Ebola (Morin 2016).

January 7, 2016 (Thursday)
Van Griensven et al. (2016) find that convalescent plasma does not significantly help Ebola patients. The fatality rate for 84 Ebola patients in Guinea transfused with 500 ml of convalescent plasma was 31%, compared to 38% for untreated patients. When the results were adjusted for patient age and Ebola virus cycle (i.e., how far along the infection was), there was even less difference. Thus, convalescent plasma does not appear to be an effective treatment for Ebola patients (Van Griensven et al. 2016).

January 10, 2016 (Sunday)
New York City will no longer monitor travelers arriving from West Africa for Ebola (Goldberg 2015).

January 14, 2016 (Thursday)
The West African Ebola outbreak is officially over (Maron 2016; Schlein 2015; World Health Organization 2016b). Two incubation periods have passed since the last known Liberian Ebola case. The WHO has declared Liberia to be Ebola-free (World Health Organization 2016b). All West African countries are now Ebola-free and there are no known Ebola cases anywhere in the world. However, additional flare-ups are likely given the nature of the disease and the ability of survivors to remain infectious (World Health Organization 2016b).

January 15, 2016 (Friday)
A new Ebola case has been confirmed in Sierra Leone (Fofana 2016; Karimi and McKenzie 2016). The victim is a 22-year-old female student named Mariatu Jalloh. She became sick in the village of Bamoi Luma near the Guinean border. She died at home on January 12, 2016. While she was infected, Jalloh had contact with at least 27 people (Fofana 2016). The case underscores the WHO's warning that there will likely be Ebola flare-ups for some time (World Health Organization 2016b).

January 18, 2016 (Monday)
Sierra Leone has placed 109 people into quarantine in response to the new Ebola case (Gaffey 2016a).

January 20, 2016 (Wednesday)

Total cases: 28,638 (1 new)   Fatalities: 11,315 (1 new)
(World Health Organization 2016c)

Fifty contacts of Sierra Leone's new Ebola case are considered at high risk of exposure (World Health Organization 2016c).

January 21, 2016 (Thursday)
A second person has developed Ebola in Sierra Leone. The new victim [Memunatu Kalokoh, Jalloh's aunt] helped prepare Mariatu Jalloh's body for burial (Roy-Macaulay 2016).

January 26, 2016 (Tuesday)
Police in Barmoi, Sierra Leone, have clashed with demonstrators protesting against Ebola restrictions. Three people were taken to the hospital with gunshot wounds (BBC 2016a).

February 3, 2016 (Wednesday)

Total cases: 28,639 (1 new)   Fatalities: 11,316 (0 new)
(World Health Organization 2016d)

February 4, 2016 (Thursday)
Fifty-five people in Sierra Leone who had contact with the most recent Ebola cases have been released from quarantine. Another 48 known contacts are missing and have not been located (Gaffey 2016b).

February 8 2016 (Monday)
Sierra Leone's last known Ebola patient, 38-year-old Memunatu Kalokoh, has recovered and been released from the hospital (Reuters 2016a).

February 18, 2016 (Thursday)
The United States has suspended Ebola screening at all airports (AFP 2016a).

February 23, 2016 (Tuesday)
Nurse Pauline Cafferkey has been admitted to the hospital again. She was initially treated at Glasgow hospital, but has been transferred to the Royal Free Hospital in London. It is unclear what is wrong with her, but she is currently in stable condition (Siddique 2016).

February 28, 2016 (Sunday)
Pauline Cafferkey has been released from the hospital after recovering from a complication related to Ebola (BBC 2016b).

March 18, 2016 (Friday)
Two people have died from Ebola in Guinea (AllAfrica 2016; BBC 2016c). The bodies of a married couple both tested positive for Ebola. Three other people may be infected (AllAfrica 2016).

March 19, 2016 (Saturday)
A young girl has died from Ebola at the Nzérékoré treatment center in Guinea (Reuters 2016b). She is the latest victim of the recent flare-up. An Ebola treatment center in southern Guinea has reopened to treat an infected woman and her child (MENAFN and AFP 2016). Both are relatives of the recent victims (MENAFN and AFP 2016).

March 22, 2016 (Tuesday)
A fifth person has died from Ebola in Guinea (Reuters 2016c). The deceased man had direct contact with the other recent victims (Reuters 2016c). A total of 816 contacts are now under quarantine in Guinea (Gaffey 2016c).

Liberia has closed its border with Guinea as a precaution (Reuters 2016c).

March 29, 2016 (Tuesday)
The WHO has downgraded the global health risk from Ebola. The WHO says the outbreak is essentially over and the agency no longer considers the outbreak to be an extraordinary health event (Roberts 2016).

March 30, 2016 (Wednesday)

Total cases: 28,646 (7 new)   Fatalities: 11,323 (7 new)
(World Health Organization 2016e)

March 31, 2016 (Thursday)
A 30-year-old woman has died from Ebola in Monrovia, Liberia. She was on her way to the hospital when she died (Sun Daily 2016).

April 2, 2016 (Saturday)
In Guinea, about 800 people who may have had contact with the recent Ebola victims have been vaccinated (Sun Daily 2016).

April 3, 2016 (Sunday)
The 5-year-old son of the latest Liberian Ebola victim has developed Ebola (Paye-Layleh 2016).

April 4, 2016 (Monday)
The woman who died from Ebola in Liberia on March 31, 2016, had traveled to Guinea. Her husband had died from the disease in Guinea. She crossed back into Liberia on March 21, 2016 (AFP 2016b).

April 7, 2016 (Thursday)
Ninety-seven people who had contact with the recent Ebola patients are under surveillance in Liberia (Parley 2016).

April 13, 2016 (Wednesday)
Mali says it is trying to locate two Guinean women who contact with the recent Ebola patients. The women are thought to have entered Mali on April 10, 2016 (Associated Press 2016).

April 20, 2016 (Wednesday)
Guinea has discharged its last known Ebola patient, an elderly man named Gbana Kalivogui (Vanguard 2016).

May 2, 2016 (Monday)
Liberia has discharged its last known Ebola patient, a 2-year-old boy. A ceremony was held to mark his release (World Health Organization 2016f).

June 9, 2016 (Thursday)
The recent Ebola flare-up in Liberia is officially over (World Health Organization 2016g). This marks the end of the 2013–2016 Ebola outbreak.

References

AAP (2015) Ebola crisis: Australian nurse airlifted to UK from Sierra Leone. AAP. The Australian. http://www.theaustralian.com.au/news/nation/ebola-crisis-australian-nurse-airlifted-to-uk-from-sierra-leone/story-e6frg6nf-1227234521866. Accessed 22 Feb 2015

AAP and Reuters (2015) Ebola: Sierra Leone, Guinea quarantine people, villages again. AAP, Reuters, The Sydney Morning Herald. http://www.smh.com.au/world/ebola-sierra-leone-guinea-quarantine-people-villages-again-20150626-ghytgy.html. Accessed 26 Jun 2015

ABC News (2015a) Clinical trial starts at Ebola center for anti-viral drug. ABC News. http://abcnews.go.com/Health/wireStory/clinical-trial-starts-ebola-center-anti-viral-drug-28022516. Accessed 6 Jan 2015

ABC News (2015b) Red Cross nurse dies of Ebola in Sierra Leone. ABC News. http://abcnews.go.com/Health/wireStory/red-cross-nurse-dies-ebola-sierra-leone-28242005. Accessed 15 Jan 2015

ABC News (2015c) Sierra Leone President predicts 0 Ebola cases by March end. ABC News. http://abcnews.go.com/Health/wireStory/sierra-leone-president-predicts-ebola-cases-march-end-28214113. Accessed 14 Jan 2015

ABC News (2015d) Sierra Leone officials confirm 3 new cases of Ebola. ABC News. http://abcnews.go.com/Health/wireStory/sierra-leone-officials-confirm-cases-ebola-33607923. Accessed 8 Sep 2015

AFP (2015a) Italy doctor with Ebola has recovered. AFP, Medical Xpress. https://medicalxpress.com/news/2015-01-italy-doctor-ebola-recovered.html. Accessed 13 Jul 2017

AFP (2015b) New Ebola lockdown in Sierra Leone as airport checks upped. AFP, The Peninsular. http://thepeninsulaqatar.com/news/international/314758/new-ebola-lockdown-in-sierra-leone-as-airport-checks-upped. Accessed 4 Jan 2015

AFP (2015c) Mob kills men in Guinea suspected of spreading Ebola. AFP, PRI. http://www.globalpost.com/dispatch/news/afp/150114/mob-kills-men-guinea-suspected-spreading-ebola. Accessed 14 Jan 2015

AFP (2015d) Sierra Leone lifts Ebola quarantines. AFP, Times of Oman. http://www.timesofoman.com/News/46181/Article-Sierra-Leone-lifts-Ebola-quarantines. Accessed 23 Jan 2015

AFP (2015e) Ebola: Liberia closes clinic. AFP, IOL. http://www.iol.co.za/news/africa/ebola-liberia-closes-clinic-1809632. Accessed 18 Jul 2017

AFP (2015f) Red Cross denounces attacks on Ebola teams. AFP, The Peninsula. http://thepeninsulaqatar.com/news/latest-news/321360/red-cross-denounces-attacks-on-ebola-teams. Accessed 11 Feb 2015

AFP (2015g) Violent protests in Ebola-hit Guinea. AFP, SBS. http://www.sbs.com.au/news/article/2015/02/10/violent-protests-ebola-hit-guinea. Accessed 11 Feb 2015

AFP (2015h) 1–3 m back in school in Ebola hit Guinea: UNICEF. AFP, Dunyanews. http://dunyanews.tv/index.php/en/World/261315-13m-back-in-school-in-Ebolahit-Guinea-UNICEF. Accessed 13 Feb 2015

AFP (2015i) Liberians rejoice as Ebola curfew is lifted. AFP, PRI. http://www.globalpost.com/dispatch/news/afp/150223/liberians-rejoice-ebola-curfew-lifted. Accessed 23 Feb 2015

AFP (2015j) U.S. wraps up its Ebola mission in Liberia. AFP, Dunyanews. http://dunyanews.tv/index.php/en/World/263993-US-wraps-up-its-ebola-mission-in-Liberia. Accessed 26 Feb 2015

AFP (2015k) Last Cuban Ebola medics leave S. Leone, new clampdown for Easter. AFP, Yahoo News. http://news.yahoo.com/last-cuban-ebola-medics-leave-leone-clampdown-easter-233542262.html;_ylt=AwrBEiLJ3RxVPlwAUlz_wgt. Accessed 2 Apr 2015

AFP (2015l) Ebola virus found in semen six months after recovery: WHO. AFP, Medical Xpress. https://medicalxpress.com/news/2015-04-ebola-virus-semen-months-recovery.html. Accessed 25 Jul 2017

AFP (2015m) Ebola-hit countries call for $8 bn for 'Marshall Plan'. AFP, Yahoo News. https://uk.news.yahoo.com/ebola-hit-countries-call-8-bn-marshall-plan-132939129.html#gytuhAm. Accessed 17 Apr 2015

AFP (2015n) US regulators recall 10-minute Ebola test. AFP, Yahoo News. http://news.yahoo.com/us-regulators-recall-10-minute-ebola-test-193530081.html. Accessed 23 Apr 2015

AFP (2015o) Lawmaker held over unsafe burial in Ebola-hit Sierra Leone. AFP, Yahoo News. http://news.yahoo.com/lawmaker-held-over-unsafe-burial-ebola-hit-sierra-171914700.html. Accessed 2 Jun 2015

AFP (2015p) Italian nurse cured of Ebola. AFP, Yahoo News. https://uk.news.yahoo.com/italian-nurse-cured-ebola-120902641.html#EVxQrgP. Accessed 10 Jun 2015

AFP (2015q) Thousands of Liberians in 'post-Ebola syndrome' study. AFP, Daily Nation. http://www.nation.co.ke/lifestyle/health/Thousands-suffer-post-Ebola-syndrome-study/-/1954202/2755946/-/s9rir6z/-/index.html. Accessed 18 Jun 2015

AFP (2015r) Sierra Leone will jail Ebola law violators. AFP, Yahoo News. http://news.yahoo.com/sierra-leone-jail-ebola-law-violators-172931252.html. Accessed 28 Jun 2015

AFP (2015s) Sierra Leone extends Ebola curfews indefinitely. AFP, The Sun Daily. http://www.thesundaily.my/news/1485096. Accessed 9 Jul 2015

AFP (2015t) Panic as Ebola patients escape in Sierra Leone. AFP, New Vision. http://www.newvision.co.ug/news/670948-panic-as-ebola-patiens-escape-in-sierra-leaone.html. Accessed 15 Jul 2015

AFP (2015u) Last four Liberian Ebola patients discharged. AFP, The Straits Times. http://www.straitstimes.com/world/africa/last-four-ebola-patients-in-liberia-discharged. Accessed 20 Jul 2015

AFP (2015v) Sierra Leone president unveils post-Ebola 'battle plan'. AFP, Yahoo News. http://news.yahoo.com/sierra-leone-president-unveils-post-ebola-battle-plan-175118537.html. Accessed 27 Jul 2015

AFP (2015w) Liberia declared free of Ebola – again: WHO. AFP, Yahoo News. http://news.yahoo.com/liberia-declared-free-ebola-again-073815188.html. Accessed 3 Sep 2015

AFP (2015x) Sierra Leone's last known Ebola patients leave hospital. AFP, Yahoo News. http://news.yahoo.com/sierra-leones-last-known-ebola-patients-leave-hospital-172438094.html. Accessed 27 Sep 2015

AFP (2015y) Liberia discharges last two Ebola cases: official. AFP, The Daily Star. http://www.thedailystar.net/backpage/liberia-discharges-last-two-ebola-cases-official-182536. Accessed 5 Dec 2015

AFP (2016a) US ends enhanced airport screening for Ebola. AFP, Yahoo News. http://news.yahoo.com/us-ends-enhanced-airport-screening-ebola-234544852.html. Accessed 19 Feb 2016

AFP (2016b) Liberia says latest Ebola fatality travelled to Guinea. AFP, The Sun Daily. http://www.thesundaily.my/news/1748599. Accessed 4 Apr 2016

AFP and Reuters (2015a) Ebola outbreak: Sierra Leone's capital deserted at start of new three-day anti-Ebola lockdown. AFP, Reuters, ABC Net. http://www.abc.net.au/news/2015-03-28/sierra-leone-in-new-anti-ebola-lockdown/6355234. Accessed 27 Mar 2015

AFP and Reuters (2015b) Liberia confirms new Ebola case as outbreak spread. AFP, Reuters, Asia One. http://yourhealth.asiaone.com/content/liberia-confirms-new-ebola-case-outbreak-spread. Accessed 14 Jul 2015

AGI (2015) Italian paramedic tests positive for Ebola virus. AGI. http://www.agi.it/en/italy/news/italian_paramedic_tests_positive_for_ebola_virus-201505122156-epp-rt10280. Accessed 12 May 2015

Aitken V (2015) Ten staff exposed to Ebola at Glasgow's Queen Elizabeth University Hospital after sample blunder. The Daily Record. http://www.dailyrecord.co.uk/news/health/ten-staff-exposed-ebola-glasgows-6801300. Accessed 10 Nov 2015

Aliyu A (2015) Liberia: Ebola – Arik resumes flight operations to Monrovia. AllAfrica, Daily Trust. http://allafrica.com/stories/201509301540.html. Accessed 1 Oct 2015

Al Jazeera (2015a) Ebola-related deaths pass 10,000 mark. Al Jazeera. http://www.aljazeera.com/news/africa/2015/03/ebola-related-deaths-pass-10000-mark-150312180128681.html. Accessed 3 Mar 2015

Al Jazeera (2015b) UN: Sierra Leone to be Ebola free in 'matter of weeks'. Al Jazeera. http://www.aljazeera.com/news/2015/06/sierra-leone-ebola-free-matter-weeks-150602044221757.html. Accessed 2 Jun 2015

Al Jazeera (2015c) Sierra Leone records two new cases of Ebola. Al Jazeera. http://www.aljazeera.com/news/2015/08/sierre-leone-records-cases-ebola-150803165143093.html. Accessed 3 Aug 2015

Al Jazeera (2015d) New Ebola death reported in northern Sierra Leone. Al Jazeera. http://america.aljazeera.com/articles/2015/9/14/new-ebola-death-reported-in-northern-sierra-leone.html. Accessed 14 Sep 2015

Al Jazeera (2015e) Fears in Liberia after new Ebola death. Al Jazeera, Yahoo News. https://en-maktoob.news.yahoo.com/fears-libera-ebola-fatality-074110657.html. Accessed 25 Nov 2015

AllAfrica (2015a) Sierra Leone: Pujehun achieves 42 days zero Ebola case. AllAfrica, Concord Times. http://allafrica.com/stories/201501091682.html. Accessed 9 Jan 2015

AllAfrica (2015b) Liberia targets February to be Ebola free. AllAfrica, The News. http://allafrica.com/stories/201501301282.html. Accessed 30 Jan 2015

AllAfrica (2015c) Gambia lifts travel ban to Ebola-affected countries. AllAfrica, The Point. http://allafrica.com/stories/201502092217.html. Accessed 10 Feb 2015

AllAfrica (2015d) Liberia: Returning to normalcy – Liberia household returns to work. AllAfrica, Front Page Africa. http://allafrica.com/stories/201502251136.html. Accessed 25 Feb 2015

AllAfrica (2015e) Liberia: No Ebola case for seven days. AllAfrica, The News. http://allafrica.com/stories/201503021915.html. Accessed 2 Mar 2015

AllAfrica (2015f) Liberia: MSF shuts Ebola care unit due to drop in cases. AllAfrica, LINA. http://allafrica.com/stories/201503261220.html. Accessed 25 Mar 2015

AllAfrica (2015g) Liberia: Kenya Airways Kq 509 Resumes Flight to Liberia. AllAfrica, Front Page Africa. http://allafrica.com/stories/201503271090.html. Accessed 27 Mar 2015

AllAfrica (2015h) Zimbabwe: Govt bans dead bodies from Ebola hit countries. AllAfrica, NewZimbabwe.com. http://allafrica.com/stories/201504200585.html. Accessed 20 Apr 2015

AllAfrica (2015i) Liberia: MSF hands over ELWA-3 to Ministry of Health. AllAfrica, Daily Observer. http://allafrica.com/stories/201504280953.html. Accessed 28 Apr 2015

AllAfrica (2015j) Sierra Leone: over 600 Ebola fighters get certificates of appreciation. AllAfrica, Government of Sierra Leone. http://allafrica.com/stories/201505071404.html. Accessed 7 May 2015

AllAfrica (2015k) Liberia: Chinese decommissions Ebola treatment unit in Liberia. AllAfrica, Front Page Africa. http://allafrica.com/stories/201505131629.html. Accessed 13 May 2015

AllAfrica (2015l) Liberia: post Ebola – Liberian bush meat sellers want ban lifted. AllAfrica, Front Page Africa. http://allafrica.com/stories/201505220586.html. Accessed 22 May 2015

AllAfrica (2015m) Liberia: U.S. revises airport screening procedures for Liberia passengers. AllAfrica, Front Page Africa. http://allafrica.com/stories/201506171551.html. Accessed 17 Jun 2015

AllAfria (2015n) Liberia: border town chiefs receive cell-phones against Ebola. AllAfrica, The New Dawn. http://allafrica.com/stories/201506221863.html. Accessed 22 Jun 2015

AllAfrica (2015o) Liberia: Govt investigates new Ebola source. AllAfrica, The New Dawn. http://allafrica.com/stories/201507011277.html. Accessed 1 Jul 2015

AllAfrica (2016) Guinea government confirms that two people have died from Ebola. AllAfrica, DW. http://allafrica.com/stories/201603180137.html. Accessed 18 Mar 2016

Andrews NM (2015) Liberia: 'We are rejected.' AllAfrica, The News. http://allafrica.com/stories/201501081205.html. Accessed 8 Jan 2015

APA (2015a) Ebola: Extra screening measures at S/Leone airport. APA, Star Africa. http://en.starafrica.com/news/ebola-extra-screening-measures-at-sleone-airport.html. Accessed 4 Jan 2015

APA (2015b) Official hails Sierra Leone's anti-Ebola operation as successful. APA, Star Africa. http://en.starafrica.com/news/official-hails-sierra-leones-anti-ebola-operation-as-successful.html. Accessed 8 Jan 2015

APA (2015c) Liberia: 12 Counties reports zero Ebola cases. APA, Star Africa. http://en.starafrica.com/news/liberia-12-counties-reports-zero-ebola-cases.html. Accessed 14 Jan 2015

APA (2015d) S Leone Journalists launch yellow ribbon Ebola awareness campaign. APA, Star Africa. http://en.starafrica.com/news/sleone-journalists-launch-yellow-ribbon-ebola-aware-ness-campaign.html. Accessed 14 Feb 2015

APA (2015e) Liberia to discharge last Ebola patient Thursday. APA, Star Africa. http://en.starafrica.com/news/liberia-to-discharge-last-ebola-patient-thursday.html. Accessed 4 Mar 2015

APA (2015f) Sierra Leone announces $1000 reward for information on Ebola suspect. APA, Star Africa. http://en.starafrica.com/news/sierra-leone-announces-1000-reward-for-information-on-ebola-suspect.html. Accessed 17 Sep 2015

APA (2015g) Guinea: Newborn tests positive for Ebola despite healthy parents. APA, Star Africa. http://en.starafrica.com/news/guinea-newborn-tests-positive-for-ebola-despite-healthy-parents.html. Accessed 2 Nov 2015

Associated Press (2015a) S Korean Ebola medic flown to Germany for anonymity. Associated Press, Waco Tribune-Herald. http://www.wacotrib.com/news/ap_nation/headlines/skorean-ebola-medic-flown-to-germany-for-anonymity/article_6e765c7d-0756-5618-97d0-dcdc941e-aba0.html. Accessed 3 Jan 2015

Associated Press (2015b) Tallmadge bridal store linked to Ebola survivor is closing. Associated Press, Hudson HUB Times. http://www.hudsonhubtimes.com/latest%20headlines/2015/01/08/tallmadge-bridal-store-linked-to-ebola-survivor-is-closing. Accessed 8 Jan 2015

Associated Press (2015c) Omaha hospital: Health care worker hasn't developed Ebola. Associated Press, The Miami Herald. http://www.miamiherald.com/living/health-fitness/article6218622.html. Accessed 13 Jan 2015

Associated Press (2015d) UN: At least 50 Ebola hotspots remain, but new cases falling. Associated Press, http://www.whas11.com/story/news/2015/01/15/50-ebola-hotspots-cases-declin-ing/21843521/. Accessed 16 Jan 2015

Associated Press (2015e) Ebola prompts mini-quarantine in Sierra Leone capital. Associated Press, USA Today. http://www.usatoday.com/story/news/2015/02/14/ebola-cases-prompt-mini-quarantine-in-sierra-leone-capital/23406259/. Accessed 13 Feb 2015

Associated Press (2015f) Last Ebola patient is released in Liberia. Associated Press, Portland Press Herald. http://www.pressherald.com/2015/03/05/last-ebola-patient-is-released-in-liberia/. Accessed 5 Mar 2015

Associated Press (2015g) American who contracted Ebola now in critical condition. Associated Press, Yahoo News. http://news.yahoo.com/american-contracted-ebola-now-critical-condi-tion-172202213.html. Accessed 16 Mar 2015

Associated Press (2015h) Families of Liberian health workers killed by Ebola get $5G. Associated Press, Fox News. http://www.foxnews.com/health/2015/03/20/families-health-workers-killed-by-ebola-in-liberia-get-5g/. Accessed 20 Mar 2015

Associated Press (2015i) AP News – Liberia investigates how most current Ebola patient got infected. Associated Press, Chronicle Bulletin. http://www.chroniclebulletin.com/world/ap-news-liberia-investigates-how-most-current-ebola-patient-got-infected-h4922.html. Accessed 21 Mar 2015

Associated Press (2015j) American who contracted Ebola improves, in serious condition. Associated Press, My Fox Dc. http://www.myfoxdc.com/story/28623374/american-who-con-tracted-ebola-improves-in-serious-condition. Accessed 26 Mar 2015

Associated Press (2015k) Guinea sees Ebola spike as families transport bodies on public buses. Associated Press, Chicago Tribune. http://www.chicagotribune.com/news/nationworld/ct-guinea-ebola-20150522-story.html. Accessed 22 May 2015

Associated Press (2015l) Liberia says 4 remaining Ebola patients have recovered. Associated Press, Hawaii News Now. http://www.hawaiinewsnow.com/story/29573258/liberia-says-4-remaining-ebola-patients-have-recovered. Accessed 17 Jul 2015

Associated Press (2015m) Sierra Leone's Ebola head says there's hope with only 4 cases. Associated Press, CTV News. http://www.ctvnews.ca/health/sierra-leone-s-ebola-head-says-there-s-hope-with-only-4-cases-1.2504854. Accessed 6 Aug 2015

Associated Press (2015n) Sierra Leone declared free of Ebola as Guinea struggles. Associated Press, Fox News. http://www.foxnews.com/health/2015/11/09/sierra-leone-declared-free-ebola-as-guinea-struggles.html. Accessed 10 Nov 2015

Associated Press (2016) Mali authorities seek 2 Guineans who had Ebola Contact. Associated Press, ABC News. http://abcnews.go.com/International/wireStory/mali-authorities-seek-guineans-ebola-contact-38359385. Accessed 14 Apr 2016

Associated Press, AFP, Macfarlan T (2015) Liberia is FREE of Ebola: Thousands gather in the streets to celebrate after country is given all clear from disease that killed 4,700. The Daily Mail. http://www.dailymail.co.uk/news/article-3077031/Liberias-government-holds-celebration-mark-Ebolas-end.html. Accessed 12 May 2015

Awareness Times (2015a) Sierra Leone news: WHH launches operation 'weed out the sick' in Tombo. Awareness Times. http://news.sl/drwebsite/publish/article_200527027.shtml. Accessed 19 Jan 2015

Awareness Times (2015b) Sierra Leone news: Ebola rages afresh in Kaffu Bullom (Lungi). Awareness Times. http://news.sl/drwebsite/publish/article_200527697.shtml. Accessed 1 Jun 2015

Awoko (2015a) Sierra Leone news: two months old survives Ebola. Awoko. http://awoko.org/2015/01/07/sierra-leone-news-two-months-old-baby-survives-ebola/. Accessed 7 Jan 2015

Awoko (2015b) Sierra Leone news: tourism drops nearly 13%. Awoko. http://awoko.org/2015/01/10/sierra-leone-news-tourism-drops-nearly-13/. Accessed 10 Jan 2015

Awoko (2015c) Sierra Leone news: as Kingtom Cemetery is now full …3 days 'sit at home' end of the month eminent. Awoko. http://awoko.org/2015/03/19/sierra-leone-news-as-kingtom-cemetery-is-now-full-3-days-sit-at-home-end-of-the-month-eminent/. Accessed 19 Mar 2015

Awoko (2015d) Sierra Leone news: as hazard pay comes to an end this month…NERC urges women to wear yellow dresses. Awoko. http://awoko.org/2015/03/26/sierra-leone-news-as-hazard-pay-comes-to-an-end-this-monthnerc-urges-women-to-wear-yellow-dresses/. Accessed 26 Mar 2015

Awoko (2015e) Sierra Leone news over 53,000 Ebola test done – Dr. Abdul Kamara. Awoko. http://awoko.org/2015/06/11/sierra-leone-news-over-53000-ebola-test-done-dr-abdul-kamara/. Accessed 12 Jun 2015

Awoko (2015f) Sierra Leone news: only 7 patients in treatment centers Awoko. http://awoko.org/2015/07/01/sierra-leone-news-only-7-patients-in-treatment-centers/

Awoko (2015g) Sierra Leone news: there is no Ebola case at present – Sidi Yaya Tunis. Awoko. http://awoko.org/2015/09/01/sierra-leone-news-there-is-no-ebola-case-at-present-sidi-yaya-tunis/. Accessed 1 Sep 2015

Baber M (2015) Football restarts in Liberia as Ebola infection rates fall. Inside World Football. http://www.insideworldfootball.com/world-football/africa/16150-football-restarts-in-liberia-as-ebola-infection-rates-fall. Accessed 8 Jan 2015

Bah Y (2015) Ebola cases reported in Guinea as people travel, worries increase with election campaigns. Associated Press, US News & World Report. http://www.usnews.com/news/world/articles/2015/06/24/ebola-cases-not-slowing-in-guinea-sierra-leone. Accessed 26 Jun 2015

Bangkok Post (2015) Sierra Leone announces new curfew to halt Ebola. Bangkok Post. http://www.bangkokpost.com/news/world/591181/sierra-leone-announces-new-curfew-to-halt-ebola. Accessed 14 Jun 2015

Banton R (2015) New model predicts end of Ebola outbreak by June. The Red & Black. http://www.redandblack.com/uganews/new-model-predicts-end-of-ebola-outbreak-by-june/article_72e66f6c-a828-11e4-8253-1f8b90dc7acb.html. Accessed 1 Feb 2015

Baysah RD (2015) Liberia: four new Ebola cases surface in Margibi. AllAfrica, LINA. http://
    allafrica.com/stories/201502251228.html. Accessed 24 Feb 2015

BBC (2015a) UK Ebola nurse Pauline Cafferkey 'in critical condition.' BBC. http://www.bbc.
    com/news/uk-30666265. Accessed 3 Jan 2015

BBC (2015b) Ebola nurse no longer critically ill. BBC. http://www.bbc.com/news/health-30783537.
    Accessed 12 Jan 2015

BBC (2015c) Ebola crisis: new cases declining in West Africa. BBC. http://www.bbc.com/news/
    world-africa-30830129. Accessed 15 Jan 2015

BBC (2015d) Ebola crisis: oxfam calls for recovery Marshall Plan. BBC. http://www.bbc.com/
    news/uk-30995631. Accessed 26 Jan 2015

BBC (2015e) Ebola crisis: first major vaccine trials in Liberia. BBC. http://www.bbc.com/news/
    world-africa-31087727. Accessed 2 Feb 2015

BBC (2015f) Second UK health worker monitored for Ebola. BBC. http://www.bbc.com/news/
    health-31091528. Accessed 2 Feb 2015

BBC (2015g) Ebola nurse infection 'down to visor.' BBC. http://www.bbc.com/news/
    health-31128964. Accessed 4 Feb 2015

BBC (2015h) Ebola crisis: Sierra Leone orphanage quarantined. BBC. http://www.bbc.com/news/
    world-africa-31587180. Accessed 24 Feb 2015

BBC (2015i) Ebola crisis: Sierra Leone's Augustine Baker dies. BBC. http://www.bbc.com/news/
    world-africa-31624149. Accessed 25 Feb 2015

BBC (2015j) Liberia Ebola doctor: 'We're going to win very soon.' BBC. http://www.bbc.com/
    news/uk-england-london-31690780. Accessed 2 Mar 2015

BBC (2015k) UK female military health worker has Ebola. BBC. http://www.bbc.com/news/
    uk-31841432. Accessed 11 Mar 2015

BBC (2015l) Ebola: British patient and four colleagues in UK hospitals. BBC. http://www.bbc.
    com/news/uk-31845947. Accessed 13 Mar 2015

BBC (2015m) Ebola crisis: Sierra Leone lockdown to hit 2.5m people. BBC. http://www.bbc.com/
    news/world-africa-31966989. Accessed 19 Mar 2015

BBC (2015n) Ebola outbreak: Sierra Leone in lockdown. BBC. http://www.bbc.com/news/world-
    africa-32083363. Accessed 27 Mar 2015

BBC (2015o) British medic declared free of Ebola. BBC. http://www.bbc.com/news/
    health-32088310. Accessed 27 Mar 2015

BBC (2015p) Ebola crisis: Guineans jailed for putting corpse in taxi. BBC. http://www.bbc.com/
    news/world-africa-32877392. Accessed 25 May 2015

BBC (2015q) Ebola crisis: UN's Ebola mission HQ in Ghana to close. BBC. http://www.bbc.com/
    news/world-africa-33063900. Accessed 8 Aug 2017

BBC (2015r) UK relaxes Ebola screening measures. BBC. http://www.bbc.com/news/
    health-33635574. Accessed 23 Jul 2015

BBC (2015s) Ebola countries record first week with no new cases. BBC. http://www.bbc.com/
    news/world-africa-34471234. Accessed 7 Oct 2015

BBC (2015t) Ebola nurse Pauline Cafferkey 'in serious condition'. BBC. http://www.bbc.com/
    news/uk-scotland-34483584. Accessed 9 Oct 2015

BBC (2015u) Ebola caused meningitis in nurse Pauline Cafferkey. BBC. http://www.bbc.com/
    news/uk-scotland-glasgow-west-34592132. Accessed 21 Oct 2015

BBC (2015v) Ebola nurse Pauline Cafferkey 'has made full recovery.' BBC. http://www.bbc.com/
    news/uk-scotland-34791692. Accessed 12 Nov 2015

BBC (2016a) Ebola outbreak: Sierra Leone clashes over market closure. BBC. http://www.bbc.
    com/news/world-africa-35409690. Accessed 27 Jan 2016

BBC (2016b) Ebola nurse Pauline Cafferkey released from hospital. BBC. http://www.bbc.com/
    news/uk-scotland-glasgow-west-35683091. Accessed 28 Feb 2016

BBC (2016c) Ebola outbreak: Guinea confirms two new cases. BBC. http://www.bbc.com/news/
    world-africa-35840782. Accessed 18 Mar 2016

Beaubien J (2015) Ebola returns to Liberia, but it's not clear how the 10-year-old got it. NPR. http://www.npr.org/sections/goatsandsoda/2015/11/20/456787852/ebola-returns-to-liberia-but-its-not-clear-how-the-10-year-old-got-it. Accessed 20 Nov 2015

Berdjis N (2015) Three new Ebola cases in Liberia. The Disease Daily. http://www.healthmap.org/site/diseasedaily/article/three-new-ebola-cases-liberia-32715. Accessed 27 Mar 2015

BERNAMA (2015) Who warns rainy season hampering Ebola response in West Africa. BERNAMA.   http://www.bernama.com.my/bernama/v8/wn/newsworld.php?id=1140994. Accessed 4 Jun 2015

Bernstein S (2015) Suspected Ebola patient admitted to California hospital. Reuters. http://www.reuters.com/article/2015/01/29/us-usa-ebola-california-idUSKBN0L22KH20150129. Accessed 29 Jan 2015

Bhutia J (2015) Pauline Cafferkey: 25 close contacts given Ebola vaccine. Yahoo News. https://uk.news.yahoo.com/pauline-cafferkey-25-close-contacts-050518628.html#wuuaT79. Accessed 13 Oct 2015

Biddle J (2015) Liberia leader thanks US as Ebola mission ends. AFP, Yahoo News. http://news.yahoo.com/us-wraps-ebola-military-mission-liberia-151753224.html. Accessed 27 Feb 2015

Booth R (2015) Passengers on flight with Scottish Ebola nurse have all been traced, say officials. The Guardian. https://www.theguardian.com/world/2015/jan/01/passengers-flight-scottish-ebola-nurse-traced. Accessed 13 Jul 2017

Boseley S (2015a) Ebola as ZMapp stocks run out doctors turn to alternative treatments. The Guardian. http://www.theguardian.com/world/2015/jan/05/ebola-zmapp-stocks-run-out-doctors-turn-alternative-treatments. Accessed 6 Jan 2015

Boseley S (2015b) WHO approves 15-minute test for Ebola. The Guardian. http://www.theguardian.com/world/2015/feb/20/who-approves-15-minute-test-for-ebola. Accessed 20 Feb 2015

Boseley S (2015c) UN special envoy says Ebola flare-ups could continue for some time. The Guardian.   http://www.theguardian.com/global-development/2015/jul/06/ebola-un-special-envoy-liberia-flare-ups-david-nabarro. Accessed 6 Jul 2015

Boseley S (2015d) Ebola nurse Pauline Cafferkey critically ill after condition deteriorates. The Guardian. http://www.theguardian.com/world/2015/oct/14/ebola-nurse-pauline-cafferkey-critically-ill. Accessed 14 Oct 2015

Brice M (2015) Ebola threat to Guinea Bissau rises as border zone heats up. Reuters, Yahoo News. http://news.yahoo.com/ebola-threat-guinea-bissau-rises-border-zone-heats-063714122.html. Accessed 2 Jun 2015

British Red Cross (2015a) Brits say "Ebola doctors are heroes, but keep away from me." British Red   Cross.   http://www.redcross.org.uk/en/About-us/News/2015/March/Brits-say-Ebola-doctors-are-heroes-but-keep-away-from-me. Accessed 18 Mar 2015

British Red Cross (2015b) Emergency Ebola appeal closes. http://www.redcross.org.uk/About-us/News/2015/December/Emergency-Ebola-appeal-closes. Accessed 11 Dec 2015

Brooks C (2015a) Liberian ambulance team joins Sierra Leone for Ebola fight. GNN Liberia. http://www.gnnliberia.com/articles/2015/01/11/liberian-ambulance-team-joins-sierra-leone-bola-fight. Accessed 11 Jan 2015

Brooks C (2015b) Liberia: new Ebola death reported In Margibi. GNN. http://www.gnnliberia.com/articles/2015/02/04/liberia-new-ebola-death-reported-margibi. Accessed 4 Feb 2015

Brooks L (2015a) Pauline Cafferkey: 58 close contacts of Ebola nurse being monitored. The Guardian.   http://www.theguardian.com/world/2015/oct/12/pauline-cafferkey-58-close-contacts-of-ebola-nurse-being-monitored. Accessed 13 Oct 2015

Brooks L (2015b) Family of Ebola nurse Pauline Cafferkey accuse doctors of 'major failings'. The Guardian. http://www.theguardian.com/world/2015/oct/11/pauline-cafferkey-family-accuses-doctors-of-major-failings. Accessed 14 Oct 2015

Brown L (2015) British aid worker evacuated from Sierra Leone in Ebola scare after patient's bodily fluids splashed in her eye as she took off protective suit. The Daily Mail. http://www.dailymail.co.uk/news/article-2957039/British-aid-worker-evacuated-Sierra-Leone-Ebola-scare-patient-s-bodily-fluids-splashed-eye-took-protective-suit.html. Accessed 17 Feb 2015

Bruz H (2015) Sierra Leone news: Ebola at Lungi airport's environs concern the NERC. Awareness Times. http://news.sl/drwebsite/publish/article_200527700.shtml. Accessed 2 Jun 2015

Butty J (2015a) Liberia awaits Ebola-free declaration to remember its victims. VOA News. http://www.voanews.com/content/liberia-awaits-ebola-free-declaration-to-remember-its-victims/2677082.html. Accessed 12 Mar 2014

Butty J (2015b) Sierra Leone schools end 8-month Ebola closure. VOA News. http://www.voanews.com/content/sierra-leone-schools-end-eight-month-ebola-closure/2719626.html. Accessed 15 Apr 2015

Butty J (2015c) Sierra Leone quarantines 50 following latest Ebola death. VOA News. http://www.voanews.com/content/sierra-leone-quarantines-50-following-latest-ebola-death/2941906.html. Accessed 2 Sep 2015

Caldwell AA (2015) US Ebola-related screening restrictions lifted for Mali. ABC News. http://abcnews.go.com/Politics/wireStory/us-ebola-related-screening-restrictions-lifted-mali-28007646. Accessed 5 Jan 2015

Canadian Press (2015) Canada drops visa ban for Liberia. Maclean's. http://www.macleans.ca/news/canada/canada-drops-visa-ban-for-liberia-now-that-country-has-been-declared-ebola-free/. Accessed 12 May 2015

CBS News (2015) New Ebola cases discovered in Sierra Leone. CBS News. http://www.cbsnews.com/news/new-ebola-cases-discovered-in-sierra-leone/. Accessed 2 Apr 2015

Centers for Disease Control and Prevention (2015a) Ebola in Liberia. What is the current situation? 4 May 2015

Centers for Disease Control and Prevention (2015b) Guidance on Personal Protective Equipment (PPE) to be used by healthcare workers during management of patients with confirmed Ebola or Persons under Investigation (PUIs) for Ebola who are clinically unstable or have bleeding, vomiting, or diarrhea in U.S. Hospitals, including procedures for donning and doffing PPE. 27 Aug 2015

Chan M (2015) Ebola kills 15-year-old boy in Liberia. Time, Reuters. http://time.com/4125786/ebola-death-liberia/. Accessed 15 Aug 2017

Cheng M (2015a) 2 leading Ebola vaccines appear safe, further tests starting. ABC News. http://abcnews.go.com/Health/wireStory/leading-ebola-vaccines-safe-tests-starting-28107527. Accessed 9 Jan 2015

Cheng M (2015b) WHO to begin large scale testing of Ebola vaccine in Guinea. Fox News. http://www.fox19.com/story/28267814/who-to-begin-large-scale-testing-of-ebola-vaccine-in-guinea. Accessed 7 Mar 2015

Cheng M (2015c) UN says it will try to identify all Ebola cases by June to stop virus. Associated Press, US News & World Report. http://www.usnews.com/news/world/articles/2015/04/28/un-says-it-will-try-to-identify-all-ebola-cases-by-june. Accessed 28 Apr 2015

Cheng M (2015d) Ailing Ebola nurse in UK may be rare case of relapse. Associated Press, ABC News. http://abcnews.go.com/Health/wireStory/ebola-nurse-uk-rare-case-relapse-34489631. Accessed 15 Oct 2015

Christie A, Davies-Wayne GJ, Cordier-Lasalle T et al (2015) Possible sexual transmission of Ebola virus – Liberia, 2015. MMWR Morb Mortal Wkly Rep 64:479–481

Clarke-Billings L (2015) British Ebola nurse Pauline Cafferkey's 'condition improves to serious but stable'. The Telegraph. http://www.telegraph.co.uk/news/uknews/11941090/British-Ebola-nurse-Pauline-Cafferkeys-condition-improves-to-serious-but-stable.html. Accessed 19 Oct 2015

Cohen E (2015) Americans exposed to Ebola return from Africa for monitoring. CNN. http://www.cnn.com/2015/03/14/health/cdc-americans-ebola/. Accessed 16 Mar 2015

Connolly AR (2015) Ebola handshake going strong as Ebola cases decrease. UPI. http://www.upi.com/Top_News/World-News/2015/01/27/Ebola-handshake-going-strong-as-Ebola-cases-decrease/5551422371260/. Accessed 27 Jan 2017

Conteh MW (2015) Kasho awards Ebola fighters. Africa Young Voices. http://africayoungvoices.com/2015/05/kasho-awards-ebola-fighters/. Accessed 12 May 2015

Cooper H, Fink S (2015) Ebola cases in 3 family members confirmed in Liberia. New York Times. http://www.nytimes.com/2015/11/21/world/africa/ebola-case-in-10-year-old-confirmed-in-liberia.html?_r=0. Accessed 20 Nov 2015

Courier (2015) Fife Ebola nurse Pauline Cafferkey in 'serious condition' after complication. The Courier, Press Association. http://www.thecourier.co.uk/news/local/fife/fife-ebola-nurse-pauline-cafferkey-in-serious-condition-after-complication-1.904221. Accessed 9 Oct 2015

Couzens G (2015) Spanish Ebola survivor whose dog was put down amid fears it had killer disease has adopted a new puppy called Alma. The Daily Mail. http://www.dailymail.co.uk/news/article-2925357/Spanish-Ebola-survivor-dog-amid-fears-killer-disease-adopted-new-puppy-called-Alma.html. Accessed 18 Jul 2017

Daily Mail (2015) ISIS fighters 'have contracted Ebola': World Health Organisation investigating reports militants showed up at Iraqi hospital with lethal disease. The Daily Mail. http://www.dailymail.co.uk/news/article-2894154/ISIS-fighters-contracted-Ebola-World-Health-Organisation-investigating-reports-Islamist-militants-disease-showed-Iraqi-hospital.html. Accessed 2 Jan 2015

Daily Record (2015) Ebola victim Pauline Cafferkey given blood from survivor Will Pooley to boost her chances of recovery. Daily Record. http://www.dailyrecord.co.uk/news/scottish-news/ebola-victim-pauline-cafferkey-given-4958932. Accessed 11 Jan 2015

David A (2015) Liberia: 'Border closure not an option'. AllAfrica, The News. http://allafrica.com/stories/201507021245.html. Accessed 1 Jul 2015

De Vries N (2015) Sierra Leone Ebola survivors help train healthcare workers. VOA News. http://www.voanews.com/content/sierra-leone-ebola-survivors-help-train-healthcare-workers/2647401.html. Accessed 17 Feb 2015

DeCapua J (2015) Ebola hits households hard. VOA News. http://www.voanews.com/content/ebola-world-bank-14jan15/2597984.html. Accessed 15 Jan 2015

Deen GF, Knust B, Broutet N et al (2015) Ebola RNA persistence in semen of Ebola virus disease survivors — preliminary report. N Engl J Med 2015

Diallo M (2015) Guinea: traditional healers support Ebola response at the risk of personal hardship. International Federation of Red Cross and Red Crescent Societies. http://www.ifrc.org/en/news-and-media/news-stories/africa/guinea/guinea-traditional-healers-support-ebola-response-at-the-risk-of-personal-hardship-68584/. Accessed 8 May 2015

Diallo B (2015a) Guinea schools reopen, but Ebola fears still keep many children at home as rumors fly. Associated Press, Daily Reporter. http://www.greenfieldreporter.com/view/story/c17974b458f04260ae2a7d63ed908af9/AF--West-Africa-Ebola. Accessed 19 Jan 2015

Diallo B (2015b) Guinea president reinforces emergency Ebola measures. Associated Press, Yahoo News. http://news.yahoo.com/guinea-president-reinforces-emergency-ebola-measures-094647285.html. Accessed 29 Mar 2015

Diallo B (2015c) Guinea shuts border with Sierra Leone in effort to end Ebola. Associated Press, ABC News. http://abcnews.go.com/Health/wireStory/guinea-shuts-border-sierra-leone-effort-end-ebola-30010952. Accessed 30 Mar 2015

DiLorenzo S (2015) Schools to reopen in Liberia, but Ebola concerns remain. USA Today. http://www.usatoday.com/story/news/world/2015/02/15/monrovia-liberia-ebola-school-opening/23456301/. Accessed 16 Feb 2015

Dixon (2015) Liberia: Nine counties report zero Ebola cases for over 21 days. AllAfrica, Liberian News Agency. http://allafrica.com/stories/201501061042.html. Accessed 14 Jul 2017

Doctor RM (2015) Last batch of Ebola contacts in Liberia finishes quarantine. Tech Times. http://www.techtimes.com/articles/115728/20151212/last-batch-of-ebola-contacts-in-liberia-finishes-quarantine.htm. Accessed 15 Aug 2015

Dosso Z (2015) World's largest Ebola unit dismantled as outbreak retreats. AFP, News 24. http://www.news24.com/Africa/News/Worlds-largest-Ebola-unit-incinerated-20150128. Accessed 28 Jan 2015

Doucleff M (2015) Ebola returns to Liberia with a mysterious case near Monrovia. NPR. http://www.npr.org/sections/goatsandsoda/2015/06/30/418913144/ebola-returns-to-liberia-with-a-mysterious-case-near-monrovia. Accessed 1 Jul 2015

Du Lac JF (2015) Guinea ground zero of the Ebola outbreak is now free of the deadly disease. The Washington Post. https://www.washingtonpost.com/news/world/wp/2015/12/29/guinea-ground-zero-of-the-ebola-outbreak-is-now-free-of-the-deadly-disease/. Accessed 29 Dec 2015

Dunn C (2015a) Ebola outbreak: quarantine 'just like a jail' in Sierra Leone. CBC News. http://www.cbc.ca/news/world/ebola-outbreak-quarantine-just-like-a-jail-in-sierra-leone-1.2890487. Accessed 6 Jan 2015

Dunn C (2015b) Ebola virus continues to fuel Sierra Leones economic freefall. CBC News. http://www.cbc.ca/news/world/ebola-virus-continues-to-fuel-sierra-leone-s-economic-freef-all-1.2896919. Accessed 11 Jan 2015

DW (2015) Ebola death in Sierra Leone leads to mass quarantine. DW. http://www.dw.com/en/ebola-death-in-sierra-leone-leads-to-mass-quarantine/a-18620558. Accessed 31 Jul 2015

Emory Medicine (2015) Emory banking plasma from Ebola survivors. Emory News Center. http://news.emory.edu/stories/2015/04/hspub_banking_ebola_plasma/campus.html. Accessed 3 Apr 2015

Executive Mansion (2015) President Sirleaf orders the nationwide curfew lifted, opening up of Liberia's main borders beginning Sunday, February 22nd, 2015. 20 Feb 2015

Fahngon JC (2015) Liberia: operation stop Ebola launched. AllAfrica. http://allafrica.com/stories/201501122231.html. Accessed 12 Jan 2015

Fallah SS (2015) Tracing 100 suspected carriers after second Ebola death. Front Page Africa. http://www.frontpageafricaonline.com/index.php/health-sci/5685-tracing-100-suspected-carriers-after-second-ebola-death. Accessed 2 Jul 2015

Farberov S (2015) Dr Nancy Snyderman resigns as NBC's chief medical editor after she sparked public outcry by violating Ebola quarantine. The Daily Mail. http://www.dailymail.co.uk/news/article-2992314/Dr-Nancy-Snyderman-resigns-NBC-s-chief-medical-editor-months-sparked-public-outcry-violating-Ebola-quarantine.html. Accessed 23 Jul 2017

Farge E (2015a) Free from Ebola, survivors complain of new syndrome. Reuters. http://www.reuters.com/article/2015/02/04/us-health-ebola-survivors-idUSKBN0L81WA20150204. Accessed 4 Feb 2015

Farge E (2015b) Sierra Leone to prosecute fraudulent Ebola "ghostworkers". Reuters. http://www.reuters.com/article/2015/02/10/us-health-ebola-fraud-idUSKBN0LE2M920150210. Accessed 10 Feb 2015

Farge E (2015c) Exclusive: Guinea says Ebola patients sent home after botched blood tests. Reuters. http://www.reuters.com/article/2015/03/02/us-health-ebola-guinea-idUSKBN-0LY20Y20150302. Accessed 2 Mar 2015

Farge E (2015d) Guinea's last Ebola case, a baby girl, leaves hospital. Reuters. http://www.reuters.com/article/2015/11/28/us-health-ebola-guinea-idUSKBN0TH0PB20151128#4ycyivucXSD MuXr0.97. Accessed 29 Nov 2015

Farge E, Fofana U (2015) How Sierra Leone is winning the battle against Ebola. Reuters, The Huffington Post. http://www.huffingtonpost.com/2015/01/21/ebola-sierra-leone_n_6514634.html. Accessed 21 Jan 2015

Farge E, Giahyue JH (2015) Female survivor may be cause of Ebola flare-up in Liberia. Reuters, EMTV. http://www.emtv.com.pg/article.aspx?slug=Female-survivor-may-be-cause-of-Ebola-flare-up-in-Liberia&subcategory=Health. Accessed 18 Dec 2015

Fink S (2015a) Ebola drug aids some in a study in West Africa. New York Times. http://www.nytimes.com/2015/02/05/science/ebola-drug-has-encouraging-early-results-and-questions-follow.html?_r=0. Accessed 4 Feb 2015

Fink S (2015b) Exposure concerns grow in Liberia after diagnosis of first Ebola case in weeks. New York Times. http://www.nytimes.com/2015/03/25/world/africa/exposure-concerns-grow-in-liberia-after-diagnosis-of-first-ebola-case-in-weeks.html?_r=0. Accessed 25 Mar 2015

Fink S (2015c) Liberia is declared free of Ebola, but officials sound note of caution. New York Times. http://www.nytimes.com/2015/05/10/world/africa/liberia-is-free-of-ebola-world-health-organization-declares.html?_r=0. Accessed 9 May 2015

Fink S (2015d) Surge of Ebola in Liberia may be linked to a survivor. New York Times. http://www.nytimes.com/2015/07/10/world/africa/surge-of-ebola-in-liberia-is-tracked-to-a-survivor.html?_r=0. Accessed 9 Jul 2015

Fitzgerald F (2015) Ebola diary: is it bouncing back? The telegraph. http://www.telegraph.co.uk/news/worldnews/ebola/11430719/Ebola-Diary-Is-it-bouncing-back.html. Accessed 24 Feb 2015

Fofana U (2015a) Sierra Leone to start laying off Ebola workers as cases fall: president. Reuters. http://www.reuters.com/article/2015/04/02/us-health-ebola-leone-idUSK-BN0MT01120150402. Accessed 2 Apr 2015

Fofana U (2015b) Sierra Leones Kailahun district records first Ebola case in months. Reuters. http://www.reuters.com/article/2015/04/04/us-health-ebola-leone-idUSKBN0MV0Q320150404. Accessed 5 Apr 2015

Fofana U (2016) Dozens feared exposed as Sierra Leone confirms new Ebola death. Reuters. http://www.reuters.com/article/us-health-ebola-leone-idUSKCN0UT0Q3. Accessed 15 Jan 2016

Fox M (2014) Blood, sweat and tears: study will watch Ebola survivors. NBC News. http://www.nbcnews.com/storyline/ebola-virus-outbreak/blood-sweat-tears-study-watch-ebola-survivors-n377256. Accessed 17 Jun 2015

Fox M (2015a) Magic blood? Emory's Ebola plasma bank. NBC News. http://www.nbcnews.com/storyline/ebola-virus-outbreak/magic-blood-emorys-ebola-plasma-bank-n285996. Accessed 14 Jan 2015

Fox M (2015b) Ebola drug ZMapp's ready for African testing. NBC News. http://www.nbc-news.com/storyline/ebola-virus-outbreak/ebola-drug-zmapps-ready-african-testing-n305981. Accessed 13 Feb 2015

Fox M (2015c) It's now 16 Americans coming back from the Ebola zone. NBC News. http://www.nbcnews.com/storyline/ebola-virus-outbreak/its-now-18-americans-coming-back-ebola-zone-n325321. Accessed 17 Mar 2015

Fox M (2015d) American with Ebola is better. NBC News. http://www.nbcnews.com/storyline/ebola-virus-outbreak/american-ebola-better-n337196. Accessed 8 Apr 2015

Fox M (2015e) Liberia's Ebola-free, but not out of the woods yet. NBC News. http://www.nbc-news.com/storyline/ebola-virus-outbreak/liberias-ebola-free-not-out-woods-yet-n357301. Accessed 12 May 2015

Fox M (2015f) Blood sweat and tears study will watch Ebola survivors. NBC News. http://www.nbcnews.com/storyline/ebola-virus-outbreak/blood-sweat-tears-study-watch-ebola-survivors-n3777256. Accessed 17 Jun 2015

Frampton W (2015) New mobile Ebola containment units unveiled at metro Atlanta air reserve base. CBS 46. http://www.cbs46.com/story/29763417/new-mobile-ebola-containment-units-unveiled-at-dobbins. Accessed 12 Aug 2015

Frankel TC (2015) The biggest threat to stopping Ebola is thinking that it's over now. The Washington Post. http://www.washingtonpost.com/blogs/wonkblog/wp/2015/03/07/the-big-gest-threat-to-stopping-ebola-is-thinking-that-its-over-now/. Accessed 7 Mar 2015

Front Page Africa (2015) A village in denial over Ebola – deaths, infections pile. Front Page Africa. http://www.frontpageafricaonline.com/index.php/news/5690-a-village-in-denial-over-ebola-deaths-infections-pile. Accessed 3 Jul 2015

Gaffey C (2016a) Sierra Leone quarantines 109 people after Ebola death. Newsweek. http://www.newsweek.com/more-100-people-quarantined-after-ebola-death-sierra-leone-416890. Accessed 18 Jan 2016

Gaffey C (2016b) Sierra Leone releases 55 people from Ebola quarantine. Newsweek. http://www.newsweek.com/sierra-leone-releases-55-people-ebola-quarantine-423007. Accessed 4 Feb 2016

Gaffey C (2016c) Ebola Guinea to quarantine 816 people in latest flare-up. Newsweek. http://www.newsweek.com/ebola-guinea-quarantine-816-people-latest-flare-439376. Accessed 23 Mar 2016

Gallagher J (2015) UK Ebola nurse Pauline Cafferkey has 'stabilised.' BBC. http://www.bbc.com/news/health-30657485. Accessed 5 Jan 2015

Ghana Business News (2015) Ghana government lifts Ebola conference ban. Ghana Business News. https://www.ghanabusinessnews.com/2015/02/19/ghana-government-lifts-ebola-conference-ban/. Accessed 19 Feb 2015

Ghanaian Times (2015) 140 suspected Ebola cases since March 2014 tested negative. Ghanaian Times. http://gbcghana.com/1.2543565. Accessed 1 Apr 2015

Giahyue JH (2015a) Bones, ashes at Liberia crematorium a reminder of Ebola trauma. Reuters. http://uk.reuters.com/article/2015/01/18/us-health-ebola-liberia-idUKKBN0KR0FB20150118. Accessed 18 Jan 2015

Giahyue JH (2015b) Liberia delays school reopening by two weeks as Ebola cases fall. Reuters. http://www.reuters.com/article/us-health-ebola-education-idUSKBN0L31PE20150130. Accessed 19 Jul 2017

Giahyue JH (2015c) Liberia confirms new Ebola case as outbreak spreads. Reuters. http://af.reuters.com/article/topNews/idAFKCN0PP0P620150715?sp=true. Accessed 15 Jul 2015

Giahyue JH (2015d) Liberia monitors over 150 Ebola contacts as virus re emerges. Reuters. http://www.reuters.com/article/2015/11/22/us-health-ebola-liberia-idUSKBN0TB0GV20151122#vHYwP3egcZJJBpHx.97. Accessed 22 Nov 2015

Gibbons B (2015) Ebola checks at Birmingham Airport scaled back. Birmingham Mail. http://www.birminghammail.co.uk/news/midlands-news/ebola-checks-birmingham-airport-scaled-9719264. Accessed 24 Jul 2015

Gill R (2015) Gambia Bird suspends all flights. Buying Business Travel. http://buyingbusinesstravel.com/news/0223586-gambia-bird-suspends-all-flights. Accessed 2 Jan 2015

GNA (2015) Ending Ebola before rainy season imperative – UNMEER. GNA, Vibe Ghana. http://vibeghana.com/2015/05/04/ending-ebola-before-rainy-season-imperative-unmeer/. Accessed 4 May 2015

Goldberg D (2015) City ends Ebola monitoring. Politico. http://www.capitalnewyork.com/article/city-hall/2016/01/8587423/city-ends-ebola-monitoring. Accessed 11 Jan 2015

Gortor W (2015a) Liberia: IMS Records 6,097 Ebola, Non-Ebola Deaths During Epidemic. AllAfrica, LINA. http://allafrica.com/stories/201503100687.html. Accessed 10 Mar 2015

Gortor W (2015b) Liberia: Guinea reopens border with Liberia. AllAfrica, LINA. http://allafrica.com/stories/201504230792.html. Accessed 23 Apr 2015

Grady D (2015) After nearly claiming his life, Ebola lurked in a doctor's eye. New York Times. http://www.nytimes.com/2015/05/08/health/weeks-after-his-recovery-ebola-lurked-in-a-doctors-eye.html?_r=0. Accessed 8 May 2015

Henao-Restrepo AM, Longini IM, Egger M et al (2015) Efficacy and effectiveness of an rVSV-vectored vaccine expressing Ebola surface glycoprotein: interim results from the Guinea ring vaccination cluster-randomised trial. Lancet 386:857–866

Heritage Liberia (2015) Liberia stands to be declared Ebola-free on May 9 if.... Heritage Liberia. http://www.heritageliberia.net/heritagenews/index.php/2014-07-17-10-02-56/other-headlines/524-liberia-stands-to-be-declared-ebola-free-on-may-9-if. Accessed 29 Apr 2015

Hirschler B (2015) Liberia Ebola vaccine trial 'challenging' as cases tumble. Reuters. http://www.reuters.com/article/2015/01/24/us-health-ebola-davos-nih-idUSKBN0KX0J320150124. Accessed 24 Jan 2015

HNGN (2015) Guinea approves wider use of anti-Ebola experimental drug. HNGN. http://www.hngn.com/articles/67593/20150207/guinea-approves-wider-use-of-anti-ebola-experimental-drug.htm. Accessed 7 Feb 2015

Hoskins N (2015) 101st Airborne Division cases colors, heads home to Fort Campbell after successful mission in Liberia. Clarksville Online. http://www.clarksvilleonline.

com/2015/02/27/101st-airborne-division-cases-colors-heads-home-to-fort-campbell-after-successful-mission-in-liberia/. Accessed 26 Feb 2015

Hussain M (2015) Mistrust and machetes thwart efforts to contain Ebola in Guinea. Reuters, PRI. http://www.globalpost.com/dispatch/news/thomson-reuters/150210/mistrust-and-machetes-thwart-efforts-contain-ebola-guinea. Accessed 10 Feb 2015

IANS (2015a) South Korean suspected of Ebola to be sent to Germany. IANS, Business Standard. http://www.business-standard.com/article/news-ians/south-korean-suspected-of-ebola-to-be-sent-to-germany-115010200505_1.html. Accessed 2 Jan 2015

IANS (2015b) 13 quarantined in Italy after Ebola virus infects nurse. IANS, Sierra Leone Times. http://www.sierraleonetimes.com/index.php/sid/232886067. Accessed 18 May 2015

IBNS (2015) Ebola: World Bank will provide seeds to farmers in West Africa to ward off hunger. India Blooms News Service. http://indiablooms.com/ibns_new/finance-details/1598/ebola-world-bank-will-provide-seeds-to-farmers-in-west-africa-to-ward-off-hunger.html. Accessed 13 Feb 2015

International Federation of Red Cross and Red Crescent Societies (2015) "I explain to these ghosts why I had to bury them this way." 11 May 2015

Irwin T (2015) Measures to safeguard schools in Ebola hit Liberia point to need for continued vigilance. UNICEF. http://www.unicef.org/infobycountry/liberia_81392.html?utm_source=unicef_news&utm_medium=rss&utm_campaign=rss_link. Accessed 30 Mar 2015

Iyengar R (2015) Priests assaulted in Guinea after being mistaken for Ebola workers. Time. http://time.com/3675775/ebola-guinea-priests-beaten-village/. 20 Jan 2015

Jabati D (2015) Back to school day 1. Africa Voices. http://africayoungvoices.com/2015/04/back-to-school-day-1/. Accessed 15 Apr 2015

Jacobson S (2015) Ebola study says a dozen more were hospitalized during Dallas outbreak than was revealed. The Dallas Morning News. http://www.dallasnews.com/news/metro/20150526-new-ebola-study-says-a-dozen-more-hospitalized-in-dallas-outbreak-than-revealed.ece. Accessed 28 May 2015

James FB (2015) Sierra Leone: staying at zero in an ex-Ebola hotspot. UNICEF. http://blogs.unicef.org/2015/02/19/sierra-leone-staying-at-zero-in-an-ex-ebola-hotspot/. Accessed 20 Feb 2015

Jansen B (2015a) Feds to end Ebola screening for air travelers from Liberia. USA Today. http://www.usatoday.com/story/news/2015/09/18/ebola-travel-airport-screening-liberia-sierra-leone-guinea-customs-border-protection/72398942/. Accessed 19 Sep 2015

Jansen B (2015b) Year of airport screening doesn't catch Ebola. USA Today. http://www.usatoday.com/story/news/2015/09/22/ebola-airport-screening-cbp-cdc/32493389/. Accessed 23 Sep 2015

Jenkins L (2015) Nurse who contracted Ebola released from hospital. The Guardian. http://www.theguardian.com/world/2015/jan/24/ebola-pauline-cafferkey-recovery-discharge. Accessed 25 Jan 2015

Jerry D (2015) 690 persons quarantined, 1 dead as Ebola resurfaces in Sierra Leone. 360 Nobs. http://www.360nobs.com/2015/09/690-persons-quarantined-1-dead-as-ebola-resurfaces-in-sierra-leone/. Accessed 15 Sep 2015

Johnson RM (2015a) Ebola-hit Sierra Leone's schools to reopen on March 30. AFP, Yahoo News. https://uk.news.yahoo.com/ebola-hit-sierra-leones-schools-reopen-march-30-174600111.html#a9SFsMN. Accessed 4 Feb 2015

Johnson RM (2015b) Sierra Leone goes door-to-door to fight Ebola surge. AFP, Interaksyon. http://www.interaksyon.com/article/105370/sierra-leone-goes-door-to-door-to-fight-ebola-surge. Accessed 19 Feb 2015

Johnson RM (2015c) WHO declares end of Ebola outbreak in Sierra Leone. AFP, Yahoo News. http://news.yahoo.com/declare-end-ebola-sierra-leone-041129310.html. Accessed 7 Nov 2015

Johnson RM, Larson N (2015) As Liberia takes stock of Ebola triumph, fleeing patients set back Sierra Leone's battle; cases rise. Mail & Guardian Africa. http://mgafrica.com/article/2015-

05-21-as-liberia-takes-stock-of-ebola-triumph-fleeing-patients-begin-to-set-back-sierra-leones-battle. Accessed 22 May 2015

K J (2015) Ebola: High mortality in young children sees four out of five dying. International Business Times. http://www.ibtimes.co.uk/ebola-high-mortality-young-children-sees-four-out-five-dying-1486989. Accessed 7 Feb 2015

Kamara K (2015a) Guinea: Poor turnout as Guinea schools reopen after Ebola break. AllAfrica, RFI. http://allafrica.com/stories/201501201308.html. Accessed 20 Jan 2015

Kamara A (2015b) Sierra Leone news: school re-opening depend on Ebola figures. Awoko. http://awoko.org/2015/01/10/sierra-leone-news-school-re-opening-depend-on-ebola-figures/. Accessed 10 Jan 2015

Kamara AM (2015c) Sierra Leone news: MSF closes Kailahun Treatment Centre today. Awoko. http://awoko.org/2015/02/20/sierra-leone-news-msf-closes-kailahun-treatment-centre-today/. Accessed 20 Feb 2015

Kamara A (2015d) Sierra Leone news: women Ebola survivors call for Health insurance scheme. Awoko. http://awoko.org/2015/03/06/sierra-leone-news-women-ebola-survivors-call-for-health-insurance-scheme/. Accessed 6 Mar 2015

Kamara AM (2015e) Sierra Leone news: as Kailahun records 182 ebola widows…KWiGN present position paper to government. Awoko. http://awoko.org/2015/03/16/sierra-leone-news-as-kailahun-records-182-ebola-widowskwign-present-position-paper-to-government/. Accessed 16 Mar 2015

Kanteh M (2015) Gambia: two charged for smuggling people from Ebola country. AllAfrica, The Daily Observer. http://allafrica.com/stories/201501191358.html. Accessed 16 Jan 2015

Karimi F, McKenzie D (2016) Ebola resurfaces in Sierra Leone hours after WHO declares outbreak over. CNN. http://www.cnn.com/2016/01/15/africa/sierra-leone-ebola-new-case/index.html. Accessed 15 Jan 2016

Karmo H (2015) Liberia: child Fund Liberia shuts down Ebola interim care center. AllAfrica, Front Page Africa. http://allafrica.com/stories/201508120991.html. Accessed 12 Aug 2015

Kenning C (2015) 101st Airborne recognized for Ebola fight. Courier-Journal. http://www.courier-journal.com/story/news/local/2015/08/25/st-airborne-recognized-ebola-fight/32322763/. Accessed 25 Aug 2015

Kime P (2015) Troops get malaria during Ebola deployment. Military Times. http://www.militarytimes.com/story/military/benefits/health-care/2015/04/23/us-military-ebola-deployment-malaria/26236769/. Accessed 24 Apr 2015

Kirby J, Cameron L (2015) Ebola nurse Pauline Cafferkey visited Scots school day before falling ill with 'reactivated' virus. Daily Record. http://www.dailyrecord.co.uk/news/scottish-news/ebola-nurse-pauline-cafferkey-visited-6608508. Accessed 10 Oct 2015

Knapton S (2015) Ebola wipes out every mother in Liberian village. The telegraph. http://www.telegraph.co.uk/news/worldnews/ebola/11304584/Ebola-wipes-out-every-mother-in-Liberian-village.html. Accessed 5 Jan 2015

Korea Times (2015) S. Korean medial worker confirmed free of Ebola virus. The Korea Times. http://www.koreatimes.co.kr/www/news/nation/2015/01/116_172043.html. Accessed 19 Jan 2015

Kroll D (2015) Chimerix ends Brincidofovir Ebola trials to focus on adenovirus and CMV. Forbes. http://www.forbes.com/sites/davidkroll/2015/01/31/chimerix-ends-brincidofovir-ebola-trials-to-focus-on-adenovirus-and-cmv/3/. Accessed 31 Jan 2015

KVUE and KCEN (2015) Dead Fort Hood soldier tests negative for Ebola. KVUE, KCEN. http://www.kvue.com/story/news/local/2015/01/13/fort-hood-soldier-found-dead-in-yard/21698101/. Accessed 14 Jan 2015

Lancaster Guardian (2015) Doctor tells of major setback in fight against Ebola. Lancaster Guardian. http://www.lancasterguardian.co.uk/news/health/local/doctor-tells-of-major-setback-in-fight-against-ebola-1-7140876. Accessed 5 Mar 2015

Levine S (2015) White House congratulates Liberia on being Ebola-free. The Huffington Post. http://www.huffingtonpost.com/2015/05/09/liberia-ebola-free_n_7248566.html. Accessed 11 May 2015

Levine AC, Shetty PP, Burbach R et al (2015) Derivation and internal validation of the Ebola prediction score for risk stratification of patients with suspected Ebola virus disease. Ann Emerg Med 66:285–293

Lewis K (2015) Guinea's Ebola numbers may be higher than reported. VOA News. http://www.voanews.com/content/ebola-irc-trust-cases-findings-lessons-government-radio-epidemic-who/2615225.html. Accessed 27 Jan 2015

Lister M (2015) Drunk jailed for Ebola cough after walking into hospital and claiming he had the deadly disease. The Mirror. http://www.mirror.co.uk/news/uk-news/drunk-jailed-ebola-cough-after-5387169. Accessed 23 Mar 2015

Lunn S (2015) Ebola doctors, nurses no longer recruited for West Africa. CBC. http://www.cbc.ca/news/canada/ebola-doctors-nurses-no-longer-recruited-for-west-africa-1.2981449. Accessed 6 Mar 2015

MacDougall C (2015) Ebola, thief of rituals, leaves no graves to decorate. New York Times. https://www.nytimes.com/2015/03/13/world/africa/ebola-thief-of-rituals-leaves-no-graves-to-decorate.html. Accessed 23 Jul 2017

Mahmud MS (2015) Liberia expands cross border screening to combat spread of Ebola. News Hour. http://www.newshour.com.bd/2015/08/12/liberia-expands-cross-border-screening-to-combat-spread-of-ebola/. Accessed 12 Aug 2015

Maron DF (2016) West Africa Ebola outbreak declared over. Scientific American. http://www.scientificamerican.com/article/west-africa-ebola-outbreak-declared-over/. Accessed 14 Jan 2016

Marrier d'Unienville A (2015) Photo feature: after Ebola, Sierra Leone's burial workers fear a bleak future. IRIN. http://www.irinnews.org/report/102164/photo-feature-after-ebola-sierra-leone-s-burial-workers-fear-a-bleak-future. Accessed 28 Oct 2015

Marteh D (2015) Liberia: Unmeer SRSG declares 'worse of Ebola behind us'. AllAfrica, Front Page Africa. http://allafrica.com/stories/201502191434.html. Accessed 19 Feb 2015

Maxmen A (2015) In Sierra Leone quarantines without food threaten Ebola response. Al Jazeera. http://america.aljazeera.com/articles/2015/2/19/in-sierra-leone-quarantined-ebola-survivors.html. Accessed 19 Feb 2015

Mazibuko K (2015) Ebola left around 10,000 orphans in West Africa. News Tonight. http://newstonight.co.za/content/ebola-left-around-10000-orphans-west-africa. Accessed 20 Jan 2015

Mazumdar T (2015a) Ebola: a day with the burial team. BBC. http://www.bbc.com/news/health-30712162. Accessed 7 Jan 2015

Mazumdar T (2015b) Ebola outbreak: virus mutating, scientists warn. BBC. http://www.bbc.com/news/health-31019097. Accessed 18 Jul 2017

Mazumdar T (2015c) Sierra Leone records zero new Ebola infections. BBC. http://www.bbc.com/news/health-33961010. Accessed 17 Aug 2015

McKay B (2015) Host of ailments plague African Ebola survivors. The Wall Street Journal. http://www.wsj.com/articles/host-of-ailments-plague-african-ebola-survivors-1430429461. Accessed 1 May 2015

McKenna M (2015) Still fighting Ebola: a view from Liberia's front line. Wired. http://www.wired.com/2015/02/ebola-liberia/. Accessed 16 Feb 2015

McNeil DG Jr. (2015) Fatality rate is falling in West African Ebola clinics. New York Times. http://www.nytimes.com/2015/02/27/health/fatality-rate-in-west-africa-ebola-clinics-is-dropping.html?_r=0. Accessed 26 Feb 2015

Médecins Sans Frontières (2015a) Ebola: ending stigma – the story of an Ebola fighter. 21 Jan 2015

Médecins Sans Frontières (2015b) Ebola crisis update – 17 July 2015. 17 Jul 2015

MENAFN and AFP (2015a) Sierra Leone back to work after Ebola lockdown. MENAFN, AFP. http://www.menafn.com/1094144513/Sierra-Leone-back-to-work-after-Ebola-lockdown. Accessed 30 Mar 2015

MENAFN and AFP (2015b) US Ebola patient's health improves again. MENAFN, AFP. http://www.menafn.com/1094144515/US-Ebola-patients-health-improves-again. Accessed 30 Mar 2015

MENAFN and AFP (2016) Ebola clinic reopens in Guinea after virus resurfaces. MENAFN, AFP. http://www.menafn.com/1094655742/Ebola-clinic-reopens-in-Guinea-after-virus-resurfaces. Accessed 19 Mar 2016

Merrifield N (2015) Government tightens Ebola screening for healthcare workers. Nursing Times. http://www.nursingtimes.net/government-tightens-ebola-screening-for-healthcare-workers/5077984.article. Accessed 6 Jan 2015

Meyer M, Garron T, Lubaki NM et al (2015) Aerosolized Ebola vaccine protects primates and elicits lung-resident T cell responses. J Clin Invest 125:3241–3255

Miles T (2015) Sex and masturbation could put Ebola recovery in jeopardy. Reuters, The Huffington Post. http://www.huffingtonpost.com/entry/sex-and-masturbation-could-put-ebola-recovery-in-jeopardy_55f072fbe4b03784e2777d07. Accessed 10 Sep 2015

Milton B (2015) Sierra Leone news: only 14 dead out of 28 Ebola infected MSF staff. Awoko. http://awoko.org/2015/04/08/sierra-leone-news-only14-dead-out-of-28-ebola-infected-msf-staff/. Accessed 9 Apr 2015

Mitchell C (2015) Rare award for returning Ebola ship. Telegraph & Argus. http://www.thetelegraphandargus.co.uk/tahistory/community_service/12902682.Rare_award_for_returning_Ebola_ship/. Accessed 21 Apr 2015

Morin M (2016) California ends Ebola monitoring of travelers returning from West Africa. The LA Times. http://www.latimes.com/local/lanow/la-me-ln-ebola-monitoring-20160107-story.html. Accessed 10 Jan 2016

Muchler B, Collins P (2015) Liberia decoration day brings back dark memories of Ebola. VOA News. https://www.voanews.com/a/decoration-day-brings-back-dark-memories-from-ebola/2676240.html. Accessed 23 Jul 2017

Mundasad S (2015) WHO: Ebola survivors at risk of eye and joint problems. BBC. http://www.bbc.com/news/health-32250515. Accessed 10 Apr 2015

Naija247 (2015) Fresh doubts over schools reopening in Ebola-hit Sierra Leone. Naija247 News. http://naija247news.com/2015/03/fresh-doubts-over-schools-reopening-in-ebola-hit-sierra-leone/. Accessed 4 Mar 2015

Nebehay S (2015) Decision on Ebola mass vaccination in August at earliest: WHO. Reuters. http://www.reuters.com/article/2015/02/27/us-health-ebola-who-vaccine-idUSKBN0LV12420150227. Accessed 27 Feb 2015

News24 (2015a) WHO: Half of all Ebola infections in S. Leone-Guinea border area. News24. http://www.news24.com/Africa/News/WHO-Half-of-all-Ebola-infections-in-S-Leone-Guinea-border-area-20150409. Accessed 9 Apr 2015

News24 (2015b) Sierra Leone lifts last major Ebola quarantine. News24. http://www.news24.com/Africa/News/Sierra-Leone-lifts-last-major-Ebola-quarantine-20150815-2. Accessed 15 Aug 2015

Ngunze M (2015) Kenya airways resumes flights To Sierra Leone. Daily Guide. http://www.dailyguideghana.com/kenya-airways-resumes-flights-to-sierra-leone/. Accessed 3 Jun 2015

Nossiter A (2015) Doctors link risky burials to Ebola rise in West Africa. New York Times. http://www.nytimes.com/2015/05/20/world/africa/ebola-cases-rise-guinea-sierra-leone-after-steep-drop.html?_r=0. Accessed 20 May 2015

O'Brien K (2015) More than 600 monitored in NJ since October for Ebola fears. NJ.com. http://www.nj.com/news/index.ssf/2015/04/njs_ebola_experience_by_the_numbers.html. Accessed 14 Apr 2015

O'Carroll L (2015a) Strike over risk pay at Sierra Leone Ebola hospital called off. The Guardian. http://www.theguardian.com/global-development/2015/jan/06/strike-sierra-leone-hospital-ebola. Accessed 6 Jan 2015

O'Carroll L (2015b) Sierra Leone declares first Ebola-free district. The Guardian. http://www.theguardian.com/world/2015/jan/10/sierra-leone-first-ebola-free-district-who. Accessed 10 Jan 2015

O'Carroll L (2015c) Ebola: Sierra Leone village in lockdown after 31 new cases recorded. The Guardian. http://www.theguardian.com/world/2015/feb/27/ebola-sierra-leone-village-lockdown-31-new-cases. Accessed 27 Feb 2015

O'Carroll L (2015d) Ebola 'leaves 12,000 orphans in Sierra Leone.' The Guardian. http://www.theguardian.com/global-development/2015/mar/04/ebola-leaves-12000-orphans-sierra-leone. Accessed 4 Mar 2015

O'Carroll L (2015e) Ebola death reported in Sierra Leone region where epidemic started. The Guardian. http://www.theguardian.com/world/2015/apr/05/ebola-death-reported-in-sierra-leone-region-where-epidemic-originated. Accessed 6 Apr 2015

O'Carroll L (2015f) International Medical Corps nurse dies of Ebola in Sierra Leone. The Guardian. http://www.theguardian.com/global-development/2015/jul/15/ebola-international-medical-corps-nurse-dies-sierra-leone-kambia. Accessed 15 Jul 2015

O'Carroll L (2015g) Sierra Leone celebrates lifting of ban on public gatherings due to Ebola. The Guardian. http://www.theguardian.com/world/2015/aug/10/sierra-leone-ebola-public-gatherings-ban-lifted-president-koroma. Accessed 10 Aug 2015

O'Carroll L (2015h) Joy as Sierra Leone's last Ebola patient ends treatment but grief and fear remain. The Guardian. http://www.theguardian.com/global-development/2015/aug/24/sierra-leone-last-ebola-patient-ends-treatment-grief-fear. Accessed 24 Aug 2015

Okafor O (2015) Kenya lifts travel ban on Liberia after country is declared Ebola-free. Pulse.ng. http://pulse.ng/health/ebola-kenya-lifts-travel-ban-on-liberia-after-country-is-declared-ebola-free-id3754650.html. Accessed 13 May 2015

Olu-Mammah J, Fofana U (2015) Police fire tear gas on crowd during Sierra Leone Ebola lockdown. Reuters. http://www.reuters.com/article/2015/03/29/us-health-ebola-leone-idUSKBN0MO0RQ20150329. Accessed 29 Mar 2015

Onishi N (2015) Empty Ebola clinics in Liberia are seen as misstep in US relief effort. New York Times. http://www.nytimes.com/2015/04/12/world/africa/idle-ebola-clinics-in-liberia-are-seen-as-misstep-in-us-relief-effort.html?_r=0. Accessed 12 Apr 2015

Osterholm MT, Moore KA, Kelley NS et al (2015) Transmission of Ebola viruses: what we know and what we do not know. MBio 6:e00137–e00115

Outbreak News Today (2015a) WHO says no Ebola in Iraq. Outbreak News Today. http://outbreaknewstoday.com/who-says-no-ebola-in-iraq-58550/. Accessed 6 Jan 2015

Outbreak News Today (2015b) GSK Ebola vaccine sent to Liberia for Phase III trials. Outbreak News Today. http://outbreaknewstoday.com/gsk-ebola-vaccine-sent-to-liberia-for-phase-iii-trials-86995/. Accessed 23 Jan 2015

Parker S, Miller N (2015) Australian nurse evacuated from Sierra Leone after Ebola scare. http://www.stuff.co.nz/manawatu-standard/news/world-news/65142439/Australian-nurse-evacuated-from-Sierra-Leone-after-Ebola-scare. Stuff, Manawatu Standard. Accessed 16 Jan 2015

Parley WW (2016) Liberia records 97 Ebola contacts. The New Dawn. http://www.thenewdawnliberia.com/news/10041-liberia-records-97-ebola-contacts. Accessed 7 Apr 2016

Paye-Layleh J (2015a) Liberia: schools reopen after 6 month Ebola closure. Associated Press, The Sentinel. http://cumberlink.com/news/health/liberia-schools-reopen-after--month-ebola-closure/article_c7881e29-c20c-51c8-99a9-bbabde3b5c6d.html. Accessed 16 Feb 2015

Paye-Layleh J (2015b) Liberia: 8 hospital staff members sent home for observation in Ebola scare in capital. Associated Press, US News & World Report. http://www.usnews.com/news/world/articles/2015/02/21/liberia-8-hospital-staff-under-observation-in-ebola-scare. Accessed 21 Feb 2015

Paye-Layleh J (2015c) Liberia removes Ebola crematorium as outbreak is contained. Associated Press, US News & World Report. http://www.usnews.com/news/world/articles/2015/03/08/liberia-removes-ebola-crematorium-as-outbreak-is-contained. Accessed 8 Mar 2015

Paye-Layleh J (2015d) Official: Ebola survivor may have infected new Liberia case. Associated Press, ABC News. http://abcnews.go.com/Health/wireStory/official-ebola-survivor-infected-liberia-case-29868478. Accessed 24 Mar 2015

Paye-Layleh J (2016) Liberia confirms 2nd new Ebola case possibly from Guinea. Associated Press, The Washington Post. https://www.washingtonpost.com/world/africa/once-ebola-free-liberia-confirms-2nd-case/2016/04/03/0f54784e-f986-11e5-813a-90ab563f0dde_story.html. Accessed 3 Apr 2016

Plucinski MM, Guilavogui T, Sidikiba S et al (2015) Effect of the Ebola-virus-disease epidemic on malaria case management in Guinea, 2014: a cross-sectional survey of health facilities. Lancet Infect Dis 15:1017–1023

Pollack A (2015) Fast track on drug for Ebola has faltered. New York Times. http://www.nytimes.com/2015/01/23/business/fast-track-on-drug-for-ebola-has-faltered.html?_r=0. Accessed 23 Jan 2015

Prescott J, Bushmaker T, Fischer R et al (2015) Postmortem stability of Ebola virus. Emerg Infect Dis 21:856–859

PRN (2015a) MSF opens new Ebola treatment centre in Freetown. PRN, News Time Africa. http://www.newstimeafrica.com/archives/37313. Accessed 9 Jan 2015

PRN (2015b) MSF: Ebola decline encouraging, but critical gaps remain. PRN, Star Africa. http://en.starafrica.com/news/msf-ebola-decline-encouraging-but-critical-gaps-remain.html. Accessed 26 Jan 2015

QMI (2015) Quebec man found dead at home may have had Ebola. QMI, Canoe.com. http://cnews.canoe.ca/CNEWS/Canada/2015/02/21/22248741.html. Accessed 21 Feb 2015

Quashie S (2015) After 169 days young girl in Sierra Leone diagnosed with Ebola. Pulse.com. http://pulse.com.gh/international/after-169-days-young-girl-in-sierra-leone-diagnosed-with-ebola-id4166322.html. Accessed 14 Sep 2015

Radio Cadena Agramonte (2015) Guinea and Sierra Leone extend health emergency on Ebola. Radio Cadena Agramonte. http://www.cadenagramonte.cu/english/index.php/show/articles/22775:guinea-and-sierra-leone-extend-health-emergency-on-ebola. Accessed 8 Jun 2015

Rampling T, Ewer K, Bowyer G et al (2015) A monovalent chimpanzee adenovirus Ebola vaccine — preliminary report. N Engl J Med 150202093719007–150202093719007

Ranosa T (2015) Tekmira stops testing Ebola drug in Sierra Leone. Tech Times. http://www.techtimes.com/articles/62237/20150620/tekmira-stops-testing-ebola-drug-in-sierra-leone.htm. Accessed 20 Jun 2015

Ravelo JL (2015) Back from Ebola's front lines, a doctor shares her experience. Devex. https://www.devex.com/news/back-from-ebola-s-front-lines-a-doctor-shares-her-experience-85628. Accessed 4 Mar 2015

Regan H (2015) 200 people are to be vaccinated in Sierra Leone after Ebola death. Time. http://time.com/4021065/ebola-sierra-leone-vaccination-death/. Accessed 2 Sep 2015

Rettner R (2015) 10,000 monitored for Ebola in US over fall & winter. Live Science. http://www.livescience.com/51428-ebola-monitoring-united-states.html. Accessed 2 Jul 2015

Reuters (2015a) Sierra Leone's President calls for week of fasting, prayer over Ebola. Reuters, VOA News. http://www.voanews.com/content/reu-sierra-leone-president-fasting-ebola-prayers/2581912.html. Accessed 1 Jan 2015

Reuters (2015b) Liberia plans to reopen schools in February as Ebola spread ebbs. Reuters. http://www.reuters.com/article/2015/01/05/us-health-ebola-liberia-idUSKBN0KE12L20150105. Accessed 5 Jan 2015

Reuters (2015c) Ebola survivors in West Africa to share stories via mobile app, to help fight stigma. Reuters. http://af.reuters.com/article/topNews/idAFKBN0KE0BZ20150105. Accessed 14 Jul 2017

Reuters (2015d) Soccer-Ebola tests for all players at Nations Cup. Reuters. http://af.reuters.com/article/africaSoccerNews/idAFL3N0UT3UA20150114?feedType=RSS&feedName=tunisiaN

ews&utm_source=feedburner&utm_medium=feed&utm_campaign=Feed%3A+reuters%2FA
fricaTunisiaNews+%28News+%2F+Africa+%2F+Tunisia+News%29. Accessed 16 Jul 2017

Reuters (2015e) Economic impact of Ebola less severe than first thought. Reuters, HR Reporter.
http://www.hrreporter.com/articleview/23302-economic-impact-of-ebola-less-severe-
than-first-thought-world-bank. Accessed 20 Jan 2015

Reuters (2015f) Sierra Leone to reopen schools in March as Ebola infections slow.
Reuters.   http://www.reuters.com/article/2015/01/21/us-health-ebola-education-idUSK-
BN0KU2N120150121. Accessed 22 Jan 2015

Reuters (2015g) Nebraska hospital releases patient found not to have Ebola. Reuters. http://
www.reuters.com/article/2015/01/22/us-usa-nebraska-ebola-idUSKBN0KV26F20150122.
Accessed 22 Jan 2015

Reuters (2015h) Just five Ebola cases left in Liberia, government says. Reuters. http://www.reuters.
com/article/2015/01/23/us-health-ebola-liberia-idUSKBN0KW27T20150123.   Accessed   23
Jan 2015

Reuters (2015i) Senegal reopens land border with Ebola-hit Guinea. Reuters. http://in.reuters.com/
article/2015/01/26/health-ebola-senegal-idINL6N0V52CW20150126. Accessed 26 Jan 2015

Reuters (2015j) Secret burials in Africa thwarting efforts to stamp out Ebola: U.N. Reuters, NBC
News.   http://www.nbcnews.com/storyline/ebola-virus-outbreak/secret-burials-africa-thwart-
ing-efforts-stamp-out-ebola-u-n-n301196. Accessed 5 Feb 2015

Reuters (2015k) In Guinea, Ebola infections double as hidden cases discovered. Reuters, VOA
News. http://www.voanews.com/content/guinea-ebola-infections-double-as-hidden-cases-dis-
covered/2631698.html. Accessed 6 Feb 2015

Reuters (2015l) Crowds attack Ebola facility health workers in Guinea. Reuters, Yahoo News.
http://news.yahoo.com/crowds-attack-ebola-facility-health-workers-guinea-141202169.html.
Accessed 13 Feb 2015

Reuters (2015m) 'S Leone Ebola funds unaccounted for.' Reuters, IOL. http://www.iol.co.za/
news/africa/s-leone-ebola-funds-unaccounted-for-1.1818214#.VN9hMbd0ziw.   Accessed   14
Feb 2015

Reuters (2015n) FDA approves Corgenix's Ebola test for emergency use. Reuters. http://www.
reuters.com/article/2015/02/26/us-health-ebola-testing-idUSKBN0LU1OO20150226.
Accessed 26 Feb 2015

Reuters (2015o) U.S., Liberia kick off trial of Ebola drug ZMapp. Reuters. http://af.reuters.com/
article/topNews/idAFKBN0LW0BW20150228?feedType=RSS&feedName=topNews&sp=t
rue. Accessed 1 Mar 2015

Reuters (2015p) At least 10 Americans being flown to U.S. after possible Ebola exposure.
Reuters, Yahoo News. http://news.yahoo.com/least-10-people-flown-u-possible-ebola-expo-
sure-195234152.html. Accessed 15 Mar 2015

Reuters (2015q) Liberia reports first Ebola case in weeks. Reuters. http://www.reuters.com/arti-
cle/2015/03/20/us-health-ebola-liberia-idUSKBN0MG2AR20150320. Accessed 20 Mar 2015

Reuters (2015r) Five US health workers released after Ebola monitoring in Nebraska. Reuters,
The Guardian. http://www.theguardian.com/world/2015/apr/01/ebola-nebraska-five-us-health-
workers-released. Accessed 1 Apr 2015

Reuters (2015s) Sierra Leone says Kailahun Ebola case report was mistaken. Reuters. http://www.
reuters.com/article/us-health-ebola-leone-idUSKBN0MY1PM20150407.   Accessed   7   Apr
2015

Reuters (2015t) Eleven handed life sentences over Guinea Ebola worker murders. Reuters. http://
uk.reuters.com/article/2015/04/22/us-health-ebola-guinea-idUKKBN0ND13A20150422.
Accessed 22 Apr 2015

Reuters (2015u) As Ebola disappears, no useful data seen from vaccine trials: WHO. Reuters,
Medical Daily. http://www.medicaldaily.com/ebola-disappears-no-useful-data-seen-vaccine-
trials-who-332934. Accessed 12 May 2015

Reuters (2015v) Guinea Ebola cases climb due to transmissions at funerals. Reuters. http://www.reuters.com/article/2015/05/15/us-health-ebola-guinea-idUSKBN0O01M220150515. Accessed 18 May 2015

Reuters (2015w) Sierra Leone imposes Ebola curfew for northern districts. Reuters, Channel News Asia.   http://www.channelnewsasia.com/news/world/sierra-leone-imposes/1912198.html. Accessed 14 Jun 2015

Reuters (2015x) Ebola returns to Sierra Leone capital after 3-week gap. Reuters. http://uk.reuters.com/article/2015/06/22/uk-health-ebola-leone-idUKKBN0P225920150622. Accessed 23 Jun 2015

Reuters (2015y) Guinea quarantines villages in reinforced bid to stamp out Ebola. Reuters, Fox News. http://www.foxnews.com/health/2015/06/25/guinea-quarantines-villages-in-reinforced-bid-to-stamp-out-ebola. Accessed 25 Jun 2015

Reuters (2015z) Liberia confirms three new Ebola cases, raising fears of remaining hidden pockets of the disease. Reuters, ABC News. http://www.abc.net.au/news/2015-07-02/liberia-finds-second-new-ebola-case-raising-fears-of-resurgence/6589818. Accessed 2 Jul 2015

Reuters (2015aa) Liberia registers second confirmed Ebola case: health official. Reuters. http://uk.reuters.com/article/2015/07/01/us-health-ebola-liberia-idUKKCN0PB47T20150701. Accessed 1 Jul 2015

Reuters (2015ab) Congo and WHO investigate possible Ebola outbreak. Reuters, The Daily Mail. http://www.dailymail.co.uk/wires/reuters/article-3147662/Congo-WHO-investigate-possible-Ebola-outbreak.html. Accessed 2 Jul 2015

Reuters (2015ac) Suspected Congo Ebola victims test negative for the virus. Reuters. http://af.reuters.com/article/topNews/idAFKCN0PF07120150705. Accessed 5 Jul 2015

Reuters (2015ad) Liberia: dog suspected in new Ebola case tests negative for the virus. Reuters, New York Times. http://www.nytimes.com/2015/07/08/world/africa/liberia-dog-suspected-in-new-ebola-case-tests-negative-for-the-virus.html?_r=0. Accessed 8 Jul 2015

Reuters (2015ae) Ebola burial teams seek bribes in Sierra Leone: health official. Reuters. http://www.reuters.com/article/2015/07/16/us-health-ebola-leone-idUSKCN0PQ1L420150716. Accessed 17 Jul 2015

Reuters (2015af) Liberia authorities track herbalist who escaped Ebola quarantine. Reuters, Yahoo News. http://news.yahoo.com/liberia-authorities-track-herbalist-escaped-ebola-quarantine-064259944.html. Accessed 17 Jul 2015

Reuters (2015ag) Trial in Africa shows Merck Ebola vaccine 100% effective. Reuters, CNBC. http://www.cnbc.com/2015/07/31/. Accessed 31 Jul 2015

Reuters (2015ah) Dead woman tests positive for Ebola in Sierra Leone. Reuters. http://www.reuters.com/article/2015/08/30/us-health-ebola-leone-idUSKCN0QZ0XZ20150830. Accessed 31 Aug 2015

Reuters (2015ai) Kenya Airways resumes West Africa flights banned due to Ebola. Reuters. http://www.reuters.com/article/2015/09/25/us-kenya-kenya-airways-idUSKCN0RP1CF20150925. Accessed 27 Sep 2015

Reuters (2015aj) Chinese firm says plans to mass produce Ebola vaccine. Reuters. http://www.reuters.com/article/2015/10/14/us-china-ebola-idUSKCN0S80M820151014. Accessed 14 Oct 2015

Reuters (2015ak) Two new Ebola cases in Guinea, WHO says. Reuters. The Daily Mail. http://www.dailymail.co.uk/wires/reuters/article-3275754/Two-new-Ebola-cases-Guinea-WHO-says.html. Accessed 16 Oct 2015

Reuters (2015al) Mystery deaths in Sierra Leone spread fear of Ebola relapses. Reuters, Fox News.   http://www.foxnews.com/health/2015/10/21/mystery-deaths-in-sierra-leone-spread-fear-ebola-relapses/. Accessed 21 Oct 2015

Reuters (2015am) Guinea records three new cases of Ebola, brings total to nine. Reuters. http://www.reuters.com/article/2015/10/29/us-health-ebola-guinea-idUSKCN0SN00X20151029. Accessed 28 Oct 2015

Reuters (2015an) Sierra Leone celebrates end of Ebola epidemic. Reuters. http://ewn. co.za/2015/11/08/Sierra-Leone-celebrates-end-of-Ebola-epidemic. Accessed 8 No 2015

Reuters (2015ao) Guinea releases last 68 people from Ebola quarantine. Reuters, Yahoo News. http://news.yahoo.com/guinea-releases-last-68-people-ebola-quarantine-143241412.html. Accessed 14 Nov 2015

Reuters (2015ap) Guinea says has no Ebola cases after last patient recovers. Reuters. http://www. reuters.com/article/2015/11/17/us-health-ebola-guinea-idUSKCN0T52OP20151117#SEICVo IIqpm3RlKa.97. Accessed 17 Nov 2015

Reuters (2015aq) Liberia monitors over 150 Ebola contacts as virus re emerges. Reuters. http:// www.reuters.com/article/2015/11/22/us-health-ebola-liberia-idUSKBN0TB0GV20151122#v HYwP3egcZJJBpHx. Accessed 22 Nov 2015

Reuters (2016a) Sierra Leone discharges last known Ebola patient. Reuters. http://www.reuters. com/article/us-health-ebola-leone-idUSKCN0VH1ZD. Accessed 8 Feb 2016

Reuters (2016b) Fourth person dies of Ebola in latest flare up in Guinea. Reuters. http://news.trust. org/item/20160319232244-ogqjg. Accessed 20 Mar 2016

Reuters (2016c) Fifth person dies in Guinea Ebola flare-up. Reuters. http://www.reuters.com/arti-cle/us-health-ebola-guinea-idUSKCN0WO2T1. Accessed 23 Mar 2016

Roberts M (2016) WHO downgrades Ebola health risk. BBC. http://www.bbc.com/news/ health-35921161. Accessed 30 Mar 2016

Roy-Macaulay C (2015) Sierra Leone releases its last Ebola patient, to start countdown to WHO Ebola-free declaration. Associated Press, US News & World Report. http://www.usnews.com/ news/world/articles/2015/08/24/sierra-leone-releases-its-last-known-ebola-patient. Accessed 24 Aug 2015

Roy-Macaulay C (2016) Sierra Leone has 2nd Ebola case after epidemic thought over. The Washington Post. https://www.washingtonpost.com/world/africa/sierra-leone-has-2nd-ebola-case-after-epidemic-thought-over/2016/01/21/537f103a-c02c-11e5-98c8-7fab78677d51_story.html. Accessed 21 Jan 2016

Roy-Macaulay C, Diallo B (2015) Guinea deploys police as Sierra Leoneans flee Ebola lockdown. Associated Press, Yahoo News. http://news.yahoo.com/sierra-leone-lockdown-aims-total-con-trol-over-ebola-132416264.html. Accessed 29 Mar 2015

RT (2015) Flight from Paris quarantined in Moscow after suspicion of Ebola on board. RT. http:// rt.com/news/224219-moscow-plane-aeroflot-ebola/. Accessed 19 Jan 2015

RTT News (2015) Red Cross releases song in solidarity with Ebola survivors in Liberia. RTT News. http://www.rttnews.com/2457055/red-cross-releases-song-in-solidarity-with-ebola-sur-vivors-in-liberia.aspx?type=pn. Accessed 16 Feb 2015

Saker A (2015) Local writer details airplane's Ebola scare. Cincinnati.com. http://www.cincinnati. com/story/news/2015/01/20/local-writer-details-airplanes-ebola-scare/22060763/. Accessed 21 Jan 2015

Samb S, Farge E (2015) Guinea Ebola cases rise three doctors infected. Reuters. http://www. reuters.com/article/2015/03/17/us-health-ebola-guinea-idUSKBN0MD1PP20150317. Accessed 17 Mar 2015

Samba A (2015a) Sierra Leone news: Kono gets Ebola laboratory treatment center. Awareness Times. http://news.sl/drwebsite/publish/article_200526955.shtml. Accessed 7 jan 2015

Samba A (2015b) Sierra Leone news: Ebola virus survivors' blood cures 35 out of sample of 40 patients. Awareness Times. http://news.sl/drwebsite/publish/article_200527015.shtml. Accessed 16 Jan 2015

Samba A (2015c) Sierra Leone news: Kailahun District clocks 42 Ebola-free days. Awareness Times. http://news.sl/drwebsite/publish/article_200527050.shtml. Accessed 22 Jan 2015

Samba A (2015d) Sierra Leone News Parliament orders the detention of NERC Coordinator. Awareness Times. http://news.sl/drwebsite/publish/article_200527266.shtml. Accessed 3 Mar 2015

Schlanger Z (2015) Roughly $1.8 billion in Ebola relief donations haven't made it to Africa. Newsweek. http://www.newsweek.com/roughly-18-billion-ebola-relief-donations-havent-made-it-africa-304083. Accessed 3 Feb 2015

Schlein L (2015) WHO: Zero Ebola cases in West Africa. VOA News. http://www.voanews.com/content/who-zero-ebola-cases-in-west-africa/3145356.html. Accessed 14 Jan 2016

Schnirring L (2015) Two more Liberia Ebola cases as Guinea, Sierra Leone log 27. Center for Infection Disease Research and Policy. http://www.cidrap.umn.edu/news-perspective/2015/07/two-more-liberia-ebola-cases-guinea-sierra-leone-log-27. Accessed 9 Jul 2015

Schogol J (2015) Air Force getting 25 isolation units for contagious patients. Air Force Times. http://www.airforcetimes.com/story/military/tech/2015/02/02/air-force-getting-25-isolation-units-for-contagious-patients/22522535/. Accessed 2 Feb 2015

Sci Dev Net (2015) Online course on Ebola for journalists developed by the WFSJ. Sci Dev Net. http://www.scidev.net/global/content/announcements_notice.29671226-3D9E-4673-B72EFFD0F90D3237.html. Accessed 7 Apr 2015

Sendolo A (2015a) Liberia: Gov't to decommission some ETUs in Monrovia. AllAfrica, The Inquirer. http://allafrica.com/stories/201502041601.html. Accessed 4 Feb 2015

Sendolo A (2015b) Liberia: following discovery of new Ebola case – 80 contacts under observation. AllAfrica, http://allafrica.com/stories/201503241498.html. Accessed 24 Mar 2015

Sesay AE (2015) Sierra Leone: GDP to Fall By 21.5 Percent in 2015. AllAfrica, Concord Times. http://allafrica.com/stories/201509171085.html. Accessed 17 Sep 2015

Shear MD, Davis JH (2015) Withdrawing troops, Obama calls for vigilance on Ebola. New York Times. https://www.nytimes.com/2015/02/12/world/africa/us-to-withdraw-nearly-all-troops-fighting-ebola.html. Accessed 20 Jul 2017

Shryock R, Bavier J (2015) Fear of Ebola's sexual transmission drives abstinence, panic. Reuters. http://af.reuters.com/article/topNews/idAFKBN0LT0JD20150225?sp=true. Accessed 25 Feb 2015

Sickles J (2015) State Dept rewards 'Ebola plane' company with multimillion dollar raise. Yahoo News. http://news.yahoo.com/state-dept-rewards-ebola-plane-company-with-multimillion-dollar-raise-163242202.html. Accessed 7 Feb 2015

Siddique H (2016) Ebola nurse Pauline Cafferkey admitted to hospital again. The Guardian. http://www.theguardian.com/world/2016/feb/23/ebola-nurse-pauline-cafferkey-returns-to-hospital. Accessed 23 Feb 2016

Siddiqui S-ur-R (2015) Sierra Leone ends Ebola bonuses for health workers. Business Recorder. http://www.brecorder.com/world/africa/218995.html. Accessed 22 Jan 2015

Sieff K (2015a) U.S.-built Ebola treatment centers in Liberia are nearly empty as outbreak fades. The Washington Post. http://www.washingtonpost.com/world/africa/us-built-ebola-treatment-centers-in-liberia-are-nearly-empty-as-disease-fades/2015/01/18/9acc3e2c-9b52-11e4-86a3-1b56f64925f6_story.html?hpid=z1. Accessed 19 Jan 2015

Sieff K (2015b) Kids in Liberia go back to school in a building where dozens died of Ebola. The Washington Post. http://www.washingtonpost.com/world/africa/kids-in-liberia-go-back-to-school--in-a-building-where-dozens-died-of-ebola/2015/01/31/71fc12e2-9c38-11e4-86a3-1b56f64925f6_story.html. Accessed 1 Feb 2015

Sierra Leone Telegraph (2015) President Koroma lifts Ebola emergency regulations. The Sierra Leone Telegraph. http://www.thesierraleonetelegraph.com/?p=10077. Accessed 8 Aug 2015

Sierra Leone Times (2015) Ebola cases rise again in Sierra Leone. Sierra Leone Times, IANS. http://www.sierraleonetimes.com/index.php/sid/230598959. Accessed 26 Feb 2015

Sifferlin A (2015a) American health worker with Ebola in 'serious condition.' Time. http://time.com/3744329/ebola-health-worker-serious-condition/. Accessed 15 Mar 2015

Sifferlin A (2015b) Ebola vaccine trial starts in Guinea. Time. http://time.com/3758011/ebola-vaccine-trial-guinea/. Accessed 23 Jul 2017

Sifferlin A (2015c) American treated for Ebola released from NIH hospital. Time. http://time.com/3816352/american-ebola-hospital-released/. Accessed 10 Apr 2015

Silva D (2015) American health worker exposed to Ebola heads to Nebraska for observation. NBC News. http://www.nbcnews.com/storyline/ebola-virus-outbreak/american-health-worker-exposed-ebola-heads-nebraska-observation-n279151. Accessed 4 Jan 2015

Sky News (2015a) Briton with Ebola cured after taking new drug. Sky News. http://news.sky.com/story/1454009/briton-with-ebola-cured-after-taking-new-drug. Accessed 27 Mar 2015

Sky News (2015b) Liberian Ebola workers protest for hazard pay. Sky News. http://www.sky-news.com.au/news/world/africa/2015/04/19/liberian-ebola-workers-protest-for-hazard-pay.html. Accessed 19 Apr 2015

Sky News (2015c) Nurse becomes Italy's second case of Ebola. Sky News. http://www.skynews.com.au/news/world/europe/2015/05/13/nurse-becomes-italy-s-second-case-of-ebola.html. Accessed 12 May 2015

South China Morning Post (2015) Liberia now urging abstinence or protected sex among Ebola survivors. South China Morning Post. http://www.scmp.com/news/world/article/1751810/liberia-now-urging-abstinence-or-protected-sex-among-ebola-survivors. Accessed 30 Mar 2015

Spy Ghana (2015) Recent Ebola patients in Liberia said to be doing well. Spy Ghana. http://www.spyghana.com/recent-ebola-patients-in-liberia-said-to-be-doing-well/. Accessed 23 Mar 2015

Starr FM Online (2015) Ebola: 42 Ghanaian health workers quarantined in Ivory Coast. Starr FM Online, Ghana News Hub. http://ghananewshub.com/ebola-42-ghanaian-health-workers-quarantined-in-ivory-coast/. Accessed 24 Jul 2017

Steenhuysen J (2015) Ebola virus sent out of high security lab was likely dead: CDC. Reuters. http://www.reuters.com/article/2015/02/04/us-health-ebola-cdc-samples-idUSKBN-0L82GI20150204. Accessed 5 Feb 2015

Stobbe M (2015) CDC lab worker remains symptom free 3 weeks after possible Ebola exposure. Associated Press, Star Tribune. http://www.startribune.com/lifestyle/health/288448121.html. Accessed 14 Jan 2015

Stout (2015) Mali is now Ebola-free. Time. http://time.com/3673242/mali-ebola-free/. Accessed 16 Jul 2017

Strum B (2015) ISIS fighters may have come down with Ebola. The New York Post. http://nypost.com/2015/01/02/isis-fighters-may-have-come-down-with-ebola-report/. Accessed 3 Jan 2015

Strunsky S (2015) Ebola scare on Newark flight as CDC holds passengers on plane. NJ.com. http://www.nj.com/news/index.ssf/2015/01/ebola_scare_on_newark_flight_as_cdc_holds_passengers_on_plane.html. Accessed 16 Jul 2017

Sun Daily (2016) New Ebola death in Liberia, hundreds vaccinated in Guinea. The Sun Daily. http://www.thesundaily.my/news/1747387. Accessed 3 Apr 2016

Susman E (2015) Study: funerals were prime places for Ebola spread. MedPage Today. http://www.medpagetoday.com/MeetingCoverage/ASTMH/54374. Accessed 30 Oct 2015

Sweeney C (2015) Partners in Health clinician diagnosed with Ebola, transferred to US. Boston Magazine. http://www.bostonmagazine.com/health/blog/2015/03/13/partners-in-health-ebola-sierra-leone/. Accessed 15 Mar 2015

Thayer RL (2015) 36th Engineers officially home from Liberia. KDH News. http://kdhnews.com/military/th-engineers-officially-home-from-liberia/article_71688372-d164-11e4-8910-8351128e80fd.html. Accessed 23 Mar 2015

The Samaya (2015) Ebola strikes again in Liberia: officials. The Samaya. http://odishasamaya.com/news/ebola-strikes-liberia-officials. Accessed 20 Mar 2015

The Star (2015) Sierra Leone reinstates Ebola restrictions after rise in cases. The Star. http://www.thestar.com/news/world/2015/02/28/restrictions-reinstated-in-sierra-leone-after-new-ebola-cases.html. Accessed 1 Mar 2015

Thomas AR (2015) Massive misappropriation of Ebola Funds uncovered in Sierra Leone. The Sierra Leone Telegraph. http://www.thesierraleonetelegraph.com/?p=8547. Accessed 14 Feb 2015

Tilghman A (2015a) More U.S. troops return from Ebola mission. Military Times. http://www.militarytimes.com/story/military/pentagon/2015/01/06/ebola-troops-return/21329133/. Accessed 6 Jan 2015

Tilghman A (2015b) Reserve mobilization canceled for Ebola mission. Military Times. http://www.militarytimes.com/story/military/guard-reserve/2015/01/23/ebola-reservists/22234951/. Accessed 23 Jan 2015

Toweh A (2015) Liberia's sole remaining known Ebola patient dies. Interaksyon. http://www.interaksyon.com/article/107865/liberias-sole-remaining-known-ebola-patient-dies. Accessed 28 Mar 2015

Toweh A, Giahyue JH (2015) Liberia investigating animal link after Ebola re-emerges. Reuters. http://www.reuters.com/article/2015/07/02/us-health-ebola-liberia-idUSKC-N0PC0WJ20150702. Accessed 2 Jul 2015

Turay SB (2015) Sierra Leone: Kroo bay quarantined homes Ebola free. AllAfrica, Concord Times. http://allafrica.com/stories/201504171048.html. Accessed 16 Apr 2015

U.S. Department of State (2015) Travel warning: Sierra Leone. 18 Sept 2015

United Nations (2015) New UN special envoy on Ebola response makes first visit to Sierra Leone. UN News Center. http://www.un.org/apps/news/story.asp?NewsID=50734#.VUI-NLd0ziw. Accessed 30 Apr 2015

Vaccine News Reports (2015) Sierra Leone reaches milestone in Ebola designation. Vaccine News Daily. http://vaccinenewsdaily.com/stories/510654529-sierra-leone-reaches-milestone-in-ebola-designation. Accessed 25 Dec 2015

Van Griensven J, Edwards T, De Lamballerie X et al (2016) Evaluation of convalescent plasma for Ebola virus disease in Guinea. N Engl J Med 374:33–42

Vanden Brook T, Locker R (2015) Tests confirm dead soldier had no Ebola. USA Today. http://www.usatoday.com/story/news/nation/2015/01/13/dead-soldier-remains-tested-ebola/21700619/. Accessed 14 Jan 2015

Vanguard (2016) Last known Ebola patient discharged in Guinea. Vanguard. http://www.vanguardngr.com/2016/04/last-known-ebola-patient-discharged-guinea/. Accessed 21 Apr 2016

Varkey JB, Shantha JG, Crozier I et al (2015) Persistence of Ebola virus in ocular fluid during convalescence. N Engl J Med 372:2423–2427

VOA News (2015a) Sierra Leone dog population rising because of Ebola crisis. VOA News. http://learningenglish.voanews.com/content/sierra-leone-dog-ebola-crisis/2730540.html. Accessed 25 Apr 2015

VOA News (2015b) US shuts Ebola treatment center in Liberia. Associated Press, VOA News. https://www.voanews.com/a/united-states-shuts-ebola-treatment-center-liberia/2744107.html. Accessed 27 Jul 2017

VOA News (2015c) Liberia ponders site for national Ebola monument. VOA News, Big News Network. http://www.bignewsnetwork.com/index.php/sid/233094491. Accessed 22 May 2015

VOA News (2015d) Ebola experts caution: vaccine still months away. VOA News. http://www.voanews.com/content/ebola-experts-caution-vaccine-still-months-away/2890566.html. Accessed 1 Aug 2015

Ward V (2015) British military nurse flown back to UK after 'needle injury' treating Ebola victim. The Telegraph. http://www.telegraph.co.uk/news/worldnews/ebola/11381496/British-military-nurse-flown-back-to-UK-after-needle-injury-treating-Ebola-victim.html. Accessed 31 Jan 2015

Watt H (2015) New medal for medical staff and military personnel who battled Ebola. The Telegraph. http://www.telegraph.co.uk/news/worldnews/ebola/11389659/New-medal-for-medical-staff-and-military-personnel-who-battled-Ebola.html. Accessed 4 Feb 2015

Waylaun RS (2015) Liberia: radio plays 93 percent in fight against Ebola – MOH & Unicef Study Reveals. AllAfrica, New Republic. http://allafrica.com/stories/201505060574.html. Accessed 6 May 2015

Weedee-Conway E (2015) Liberia: land owners block road to Ebola burial site. AllAfrica, Heritage. http://allafrica.com/stories/201504090797.html. Accessed 8 Apr 2015

Weekend Edition (2015) Death becomes disturbingly routine: The diary of an Ebola doctor. NPR. http://www.npr.org/blogs/goatsandsoda/2015/01/11/376362000/death-becomes-disturbingly-routine-the-diary-of-an-ebola-doctor. Accessed 11 Jan 2015

Whitman E (2015) UK Ebola nurse update: 4 came into contact with infected worker; Medic And 2 Others Evacuated. International Business Times. http://www.ibtimes.com/uk-ebola-nurse-update-4-came-contact-infected-worker-medic-2-others-evacuated-1844740. Accessed 12 Mar 2015

Wild F, Camara O (2015) Guinea's government expects an end to Ebola epidemic by November. Bloomberg.   http://www.bloomberg.com/news/articles/2015-09-21/guinea-s-government-expects-an-end-to-ebola-epidemic-by-november. Accessed 21 Sep 2015

Williams A (2015a) Sierra Leone's President has ordered a three day lock down forcing the country's entire population to stay in their homes to try and stop the spread of deadly Ebola. The Daily Mail. http://www.dailymail.co.uk/news/article-3006276/Sierra-Leone-s-President-ordered-three-day-lock-forcing-country-s-entire-population-stay-homes-try-stop-spread-deadly-Ebola.html. Accessed 22 Mar 2015

Williams SCP (2015b) Fingerprick test quickly diagnoses Ebola. Science. http://news.sciencemag.org/health/2015/06/fingerprick-test-quickly-diagnoses-ebola. Accessed 26 Jun 2015

Williams WCL (2015c) Liberia: last patient Liberia on track to being Ebola free? AllAfrica, Front Page Africa. http://allafrica.com/stories/201503051219.html. Accessed 5 Mar 2015

Williams WCL (2015d) Liberia: 'Gross disrespect' – Ebola victims getting fitting burial. AllAfrica, Front Page Africa. http://allafrica.com/stories/201503091078.html. Accessed 9 Mar 2015

Wilson J (2015) Worcestershire medal service to make medal for more than 3000 heroes of Ebola. Malvern Gazette. http://www.malverngazette.co.uk/news/13327510.Worcestershire_firm_to_make_medal_for_more_than_3_000_heroes_of_Ebola/. Accessed 12 Jun 2015

Wintercross W (2015) Ebola crisis: Sierra Leone's cemetery full of children. The Telegraph. http://www.telegraph.co.uk/news/worldnews/ebola/11352429/Ebola-crisis-Sierra-Leones-cemetary-full-of-children.html. Accessed 17 Jan 2015

WLTZ (2015) More soldiers to deploy to West Africa. WLTZ. http://www.wltz.com/story/28606523/more-soldiers-to-deploy-to-west-africa. Accessed 25 Mar 2015

WNCN (2015) Troops released from Ebola-watch isolation on Ft. Bragg. CBS North Carolina, WNCN. http://www.wncn.com/story/28359775/troops-released-from-ebola-watch-isolation-on-ft-bragg?clienttype=mobile. Accessed 11 Mar 2015

World Bulletin (2015) S. Leoneans fined for handshakes, hiding Ebola patients. World Bulletin. http://www.worldbulletin.net/world/152786/s-leoneans-fined-for-handshakes-hiding-ebola-patients. Accessed 12 Jan 2015

World Health Organization (2015a) Ebola situation report. 7 Jan 2015

World Health Organization (2015b) Ebola situation report. 14 Jan 2015

World Health Organization (2015c) One year into the Ebola epidemic: a deadly, tenacious and unforgiving virus. January 2015

World Health Organization (2015d) Ebola situation report. 21 Jan 2015

World Health Organization (2015e) Ebola situation report. 28 Jan 2015

World Health Organization (2015f) Ebola situation report. 4 Feb 2015

World Health Organization (2015g) Ebola situation report. 11 Feb 2015

World Health Organization (2015h) Ebola situation report. 18 Feb 2015

World Health Organization (2015i) Ebola situation report. 25 Feb 2015

World Health Organization (2015j) Ebola situation report. 4 Mar 2015

World Health Organization (2015k) Ebola situation report. 11 Mar 2015

World Health Organization (2015l) Ebola situation report. 18 Mar 2015

World Health Organization (2015m) Ebola situation report. 25 Mar 2015

World Health Organization (2015n) World on the verge of an effective Ebola vaccine. 31 Jul 2015

World Health Organization (2015o) Ebola situation report. 1 Apr 2015

World Health Organization (2015p) Ebola situation report. 8 Apr 2015

World Health Organization (2015q) Ebola situation report. 15 Apr 2015

World Health Organization (2015r) Ebola situation report. 22 Apr 2015

World Health Organization (2015s) Ebola situation report. 29 Apr 2015

World Health Organization (2015t) Ebola situation report. 6 May 2015

World Health Organization (2015u) The Ebola outbreak in Liberia is over. 9 May 2015

World Health Organization (2015v) Ebola situation report. 13 May 2015

World Health Organization (2015w) Ebola virus disease – Italy. 13 May 2015

World Health Organization (2015y) The last Ebola survivor of his team. May 2015

World Heath Organization (2015x) Ebola situation report. 20 May 2015

World Heath Organization (2015z) Ebola situation report. 27 May 2015

World Health Organization (2015aa) Ebola situation report. 3 Jun 2015

World Heath Organization (2015ab) Ebola situation report. 10 Jun 2015

World Heath Organization (2015ac) Ebola situation report. 17 Jun 2015

World Heath Organization (2015ad) Ebola situation report. 24 Jun 2015

World Heath Organization (2015ae) Ebola situation report. 1 Jul 2015

World Heath Organization (2015af) Ebola situation report. 8 Jul 2015

World Heath Organization (2015ag) Ebola situation report. 15 Jul 2015

World Heath Organization (2015ah) Ebola situation report. 22 Jul 2015

World Heath Organization (2015ai) Ebola situation report. 29 Jul 2015

World Heath Organization (2015aj). World on the verge of an effective Ebola vaccine. 31 Jul 2015

World Heath Organization(2015ak) Ebola situation report. 5 Aug 2015

World Health Organization (2015al) Ebola situation report. 12 Aug 2015

World Heath Organization (2015am) Sierra Leone down to the last chain of Ebola virus transmission. 17 Aug 2015

World Heath Organization (2015an) Ebola situation report. 19 Aug 2015

World Heath Organization (2015ao) Ebola situation report. 26 Aug 2015

World Heath Organization (2015ap) Ebola situation report. 2 Sep 2015

World Heath Organization (2015aq) Ebola situation report. 9 Sep 2015

World Heath Organization (2015ar) Ebola situation report. 16 Sep 2015

World Heath Organization (2015as) Ebola situation report. 23 Sep 2015

World Health Organization (2015at) Ebola situation report. 30 Sep 2015

World Health Organization (2015au) Ebola situation report. 7 Oct 2015

World Heath Organization (2015av) Ebola situation report. 14 Oct 2015

World Heath Organization (2015aw) Ebola situation report. 21 Oct 2015

World Heath Organization (2015ax) Ebola situation report. 28 Oct 2015

World Heath Organization (2015ay) Ebola situation report. 4 Nov 2015

World Heath Organization (2015az) Statement on the end of the Ebola outbreak in Sierra Leone. 7 Nov 2015

World Heath Organization (2015ba) Ebola situation report. 11 Nov 2015

World Heath Organization (2015bb) Ebola situation report. 18 Nov 2015

World Heath Organization (2015bc) Ebola situation report. 25 Nov 2015

World Heath Organization (2015bd) Ebola situation report. 2 Dec 2015

World Heath Organization (2015be) Ebola situation report. 9 Dec 2015

World Heath Organization (2015bf) Ebola situation report. 16 Dec 2015

World Health Organization (2015bg) Ebola situation report. 23 Dec 2015

World Health Organization (2015bh) End of Ebola transmission in Guinea. 29 Dec 2015

World Heath Organization (2015bi) Ebola situation report. 30 Dec 2015

World Health Organization (2016a) Ebola situation report. 3 Jan 2016

World Health Organization (2016b) Latest Ebola outbreak over in Liberia; West Africa is at zero, but new flare-ups are likely to occur. 14 Jan 2016

World Health Organization (2016c) Ebola situation report. 20 Jan 2016

World Health Organization (2016d) Ebola situation report. 3 Feb 2016

World Health Organization (2016e) Ebola situation report. 30 Mar 2016

World Health Organization (2016f) Liberia and Guinea discharge final Ebola patients in latest flare-up and begin 42 days of heightened surveillance. 2 May 2016

World Health Organization (2016g) End of the most recent Ebola virus disease outbreak in Liberia. 9 Jun 2016

WRAL (2015) Bragg soldiers who fought Ebola coming home Thursday following medical quarantine. WRAL. http://www.wral.com/bragg-soldiers-coming-home-thursday-following-medical-quarantine/14377390/. Accessed 22 Jan 2015

WRIC (2015) 103 being monitored for Ebola symptoms in Virginia. WRIC. http://wric.com/2015/06/03/103-being-monitored-for-ebola-symptoms-in-virginia/. Accessed 4 Jun 2015

Wulfhorst E (2015) New York Times wins Pulitzers for West Africa Ebola coverage. Reuters. http://www.reuters.com/article/2015/04/20/us-usa-pulitzers-winners-idUSKBN0NB29D20150420. Accessed 20 Apr 2015

Xinhua (2015a) Sierra Leone launches campaign for zero Ebola infection. Xinhua, Global Times. http://globaltimes.cn/content/914286.shtml. Accessed 27 Mar 2015

Xinhua (2015b) 13 people detained for unsafe burials in Ebola hit Sierra Leone. Xinhua, Global Times. http://www.globaltimes.cn/content/915737.shtml. Accessed 8 Apr 2015

Xinhua and NAN (2015) Liberia Cremates 2,800 Ebola Bodies. Xinhua, NAN, Leadership. http://leadership.ng/news/405831/liberia-cremates-2800-ebola-bodies. Accessed 22 Jan 2015

Xinhua News Agency (2015a) China-team cures three Liberian Ebola patients. Xinhua News Agency, PRI. http://www.globalpost.com/dispatch/news/xinhua-news-agency/150113/china-team-cures-three-liberian-ebola-patients. Accessed 13 Jan 2015

Xinhua News Agency (2015b) Blood samples at Sierra Leones airport "safe": authority. Xinhua News Agency, PRI. http://www.globalpost.com/dispatch/news/xinhua-news-agency/150227/blood-samples-at-sierra-leones-airport-safe-authority. Accessed 27 Feb 2015

Yenko A (2015) Bishop confirms Ebola patient released from Australian funded clinic. International Business Times. http://au.ibtimes.com/articles/578334/20150107/ebola-sierra-leone-julie-bishop.htm#.VK1Mt7d0ziw. Accessed 7 Jan 2015

Yorkshire Post (2015) 'Ebola' package sent to George Galloway declared safe. The Yorkshire Post. http://www.yorkshirepost.co.uk/news/main-topics/general-news/ebola-package-sent-to-george-galloway-declared-safe-1-7275551. Accessed 22 May 2015

Zoroya G (2015a) Downward Ebola trend suddenly reverses itself. USA Today. http://www.usatoday.com/story/news/world/2015/02/05/ebola-liberia-sierra-leone-guinea-infections-increase/22935171/. Accessed 6 Feb 2015

Zoroya G (2015b) Military Ebola mission in Liberia coming to an end. USA Today. http://www.usatoday.com/story/news/world/2015/02/04/ebola-army-troops-liberia-usaid/22694031/. Accessed 5 Feb 2015

Zoroya G (2015c) Last known Ebola patient in West Africa recovers. USA Today. http://www.usatoday.com/story/news/world/2015/11/17/last-known-ebola-patient-baby-girl-recovers/75916410/. Accessed 18 Nov 2015

Chapter 8
Outbreak Data

Abstract The 2013–2016 Ebola outbreak was a worldwide event with global impacts. It was also the largest disease event in the modern era to involve a BSL-4 pathogen. The outbreak lasted 920 days, from December 2, 2013, to June 9, 2016. During this time, almost 29,000 people were infected and more than 11,000 people died. With the advent of an effective vaccine, it is hoped that this will be the world's last large-scale Ebola outbreak. The lessons learned from the outbreak will help shape public health protocols and policies for years to come.

8.1 Chapter Overview

This chapter includes a timeline of the 2013–2016 Ebola outbreak, a list of travel restrictions imposed during the outbreak, a list of people associated with the outbreak, a casualty table (Table 8.1), and maps of the affected regions (Figs. 8.1–8.5).

8.2 Timeline of the 2013–2016 Ebola Outbreak

2013

Dec 2   Emile Ouamouno, the first known victim of the 2013–2016
        Ebola outbreak, becomes ill
Dec 6   Emile Ouamouno dies

2014

Mar 10 The Guinean Ministry of Health is notified about the outbreak of an
        unidentified, highly fatal disease in south-central Guinea
Mar 22 Ebola is identified as the disease causing the outbreak in Guinea
Mar 29 *Zaire ebolavirus* is identified as the species
        of Ebola causing the outbreak

© Springer International Publishing AG, part of Springer Nature 2018
S. G. Bullard, *A Day-by-Day Chronicle of the 2013-2016 Ebola Outbreak*,
https://doi.org/10.1007/978-3-319-76565-5_8

Mar 30	Ebola is found in Liberia. The WHO confirms that two blood samples from Liberia have tested positive for Ebola
Apr 28	Faith healer Finda Nyuma (known as Mendinor) becomes ill
May 14	The Ebola outbreak appears to be nearly over. No new cases have occurred in Guinea since April 2014
May 23	Two new Ebola cases are confirmed in Guinea
May 25	Ebola is found in Sierra Leone. The first two Ebola cases are confirmed in Sierra Leone
Jun 28	Liberia declares that the Ebola outbreak is a national public health emergency
Jul 25	Nigeria confirms an Ebola case. The body of a Liberian man (Patrick Sawyer) has tested positive for Ebola. Sawyer arrived in Nigeria on July 20
Jul 26	US workers Nancy Writebol and Dr. Kent Brantly test positive for Ebola in Liberia. They are the first Americans to contract Ebola during the outbreak
Jul 30	Sierra Leone declares are state of emergency
Jul 31	The experimental drug ZMapp is used on Dr. Kent Brantly and Nancy Writebol
Aug 2	Dr. Kent Brantly arrives in the United States. He is the first Ebola patient to arrive in the United States
Aug 5	Spanish priest Miguel Pajares tests positive for Ebola in Liberia. He is the first European to contract the disease during the outbreak
Aug 6	Liberia declares a state of emergency
Aug 7	Spanish priest Miguel Pajares arrives in Spain. He is the first Ebola patient to arrive in Europe
Aug 8	The WHO declares the Ebola outbreak a public health emergency of international concern
Aug 12	Spanish priest Miguel Pajares dies in Spain
Aug 13	Guinea declares the Ebola outbreak a public health emergency
Aug 19	The West Point slum in Monrovia, Liberia, is quarantined
Aug 23	British volunteer nurse William Pooley tests positive for Ebola in Sierra Leone
Aug 24	William Pooley arrives in the United Kingdom. He is the first Ebola patient to arrive in the United Kingdom
Aug 27	An infected Senegalese doctor working for the WHO has been evacuated to Germany. This is the first Ebola patient to arrive in Germany
Aug 28	The WHO releases its Ebola roadmap
Aug 29	Senegal confirms its first Ebola case
Aug 30	The quarantine of West Point, Liberia, is lifted
Sep 6	Sierra Leone announces plans for a 3-day, nationwide lockdown
Sep 16	The United States pledges to take a leading role in dealing with the Ebola outbreak

Sep 18	The UN Security Council unanimously passes a resolution that declares the Ebola outbreak is a threat to world peace and security. UNMEER is created. The first US military aid arrives in Liberia
Sep 19	The 3-day, nationwide lockdown begins in Sierra Leone
Sep 22	The nationwide lockdown ends in Sierra Leone
Sep 30	Thomas Duncan is diagnosed with Ebola in Dallas, Texas. He is the first active Ebola case in the United States
Oct 6	María Teresa Romero Ramos is diagnosed with Ebola in Spain. She is the first active Ebola case in Europe
Oct 12	Nurse Nina Pham tests positive for Ebola in Dallas, Texas. Pham helped treat Thomas Duncan
Oct 15	A second Dallas nurse, Amber Vinson, tests positive for Ebola. She also worked with Thomas Duncan. Vinson had traveled to Tallmadge, Ohio, before being diagnosed
Oct 17	The Ebola outbreak in Senegal is officially over. Ron Klain is appointed US Ebola response coordinator (i.e., Ebola Czar)
Oct 20	The Ebola outbreak in Nigeria is officially over
Oct 23	Dr. Craig Spencer tests positive for Ebola in New York City. Two-year-old Fanta Condé tests positive for Ebola in the West African country of Mali
Oct 24	New York and New Jersey employ enhanced Ebola-containment protocols
Nov 7	MSF confirms that the number of Ebola cases in Liberia is declining
Nov 12	A new Ebola case has been confirmed in Mali. This new case is unrelated to Fanta Condé
Nov 13	Liberia allows its state of emergency to expire
Dec 2	The Ebola outbreak in Spain is officially over
Dec 22	An accident occurs in a CDC lab in Atlanta. A technician in a BLS-2 laboratory may have been exposed to live Ebola samples
Dec 29	Nurse Pauline Cafferkey is diagnosed with Ebola in Scotland. She is first active Ebola case in the United Kingdom

2015

Jan 8	Pujehun District in Sierra Leone is declared Ebola-free. It is the first district in Sierra Leone to be free of Ebola
Jan 18	Mali is officially Ebola-free
Jan 23	All district quarantines in Sierra Leone are lifted
Feb 11	President Obama announces that he is withdrawing most US troops from West Africa
Mar 5	Liberia releases its last Ebola patient
Mar 20	A new Ebola case is confirmed in Liberia
Mar 27	A new 3-day, nationwide lockdown has begun in Sierra Leone

Mar 30	The nationwide lockdown has ended in Sierra Leone
May 9	Liberia is officially Ebola-free
May 12	An Italian nurse tests positive for Ebola in Sardinia
Jun 30	A new Ebola case is confirmed in Liberia
Aug 24	Sierra Leone releases its last Ebola patient
Aug 30	A new Ebola case is confirmed in Sierra Leone
Sep 3	Liberia is officially Ebola-free after its recent flare-up
Sep 27	Sierra Leone releases its last two Ebola patients
Oct 4	There are no new confirmed Ebola cases during the week ending October 4, 2015
Oct 9	The Scottish nurse who recovered from Ebola in Jan 2015 is hospitalized with a late complication of Ebola
Nov 7	Sierra Leone is officially Ebola-free
Nov 17	Guinea releases its last Ebola patient
Nov 19	A new Ebola case is confirmed in Liberia
Dec 3	Liberia releases its last two Ebola patients
Dec 29	Guinea is officially Ebola-free

2016

Jan 14	The West African Ebola outbreak is declared officially over. Liberia is officially Ebola-free
Jan 15	A new Ebola case is confirmed in Sierra Leone
Feb 8	Sierra Leone releases its last Ebola patient
Feb 23	The Scottish nurse who recovered from Ebola in Jan 2015 is hospitalized again with another late complication of Ebola
Mar 18	Guinea confirms two new Ebola deaths
Mar 31	Liberia confirms a new Ebola death
Apr 20	Guinea releases its last Ebola patient
May 2	Liberia releases its last Ebola patient
Jun 9	The West African Ebola outbreak is officially over

8.3   Border Closings

During the 2013–2016 Ebola outbreak, many countries imposed border closings or travel bans to prevent the spread of Ebola. The following are restrictions known to have been implemented during the outbreak.

2014

Mar 29	Senegal closes its border with Guinea
Apr 15	The Gambia bans flights from Guinea, Sierra Leone, and Liberia
May 6	Senegal reopens its border with Guinea

May 14	The Gambia lifts its flight ban for Sierra Leone and Liberia; Guinea is not mentioned
Jun 11	Sierra Leone closes its borders with Guinea and Liberia
Jul 27	Liberia closes its borders with Sierra Leone and Guinea. Nigeria's Arik Air suspends flights to Liberia and Sierra Leone
Aug 2	Emirates airline from Dubai suspends flights to Guinea
Aug 4	Saudi Arabia bans Haj pilgrims from Ebola-affected countries
Aug 6	British Airways suspends flights to Liberia and Sierra Leone
Aug 9	Guinea closes its borders with Sierra Leone and Liberia. Zambia will deny entry to travelers from Ebola-affected countries and will prevent Zambian citizens from traveling to countries with Ebola outbreaks
Aug 12	Guinea-Bissau closes its borders with Guinea
Aug 19	Kenya will not admit travelers from Sierra Leone, Guinea, or Liberia
Aug 21	South Africa has issued an entry ban for all noncitizens from Ebola-affected countries. Senegal closes its border with Guinea. Senegal blocks a UN flight carrying aid workers from landing in Dakar; it also bans all further flights and ship traffic from Ebola-affected countries
Aug 22	Ivory Coast closes its borders with Liberia and Guinea
Aug 27	Air France suspends flights to Freetown, Sierra Leone. British Airways suspends flights to Sierra Leone and Liberia until Dec 31, 2014. Brussels Airlines resumes flights to Guinea, Liberia, and Sierra Leone
Aug 28	The United Kingdom says that all nonessential travel to Sierra Leone, Guinea, and Liberia should be avoided
Aug 30	Liberia will not allow crew members to disembark from ships at the country's seaports
Sep 15	Mumbai, India, will no longer allow passengers to disembark from ships coming from West Africa. Crew members will be screened for Ebola
Sep 23	Sierra Leone sends troops to its borders with Guinea and Liberia to better seal the boundaries
Sep 25	Ivory Coast announces it will resume flights to Ebola-affected countries next week
Oct 1	Mauritius will not allow foreign nationals to enter the country if they have visited an Ebola-affected country 2 months before their arrival
Oct 7	Gambia Bird Airlines will resume flights to Freetown, Sierra Leone, starting October 17, 2014
Oct 11	The United States starts screening travelers from West Africa at JFK airport
Oct 17	Belize will not issue visas to travelers from West African countries
Oct 18	France starts screening airport passengers arriving from Guinea
Oct 19	Rwanda starts screening passengers arriving from the United States and Spain

Oct 23	Rwanda stops screening passengers arriving from the United States and Spain
Oct 25	Mauritania has closed its border with Mali.
Oct 27	Australia stops issuing visas to travelers from Ebola-affected countries
Oct 31	Canada will no longer process visa applications for residents and nationals of countries with widespread and persistent-intense Ebola transmission
Nov 11	The Gambia has reopened its borders with Sierra Leone
Nov 14	Senegal has reopened its transportation links with Ebola-affected countries and will allow planes and ships to arrive from West Africa. France says citizens should avoid nonessential travel to Bamako and Kayes, Mali

2015

Jan 6	The United States will no longer screen travelers from Mali
Jan 26	Senegal reopens its land border with Guinea
Feb 9	The Gambia has lifted all of its travel bans to Ebola-affected countries
Feb 22	Liberia reopens its borders
Mar 30	Guinea closes its border with Sierra Leone
Apr 21	Guinea reopens its border with Liberia
May 11	Canada has ended its visa ban for Liberia and will resume processing visas for Liberian residents
May 13	Kenya lifts its travel ban on Liberia
Jun 2	Kenya Airways has resumed flights to Sierra Leone
Jul 23	The United Kingdom will no longer conduct on-site screenings at the Birmingham or Manchester airports or at the Eurostar terminal in St. Pancras. Travelers arriving at these sites will still be screened over the phone
Sep 21	The United States has ended Ebola screening for travelers from Liberia
Sep 25	Kenya Airways resumes flights to Liberia and Sierra Leone
Oct 5	Nigeria's Arik Air will resume flights to Liberia
Dec 22	Sierra Leone is removed from the CDC's list of nations subject to enhanced screening for health conditions and diseases

2016

| Feb 18 | The United States suspends Ebola screening at all airports |
| Mar 22 | Liberia closes its border with Guinea as a precaution against the current flare-up |

8.4   People Involved with the Ebola Outbreak

A very large number of people were affected by the 2013–2016 Ebola outbreak. It is not possible to acknowledge everyone who was impacted by the disease. The following are some of the people who played prominent roles during the outbreak:

Ahmed, Ismail Ould Cheikh – Special Representative for UNMEER.

Baez, Felix – Ebola survivor. Cuban doctor infected in Sierra Leone. Treated at Geneva University Hospital, Switzerland.

Bai, Ernest – President of Sierra Leone.

Banbury, Anthony – Special Representative for UNMEER.

Borbor, Abraham – Deceased Ebola victim. Liberian doctor. Treated with ZMapp.

Brantly, Kent – Ebola survivor. US doctor infected in Liberia. Worked for Samaritan's Purse. Treated with ZMapp. Treated at Emory University Hospital.

Brisbane, Samuel – Deceased Ebola victim. Liberian doctor. Chief Medical Doctor at JFK Medical Center in Monrovia.

Cafferkey, Pauline – Ebola survivor. Scottish nurse. Infected in, Sierra Leone. Treated at the Royal Free Hospital in London. After recovery, hospitalization several times for Ebola-related complications.

Chan, Margaret – Director-General of the WHO.

Condé, Alpha – President of Guinea.

Condé, Fanta – Deceased Ebola victim. Two-year-old girl. First Ebola victim in Mali.

Conteh, Alfred Palo – Sierra Leone Ebola Czar.

Cross, Anna – Ebola survivor. British military healthcare worker infected in Sierra Leone.

Crozier, Ian – Ebola survivor. US doctor infected in Kenema, Sierra Leone. Treated at Emory University Hospital.

Diallo, Mamadou Alimuo – Ebola survivor. Guinean student who brought Ebola to Senegal.

Dixon, Morgan – Dr. Craig Spencer's fiancée.

Duncan, Thomas Eric – Deceased Ebola victim. Liberian. Confirmed Ebola-positive in Dallas, Texas, September 30, 2014. First Ebola victim diagnosed in the United States.

Fallah, Mosoka – Liberian doctor. Helped coordinate community action against Ebola.

Fonnie, Mbalu – Deceased Ebola victim. Nurse. Head of the Lassa fever unit and Ebola management center at Kenema hospital in Sierra Leone.

Frieden, Thomas – Director of the CDC.

Gbotoe, Nathan – Deceased Ebola victim. Confirmed to have Ebola November 19, 2015. First Ebola patient in Liberia after Liberia was declared Ebola-free September 3, 2015.

Graaff, Peter Jan – Special Representative for UNMEER.

Hickox, Kaci – US nurse. Quarantined in New Jersey after returning from Sierra Leone.

Ireland, Zukunis – Ebola survivor. Liberian doctor treated with ZMapp.

Jalloh, Mariatu – Deceased Ebola victim. Died January 12, 2016, in Sierra Leone. Confirmed to have Ebola January 15, 2016. First Ebola victim after the West African Ebola outbreak was officially declared over January 14, 2016.

Janssens, Bart – MSF director of operations.

Kamara, Shakie – Deceased. Fifteen-year-old boy shot during riot in West Point, Liberia.

Kekula, Fatu – Liberian nursing student. Developed homemade PPE known as the "trash bag method."

Khan, Sheik Umar – Deceased Ebola victim. Sierra Leone doctor.

Ki-moon, Ban – UN Secretary-General.

Klain, Ron – US Ebola response coordinator. Often referred to as the US Ebola Czar.

Kalivogui, Gbana – Ebola survivor. Last Guinean Ebola patient. Released April 20, 2016.

Komano, Rose – Ebola survivor. First Guinean survivor.

Konneh, Messie – Deceased Ebola victim. Sierra Leone nurse.

Koroma, Ernest Bai – President of Sierra Leone.

Koye, Olubukun – Ebola survivor. Nigerian diplomat. Brought Ebola to Port Harcourt, Nigeria.

Liu, Joanne – International president of MSF.

Logan, Gobee – Liberian doctor.

Marongiu, Stefano – Ebola survivor. Italian nurse infected in Sierra Leone. Treated in Lazzaro Spallanzani Hospital, Italy.

Mawanda, Michael – Ebola survivor. Ugandan doctor infected in Sierra Leone. Treated in Germany.

Memaigar, Abraham – Deceased Ebola victim. Died in Liberia on June 28, 2015. He was the first Ebola victim after Liberia had been declared Ebola-free on May 9, 2015.

Mendinor – Pseudonym of faith healer Finda Nyuma.

Meyler, Katie – Founder of the Liberian charity More Than Me.

Michalsen, Silje – Ebola survivor. Norwegian doctor infected in Sierra Leone. Treated at Ulleval Hospital, Oslo.

Monnig, Michael – Dallas county sheriff's deputy.

Moore, John – Photojournalist.

Mukpo, Ashoka – Ebola survivor. Infected in Liberia while working as a cameraman for NBC News. Treated at Nebraska Medical Center.

Mutoro, Samuel Muhumuza – Deceased Ebola victim. Ugandan doctor infected in Liberia.

Nabarro, David – UN Special Envoy for Ebola.

Nubia – Ebola survivor. Born to an infected mother on October 27, 2014. Released November 17, 2015, as Guinea's "last" Ebola patient. First newborn known to survive Ebola.

Nyuma, Finda – Deceased Ebola victim. Faith healer who used the pseudonym Mendinor. Worked near the border of Sierra Leone and Guinea.

Ouamouno, Emile – Deceased Ebola victim. The first known victim of the 2013–2016 Ebola outbreak. Two-year-old boy who lived in the village of Meliandou near the town of Guéckédou, Guinea.

Pajares, Miguel – Deceased Ebola victim. Spanish priest infected in Liberia. Treated in Carlos III Hospital, Spain.

Pham, Nina – Ebola survivor. US nurse infected while treating Thomas Duncan in Dallas, Texas. First known case of person-to-person Ebola transmission in the United States.

Piot, Peter – Belgian doctor. Co-discovered of the Ebola virus.

Pooley, William – Ebola survivor. British nurse infected in Sierra Leone. Treated at the Royal Free Hospital in Hampstead, London.

Poncin, Marc – Ebola response coordinator for MSF.

Pulvirenti, Fabrizio – Ebola survivor. Italian doctor infected in Sierra Leone. Treated at Spallanzani Institute, Italy.

Ramos, María Teresa Romero – Ebola survivor. Spanish nursing assistant infected while treating Priest Manuel Garcia Viejo in Spain.

Rodriguez, David – American General. Commander of US Africa Command.

Sacra, Richard – Ebola survivor. American doctor infected in Liberia while working with Serving in Mission. Treated at Nebraska Medical Center.

Salia, Martin – Deceased Ebola victim. Sierra Leone doctor. Permanent US resident. Infected in Sierra Leone. Treated at Nebraska Medical Center.

Samura, Fasineh – Doctor. Coordinator of Koinadugu District Ebola response center, Sierra Leone.

Sankoh, Adama – Ebola survivor. "Last" Sierra Leone Ebola patient. Released August 24, 2015.

Sawyer, Patrick – Deceased Ebola victim. Liberia. Introduced Ebola to Nigeria.

Sellu, Josephine Finda – Senior nurse at government hospital in Kenema, Sierra Leone.

Sesay, Mohamed – Ebola survivor. Sole survivor from an eight-person laboratory unit in Sierra Leone.

Shuaib, Faisal – Head of Nigeria's Ebola Emergency Operation Center.

Sirleaf, Ellen Johnson – President of Liberia.

Snyderman, Nancy – American doctor. Chief medical editor and correspondent for NBC News.

Spencer, Craig – Ebola survivor. American doctor infected in Guinea. Diagnosed with Ebola after he returned to New York City. Treated at Bellevue Hospital.

Stylianides, Christos – EU Ebola coordinator. Often referred to as the EU Ebola Czar.

Troh, Louise – Fiancée of Thomas Eric Duncan.

Tugbah, Ruth – Deceased Ebola victim. Confirmed Ebola-positive on March 20, 2015. First Liberian Ebola patient after Liberia had released its "last" Ebola patient. Most likely infected through sexual contact with an Ebola survivor.

Viejo, Manuel Garcia – Deceased Ebola victim. Spanish priest infected in Sierra Leone. Treated at Carlos III Hospital, Spain.

Vinson, Amber Joy – Ebola survivor. US nurse infected while treating Thomas Duncan in Dallas, Texas. Traveled to Ohio before being diagnosed with Ebola. Treated at Emory University Hospital.

Wiah, Shurina Rose – Deceased. Miss Liberia in 2009–2010. Rumored to have died from Ebola.

Williams, Darryl – American Major General.

Willoughby, Victor – Deceased Ebola victim. Sierra Leone doctor. Considered one of Sierra Leone's most senior doctor.

Writebol, Nancy – Ebola survivor. American missionary infected in Liberia. Worked for Samaritan's Purse. Treated with ZMapp. Treated at Emory University Hospital.

Yardolo Beatrice – Ebola survivor. Liberia's "last" Ebola patient released March 5, 2015.

Yillah, Victoria – Ebola survivor. Sierra Leone's first Ebola survivor. Released June 14, 2014.

8.5   Casualty Table and Maps

Table 8.1 Total number of Ebola cases and fatalities during the 2013–2016 Ebola outbreak

Country	Cases[a]	Deaths[a]
Guinea	3811[a]	2543[a]
Italy	1	0
Liberia	10,675[a]	4809[a]
Mali	8	6
Nigeria	20	8
Senegal	1	0
Sierra Leone	14,124[a]	3956[a]
Spain	1	0
United Kingdom	1	0
United States	4	1
Total	28,646[a]	11,323[a]

Derived from World Health Organization (2017)
[a]Includes suspect, probable, and confirmed cases

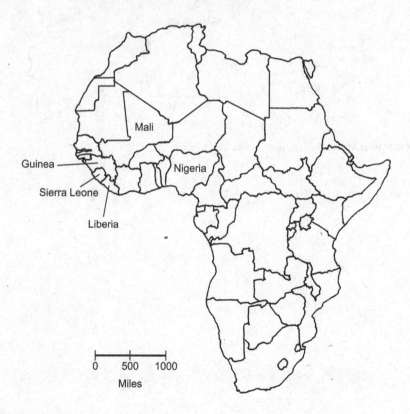

Fig. 8.1 Africa

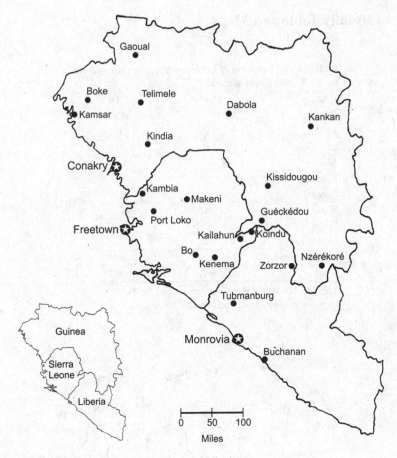

Fig. 8.2 West Africa. Guinea, Sierra Leone, and Liberia

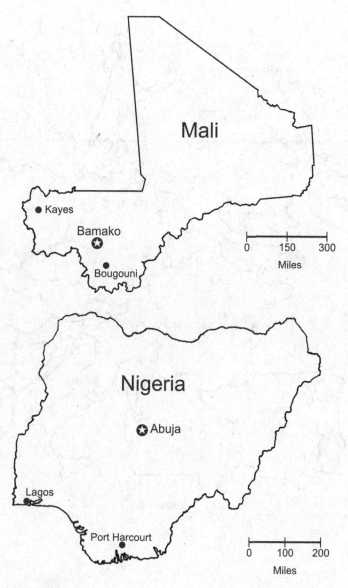

Fig. 8.3 Nigeria and Mali

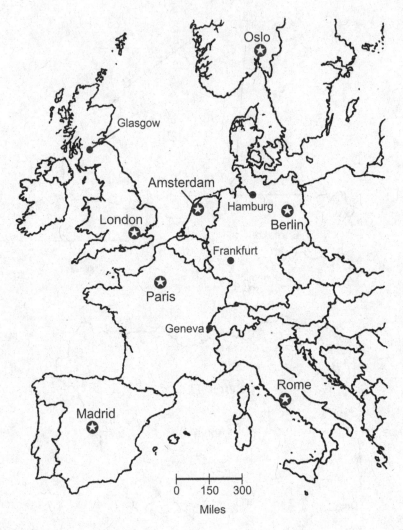

Fig. 8.4 Europe

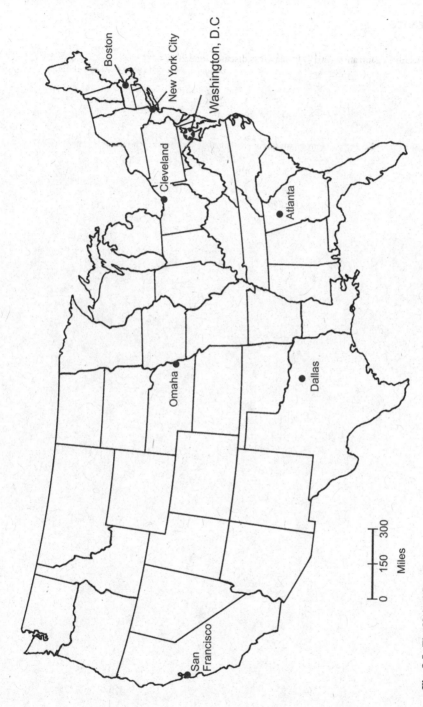

Fig. 8.5 The United States

Reference

World Health Organization (2017) Ebola virus disease. June 2017

Index

© Springer International Publishing AG, part of Springer Nature 2018
S. G. Bullard, *A Day-by-Day Chronicle of the 2013-2016 Ebola Outbreak*,
https://doi.org/10.1007/978-3-319-76565-5

Printed in the United States
By Bookmasters